GETTING PREGNANT

When You Thought You Couldn't

REVISED EDITION

THE INTERACTIVE GUIDE THAT HELPS YOU UP THE ODDS

HELANE S. ROSENBERG, PH.D.
and YAKOV M. EPSTEIN, PH.D.

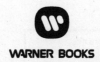

WARNER BOOKS

A Time Warner Company

PUBLISHER'S NOTE: The information and advice herein is not intended to replace the services of trained health professionals or be a substitute for medical advice. You are advised to consult with your health care professional with regard to matters relating to your health, and in particular regarding matters that may require diagnosis or medical attention.

Copyright © 1993, 2001 by Helane S. Rosenberg and Yakov M. Epstein
All rights reserved.

Visit our Web site at www.twbookmark.com.
For information on Time Warner Trade Publishing's online program, visit www.ipublish.com.

A Time Warner Company

Printed in the United States of America

First Warner Books Revised and Updated Edition: September 2001
10 9 8 7 6 5 4 3 2 1

Library of Congress Cataloging-in-Publication Data

Rosenberg, Helane S.
    Getting pregnant when you thought you couldn't : the interactive guide that helps you up the odds / Helane S. Rosenberg and Yakov M. Epstein—[Rev. and updated ed.].
        p. cm.
    Includes bibliographical references and index.
    ISBN 0-446-67683-7
    1. Infertility, Female—Popular works. 2. Infertility, Female—Psychological aspects—Popular works. 3. Human reproductive technology—Popular works. I. Epstein, Yakov M. II. Title.

RG201 .R67 2001
618. 1'78—dc21   2001026246

Book design and text composition by L&G McRee
Cover design by Robin Locke Monda

AT LAST! HERE IS A BOOK THAT TELLS YOU WHAT CHOICES ARE AVAILABLE, WHERE YOU CAN TURN TO, AND HOW TO COPE—EMOTIONALLY AND PHYSICALLY—WITH TRYING TO HAVE A BABY.

Written by two nationally recognized authors on the subject, a married couple who have themselves struggled to have a child, this book uses a total approach to overcoming infertility—helping you to deal with all the medical and psychological challenges as it pulls together the latest research to lead you every step of the way through this swiftly changing field.

GETTING PREGNANT WHEN YOU THOUGHT YOU COULDN'T

"Tempered by their own personal experience, Drs. Rosenberg and Epstein offer a multitude of practical strategies that have helped thousands of others understand, manage, and thrive."

—SAMUEL THATCHER, M.D., Ph.D., director,
Center for Applied Reproductive Science, professor of obstetrics and gynecology, East Tennessee Medical School, and coauthor of *Making a Baby: Everything You Need to Know to Get Pregnant*

"This is the most compassionate and useful resource for infertile couples. It is filled with sound advice and helpful information."

—Arnold A. Lazarus, Ph.D., distinguished professor,
Graduate School of Applied and Professional Psychology,
Rutgers University

To our families: past, present, and future

ACKNOWLEDGMENTS

The revised edition of *Getting Pregnant When You Thought You Couldn't* reflects not only the changes in the medical treatment of infertility but the changes in our life as well. We now have had eight more years of experience working with infertile couples and raising our twins, Nathaniel and Allegra. All of these experiences have involved people whose contributions have enhanced this book. We gratefully acknowledge the contributions of the following people:

Amy Einhorn, our enthusiastic, energetic editor at Warner Books, who helped to shape and fine-tune this book. Jamie Raab, our first editor and now Publisher of Warner Books, who believed in us and in the merits of our project then and now and whom we consider to be the true "mother" of this book. Shannon Beatty, Editorial Assistant at Warner Books, listened to us and paid attention to every detail in the project. Barbara Lowenstein, our agent, encouraged us to revise and update this book.

The wonderful physicians who helped educate us about infertility, read our manuscript, and provided helpful feedback and advice: Susan Treiser, M.D., Ph.D., of IVF New Jersey (Somerset, New Jersey); Annette Lee, M.D., of Reproductive Medicine Associates (Morristown, New Jersey); Samuel Thatcher, M.D., Ph.D., of the Center for Applied Reproductive Science (Johnson City, Tennessee); Gary S. Berger, M.D., of the Chapel Hill Fertility Center (Chapel Hill, North Carolina); and

Walid Saleh, of the Center for Reproductive Endocrinology (Bedminster, New Jersey).

Other medical professionals, scientists, and lawyers also provided much needed information. Cindy Comito and Greg Ryan, embryologists at IVF New Jersey, allowed us to watch as they handled sperm and eggs and permitted us to look at these gametes under the microscope. Bill Sofer, Ph.D., Professor of Genetics at the Waksman Institute of Rutgers University, helped educate us in molecular biology and genetics. Attorneys Andrew Vorzimer and Melissa Brisman provided legal expertise about insurance matters and legal aspects of third-party procedures.

We are also indebted to the behavioral scientists and researchers who offered feedback about our psychological material, both original and adapted: Sandra Leiblum of the Department of Psychiatry, Robert Wood Johnson Medical School; Lee Jussim, Professor of Psychology, Rutgers University; and Arthur L. Greil, Department of Sociology, Alfred University.

We want to give special thanks to the International Council on Infertility Information Dissemination (INCIID) and to their president, Theresa Venet Grant, and their vice president, Nancy Hemenway. From its inception, INCIID encouraged us to join their organization and honored us with appointments to their advisory board and board of directors. They encouraged us to moderate on-line discussion forums, featured us as guests in special chat sessions, and, with support from Ferring Pharmaceuticals, honored us with the Online Angel award for these efforts. These interactions with patients from all over the world taught us invaluable lessons, which we incorporated into this book.

Rutgers University provided us with an opportunity to work on this project and allowed us to teach a Rutgers College honors seminar titled "Fertility and Infertility in Contemporary American Society." Students in this course asked probing questions and stimulated us to consider many of the issues discussed in this book.

Members of our household, Nathaniel Henry Epstein, our eight-year-old comedian, and Allegra Heart Epstein, his twin sister and our resident artist, and even Toronto, our favorite parakeet, generously gave us the time to work on this book and provided us with constant stimulation and song. Danielle Bray, baby-sitter extraordinaire, entertained our children while we worked on the manuscript at our summer home in "Blueberry Hill."

Finally, we offer our gratitude to God, our silent partner, who guided us throughout this project and is helping us raise our two wonderful and healthy children.

—HELANE S. ROSENBERG and YAKOV M. EPSTEIN
New York City
October 2000

CONTENTS

AUTHORS' NOTE

Throughout this book we will provide examples drawn from the experience of clients with whom we have worked. In all cases we have changed names and other identifying information to conceal the identity of these persons.

FOREWORD

Anyone dealing with infertility will benefit greatly from reading *Getting Pregnant When You Thought You Couldn't*. This practical and informative guide is written from a unique perspective. Drs. Helane Rosenberg and Yakov Epstein are a married couple who overcame their own infertility through egg donation, and every day, as practicing mental-health professionals, they help other couples undergoing advanced reproductive treatments. Based on extensive professional knowledge and personal experience, they have succeeded in providing an easy-to-understand, up-to-date, and accurate guide on how to overcome the emotional and medical challenges of infertility. Their explanations of and links to useful Internet resources add a timely and dynamic dimension to this outstanding book.

Getting Pregnant When You Thought You Couldn't will help you become well informed about all of your options, work together as active partners with your doctor, and maintain a positive approach even if you fear you might not *ever* have a baby. The Ten Pointers provided in Chapter 1 set the theme of the book. This book is about hopefulness and overcoming negative emotions through education, discussion, exercises, and realistic assessment of your situation. This insightful approach will help you face difficult issues not only about infertility, but also many of life's challenges. This sets the book apart from other popular books about infertility and makes it a "must read" text. If you are a newcomer to the issues of infertility and are looking for a thorough, thoughtful, and sensitive guide to what you might face, start here. If you are already experienced with infertility treatments that haven't succeeded and you feel like giving up, this book will give you new skills, strength, and inspiration.

In the end, this book is about Hope . . .

> . . . the thing with feathers—
> That perches in the soul—
> And sings the tune, without the words—
> And never stops—at all—
> —EMILY DICKINSON

—GARY S. BERGER, M.D.
Director, Chapel Hill Fertility Center
Clinical Associate Professor of Obstetrics,
University of North Carolina
Co-author, *The Couple's Guide to Fertility*

PROLOGUE

We are a married couple. We have several current and past careers. In her "past" life, Helane acted in plays and on television. She obtained a Ph.D. in children's theater, directed theater productions at the University of North Dakota, and then moved east to Rutgers University in New Jersey. At Rutgers she headed the Creative Arts Education program in the Rutgers Graduate School of Education. From 1978 until 1989 she spent her time conducting research on the development of imagination and creativity. Her work was fruitful and multiplied, but she remained single and childless. Helane was certain that once she had established her research career she could concentrate on marriage and starting her family.

Yakov's path differed from Helane's. Upon completing graduate school, he married and accepted an appointment in the Psychology Department at Rutgers. His first daughter, Deborah, was born in 1970 and his second, Jennifer, in 1977. In 1980 he became licensed as a clinical psychologist specializing in the treatment of children and families. His first marriage ended in 1987, and he subsequently obtained custody of his youngest daughter. Shortly thereafter, he met Helane. We married in 1989, parented Jennifer, and began trying to have a baby. That's when our lives changed drastically.

Up to this point, Helane had experienced success in most of her endeavors. She had learned that with hard work and perseverance she could achieve almost anything she wanted. Similarly, Yakov never assumed that having children would be a problem. His two daughters from his first marriage were conceived without difficulty. Both of us were completely unprepared for the shock of infertility. Since Helane was ovulating on our wedding night, we assumed we would have a baby nine months later. Though we were both fairly well informed about many things, we quickly realized how uninformed we were about fertility and infertility.

We learned that infertility is much more widespread than we ever imagined, affecting one out of six couples in the United States. Of course we knew that some people have trouble conceiving, but we never imagined that *so many* people had trouble. And we never realized how many of the people we knew personally had experienced a fertility problem. Both of us had known one or two individuals who never had children and a few people who had adopted. But we had no idea how profoundly their lives had been affected by infertility until we experienced it ourselves. We soon became aware of how great the stigma attached to infertility is. Because of this stigma, people go to great lengths to conceal their fertility problems from others. We learned that there was a national organization of infertile people called RESOLVE Inc., who met monthly, held educational seminars, offered support groups, and engaged in advocacy to increase awareness of the problem and support for medical interventions to treat it.

We tried to make our way through infertility. We explored many treatments, suffered two miscarriages, and had many unpleasant and debilitating encounters along the way. Luckily, we put our Ten Pointers into practice even before we created them. (These Pointers are discussed in detail throughout the book.) We read everything we could get our hands on, talked to other couples who were experiencing infertility, became support-group leaders for RESOLVE Inc., and began educating and counseling couples at IVF New Jersey, an infertility medical practice in Somerset, New Jersey. As we researched the first edition of *Getting Pregnant When You Thought You Couldn't*, we started the egg-donor program at IVF-NJ and had the first successful egg-donation birth in New Jersey. As we write this preface, our twins, Allegra and Nathaniel, are 7½ years old and are about to enter second grade.

Since the first edition of *Getting Pregnant* came out, many things have changed in the treatment of infertility and for us personally. Treatment is now more successful and more costly. More and more people—even those without infertility problems—know about infertility because so many stories (both good and bad) have made the news. For those of you reading this prologue who are trying to become pregnant, the past is not as important as what is happening today. What *was* eight years ago is not nearly as important as what *is* today.

That's why we wrote this new edition. We feel that our knowledge of cutting-edge treatment, coupled with our eight additional years of working with infertile couples, has provided us with a depth and breadth of understanding of the situation as it is now. Our book presents a coherent picture of the causes and the treatments; the problems, medical and emotional; and ways to cope with them—today.

But the "complete picture" that a book can offer is offset by the fact that it is frozen in time. What is current as this book goes to press may be outdated by the time it hits the shelves. The latest information, constantly changing, is readily available on the Internet—if you know where to look and how to find and assess that information. This book will show you where to go on the Internet. Also, we have our own Web site—www.gettingpregnantbook.com—which supplements this book and provides useful forms and information. The Internet provides up-to-date pieces of the picture. But you need both a book that provides a total picture and access to newly available, discrete pieces of information. Armed with our book and the resources it provides, you can have the best of both worlds.

As we write this new edition, we see and hear the real evidence of our personal success: our energetic twins, who were not born until the first edition was already in press. We know firsthand what an infertility success can be.

August 2000
New York City

CHAPTER 1

Ten Pointers to Help You Get Pregnant When You Thought You Couldn't

etting Pregnant When You Thought You Couldn't, revised edition, presents our unique and recently updated approach to helping couples cope with infertility. Our method is based upon Ten Pointers. The Pointers stem from experience with scores of infertile couples we have counseled, as well as from our experiences with our own infertility. Since these Pointers are an outgrowth of a healthy approach to any kind of problem-solving, you instinctively may have incorporated some of them into your daily life already. Interestingly, people who read our first edition wrote to us to tell us that they had indeed already embraced much of our advice. They were then able to incorporate other new ideas into their planning and decision-making.

We begin with The Getting Pregnant Quiz, a ten-item questionnaire that can help you find out how *you* deal with your infertility. Your answers to the quiz will help you map out your Psychological Getting Pregnant Profile. Using this information, you can pinpoint any attitudes and behaviors that stand in your way.[1]

Please take a few minutes now to complete the quiz. Then score your answers. Before you begin, we recommend that you photocopy the quiz so you can retake it after you have completed the book and have begun to incorporate the Pointers into your life. By the time you finish this book, you will have two books: the one you bought and the one you create as you photocopy pages and make your own personal notebook.

THE GETTING PREGNANT QUIZ

Directions: The Getting Pregnant Quiz allows you to examine how you deal with your infertility. *There are no right or wrong answers.* Each question has four choices. Pick the one that best represents how you act or what you believe. Read the questions carefully. Then circle the number of the response that best represents your choice. If you feel that an item does not apply to you (e.g., the item asks about how you and your partner work as a team and you are a single woman with no partner), just skip the item.

1. How educated are you about the diagnostic tests, medications, side effects, and treatments for infertility?
   1. Extremely well educated
   2. Moderately well educated
   3. Slightly educated
   4. Not at all educated

2. How well are you able to identify your feelings about infertility and accept them as "okay"?
   1. Extremely able to do this
   2. Moderately able to do this
   3. Slightly able to do this
   4. Not at all able to do this

3. If you ever find yourself having unrealistic or unreasonable ideas about infertility (such as "My infertility is a punishment for an affair I had five years ago"), how well are you able to *challenge* these unrealistic or unreasonable views?
   1. Extremely able to do this
   2. Moderately able to do this
   3. Slightly able to do this
   4. Not at all able to do this

4. How able are you and your partner to work together as a team and support one another through infertility?

1. Extremely able to do this
2. Moderately able to do this
3. Slightly able to do this
4. Not at all able to do this

5. How able are you to give yourself permission to avoid stressful family and social situations, and to organize your social life accordingly?
   1. Extremely able to do this
   2. Moderately able to do this
   3. Slightly able to do this
   4. Not at all able to do this

6. How able are you to be an active consumer and a partner to your physician in your infertility treatment?
   1. Extremely able to do this
   2. Moderately able to do this
   3. Slightly able to do this
   4. Not at all able to do this

7. How able are you to organize your record-keeping of treatment, insurance payments, and receipts?
   1. Extremely able to do this
   2. Moderately able to do this
   3. Slightly able to do this
   4. Not at all able to do this

8. How able are you to develop a long-range plan (six months or so) that identifies how much money you are willing to spend on treatment, how long you want to remain in treatment, and how much physical and emotional trauma you are willing to withstand, and how able are you to reassess this plan after six months?
   1. Extremely able to do this
   2. Moderately able to do this
   3. Slightly able to do this
   4. Not at all able to do this

9. When faced with an either/or decision in terms of treatment options, doctor or clinic selection, or moral, legal, or insurance

choices, how able are you and your partner to make a decision in a timely manner?
1. Extremely able to do this
2. Moderately able to do this
3. Slightly able to do this
4. Not at all able to do this

10. To what extent are you able to "hang in" despite setbacks so long as you have the resources to do so and your goal is still to get pregnant? (While it is important to maintain a stance of cautious and realistic optimism, it is equally important to confront the emotional, physical, and psychological costs of pursuing a goal that may appear, and might actually be, elusive and unrealistic.)
1. Extremely able to do this
2. Moderately able to do this
3. Slightly able to do this
4. Not at all able to do this

Scoring Sheet

Each of the ten items corresponds to one of our Ten Pointers. On the scoring sheet below, enter your score for each of the ten items in the column labeled "Pretest." After reading this book and practicing the activities in it, try taking the quiz again and then entering your score in the column labeled "Posttest."

POINTER	PRETEST	POSTTEST
1. Educate Yourself About Infertility		
2. Get in Touch with Your Feelings		
3. Change Your Thinking		
4. Work as a Team		

POINTER	PRETEST	POSTTEST
5. Manage Your Social Life		
6. Be a Partner in Treatment		
7. Get Organized		
8. Make a Plan		
9. Make Decisions		
10. Don't Give Up		
TOTAL (add up the points from all 10 items)		

Put a bookmark on the page that contains your Total Score. Refer back to this page as you read about each of the Ten Pointers. As you make your way through the infertility maze, keep in mind that your job is to help yourself through your infertility. By incorporating these Ten Pointers into your daily life, you can gain some control over a situation that is often considered uncontrollable. You can help yourself stay strong, active, and optimistic as you seek and undergo treatment. You can empower yourself.

1. EDUCATE YOURSELF ABOUT INFERTILITY

Familiarize yourself with the nature and use of diagnostic tests, procedures, and medications typical in infertility treatment. You need to understand what's happening to you. Most adults think they already know how to make babies. For infertile couples, making babies demands knowledge far beyond what the average person knows. There is much to learn, but not so much as to be daunting. You need to learn about basal body thermometers, ovulation kits, laparoscopies, and infertility drugs. (All of these topics are detailed in later chapters.)

Make all the important infertility terms part of your vocabulary. Let the glossary at the end of this book be your guide. The glossary includes explanations of the alphabet soup of high-tech infertility treatment: *IVF, ICSI, TESA, MESA, PCT, HSG, IUI.* It also covers procedures that sound more akin to construction or animal husbandry than to the lexicon of human medical care: *cryopreservation, egg retrieval, assisted hatching, embryo transfer.* Terms such as *luteal phase defect, endometrial biopsy, sperm morphology, varicocelectomy, and anticardiolipin antibodies* sound ominous but are less frightening when you know their meaning. Couples who are successful arm themselves with as much information as possible so they can feel confident, make informed decisions, and converse fruitfully with their physicians.

We encourage you to be a voracious reader. Read *everything* written about infertility in books, magazines, and newspapers and on the Internet. You'll probably be surprised at the huge volume of information out there. Add to your rapidly expanding knowledge by focusing on the chapters in *Getting Pregnant When You Thought You Couldn't* that explain and describe diagnosis and treatment. Also, watch for talk shows and news programs both on broadcast television and on Web sites (such as MSNBC.com or CNN.com) with infertility segments. Remember, you don't have to go to medical school to understand what's happening to you.

Others can help you, too. Talk to everybody you know who has experienced infertility. One way to meet these individuals is to join RESOLVE Inc., founded by Barbara Eck Menning[2] in 1973. Through RESOLVE, you can join a support group in your area or call a hot line. RESOLVE meetings, besides providing emotional support, give members opportunities to trade medical information (How should you prepare for an endometrial biopsy?), practical information (Where do you stick the needle when performing a Humegon injection so that it hurts less?), and even financial information (What's the best way to submit an insurance claim to receive the optimum reimbursement?). By educating yourself you'll not only feel calmer, but you'll also increase your chances of getting pregnant when you thought you couldn't.

Maybe you live in an area of the United States where there is no RESOLVE chapter within driving distance. Or maybe you live in a country that does not have an organization like RESOLVE. If you have access to a personal computer, you have an opportunity to visit any of several excellent on-line infertility-related resources. These resources provide educational information and the opportunity to converse either asynchronously or to "chat" in "real time" with folks from the four corners of the earth who themselves are facing infertility.

2. GET IN TOUCH WITH YOUR FEELINGS

The most overwhelming characteristic of infertility is how stressful it is. It's stressful because you never know how long it will last. It's stressful because it's unexpected. It's stressful because it makes you feel different and because treatments are physically demanding and often very expensive.

Different people respond differently to infertility-related stress. A rich collection of reactions can be found in infertility bulletin board discussions. Throughout this book we will share some illustrative "postings." We encourage you to visit some of these forums whose addresses can be found in this book.

Researcher Margarete Sandelowski, a professor in the School of Nursing at the University of North Carolina at Chapel Hill, has investigated the emotional responses of infertile women. She reports that some infertile women describe the central experience of infertility to be one of ambiguity.[3] They are not sure why they are infertile. They aren't clear about whether they should try a different treatment or change doctors. They don't know when or even if they will ever have a baby. They are *confused*.

One executive sent this posting to participants on the International Council on Infertility Information Dissemination (INCIID) emotional issues bulletin board, which we moderate:[4] "I cannot believe what infertility treatment has done to my mind. I just got started (this is my first medicated cycle), and I find that I have a hard time thinking about anything else. I mean, today I was sitting in a board of directors meeting and caught myself thinking, 'I don't feel any side effects from the meds. My breasts are not tender.' and on and on. Then I thought, 'Oh my God, I have really lost it! What would these people think?'"

One of our clients, Phyllis, also fits the "confused" profile perfectly. The thoughts that wind through her mind reflect her confusion: "Every month I can't stand the wait. Maybe this insemination will work. Should I have a laparoscopy? Should we just go on vacation? Should I forget about having my own baby and adopt?"

Nobody knows why Phyllis can't conceive. She just wishes that some doctor would tell her that she'll never get pregnant. Then she thinks she would know what to do next. But maybe not. Other infertile women focus on the alienation of their experience.[5] They feel different from all the other women who get pregnant and have babies. They feel singled out and stigmatized by the infertility label. They can't talk to women with children; they can't talk to single women; they can't talk to voluntarily childless women. They feel like they just don't fit in. They feel *isolated and alone.*

Maya expresses her feelings of stigmatization poignantly in this bulletin board posting: "I've just come back from the hairdresser's. The lady in the chair next to me was pg [Internet shorthand for pregnant].[6] I was the only non-mother, they kept saying 'You'll understand someday.' It was only that I had a highlighting cap on my head that stopped me from walking out of the hairdresser's then and there, and I found it so hard not to burst into tears and to sound interested and happy for the lady. Apart from feeling the obvious jealousy towards this woman, although I wish her every luck with her pg, I just felt so alone and excluded. It feels like there is this magical club that once you become a mother you suddenly become enlightened. . . . I can't help but feel like I'm an outsider. Am I strange to be feeling like this?"[7]

Arlene is another one of those who feel "desperately different." Everyone around her seems to be pregnant or wheeling a baby carriage. Every weekend at her synagogue there's another baby naming. Arlene feels left out. "I am not like my sisters," she says. "They both got pregnant. I'm not like anyone in the whole world."

Time is the overwhelming aspect of other women's infertility experiences. They feel that their biological clock is running out. They respond by rushing through treatments or by changing doctors. They dwell on the past and are anxiety-ridden about the future. They think about themselves only as "ovulators" and "menstruators." Nothing else counts for them. All they can focus on is that they'd better get pregnant soon because time is slipping away.

Debby can't seem to think of anything else but the fact that she is forty-one and not yet pregnant. She laments her five-year relationship with Freddie. "I wasted so much time," she says. "I don't have many months left." She explains that she is going to two different doctors this week to get their opinions. She is overwhelmed by her sense of impending doom—menopause and the end of the road. Time is her primary stressor.

Infertile people say they feel anger, jealousy, repulsion, or disgust. Misty's posting on the INCIID emotions bulletin board says it all:[8] "It's really uncomfortable for me to face my own feelings in my own life. This weekend I saw my two best friends. It was just the five of us—they brought their adorable sons, born five days apart, now nine months old. Of course those sweet little boys were the center of attention! Why shouldn't they be—they are adorable. Lots of photos and videos of the two boys together. My friends are the souls of consideration, kindly asking about my fertility treatments, purposefully turning the conversation away from the babies so that I wouldn't feel bad. I felt like a freak, weird and childless. I also felt so jealous that they had their sons together—though they both have always been very loving and inclusive toward me. But even so, I felt bad! At one point, my closest friend said—trying to make me feel better: 'Why are you putting yourself through all this stress—you don't need a baby to have a meaningful life,' as she bounced her son on her knee. She gets pg without even trying, and has three children. She doesn't understand what it's like for me to wonder if I'll ever have the chance to be a mother—her babies were all unplanned." You too may feel like Misty does. In fact, you may feel grief, depression, loss, confusion—all sorts of negative and potentially debilitating emotions. Despite the difficulty, *you must face your emotions and acknowledge them.*

Often the shock of infertility can make people report that they are disconnected from themselves, or completely unaware of their feelings. Find and acknowledge your innermost emotions, for these feelings may be preventing you from getting beyond the obvious sadness and grief of infertility. Author Niravi B. Payne, M.S., in her 1997 book *The Language of Fertility,*[9] suggests that women experiencing infertility become aware of these negative emotional issues and work to counteract them. Remember, in terms of infertility, all emotions are valid, even though you may never have experienced feelings like these before. At one time or other, everyone experiences emotions that surprise them.

You might feel *angry*. At whom are you angry? There may be no clear target. People who believe in God may feel angry at Him. Others focus their anger on abusive or neglectful parents or on women who choose to abort their pregnancies. Others prefer not to focus their anger on an external target. Instead, they turn their anger inward. They get angry at their bodies for failing to make babies. When people turn their anger inward, they become *depressed*.

You might feel *jealous*. Some people say they feel jealous of parents or pregnant women. They envy the ease with which friends get pregnant. They are even jealous of their previously infertile friends, even though they truly want their friend to have a baby. Your feelings may confuse you. You may feel *repulsed* when your friend asks you to hold her baby. You wonder, "How can I, who so much loves babies and wants one, feel repulsed by this innocent little creature in my arms?"

Also, you may feel *disgusted* with yourself because you feel so inadequate. Month after month you fail to get pregnant. Looking in the mirror, you notice how the fertility drugs make you appear pregnant. What a shame. You have a body that looks pregnant but isn't.

All, or at least some, of these and other emotions will be part of your life. Getting in touch with these feelings ultimately will help you become a happier person despite your infertility. You can begin to combat negative feelings by learning to relax. The progressive relaxation and breathing exercises in the Getting Pregnant Workout in Chapter 2 are designed to help you feel calmer. The Workout's guided imagery exercises can help you "go away" from your problem and give your mind time to heal itself.

Dr. Alice Domar, who directs the Women's Health Program in the Division of Behavioral Medicine at Harvard Medical School, has created the *Mind-Body Program for Infertility* with branches throughout the United States. The Mind-Body Program's approach is very similar to the one we advocate in this book. Domar's program does an excellent job of helping her clients cope with the stress of infertility. For those of you who cannot get to the location of her program, we offer the activities in this book to achieve the same goal.[10]

After you get in touch with your negative emotions, realize that there comes a time to move beyond them and eventually replace them with positive feelings. Emotions that are perfectly valid at one time may hinder you from exploring options at another time. Of course, there is no rule about how long you can expect to feel overwhelming sadness or anger or jealousy (and these emotions will probably never leave you entirely), but at a certain point in your infertility diagnosis and treatment, you must allow yourself to get past what you are feeling so you can move on.

Some clients who come to us are already in touch with their emotions, so much so that it backfires and prevents them from seeking proper, productive treatment. They are grieving and feel helpless about their loss. "This isn't my fault," they say to themselves. "I'm not responsible for what is happening to me." While it's true that the fault is not theirs nor are they responsible for their condition, they nevertheless feel trapped by their debilitating emotions. They are fixated on negative thoughts, and their non-action triggers a form of guilt for failing to become more involved in their treatment. This, in turn, makes their negative feelings more intense.

Either case—failing to acknowledge your feelings or feeling your emotions too much—has a strong effect on whether you will allow yourself to try to conquer your infertility and get pregnant when you thought (and felt) that you couldn't. Getting in touch with your feelings, giving yourself time to experience them, and then moving past your pain into a new, more empowered phase of coping with your infertility is the goal of the Getting in Touch with Your Feelings Pointer.

3. CHANGE YOUR THINKING

Infertility puts a strain on so many parts of your life: marriage, career, family, friendships, as well as your own identity and self-worth. We hear so many statements like "I am a failure because I will not carry on my family line" or "I'm defective because I have a body that doesn't work right" or "I deserve this infertility because I wanted too much. I have a husband and a house and a job. I'm too greedy."

You must dispute your irrational beliefs. You are *not a failure* because you may not carry on the family line. It's not your fault. You are doing more than most people do to have a baby. Instead of berating yourself, pat yourself on the back for the effort you are making. You are *not defective* because your body can't get pregnant. Your mind works extremely well. And your soul is gentle and kind. You are *not greedy* because you want your life to go as planned. And, as you know, babies don't always go to the ones who want or deserve them most.

The so-called rational/emotive approach[11] is a form of psychotherapy that focuses on restructuring thoughts and feelings to foster adaptive behavior. This approach, modified for use with infertility, can provide you with the ABCs of getting pregnant when you thought you couldn't. The A (the *a*ctivating experience) refers to some real external event to which you are exposed. Your A is called infertility. The B (*b*elief) refers to the chain of thoughts about A. Your B might be, "I'm defective." C symbolizes the *c*onsequences, which are those emotions that result from B. For example, you may want to stay home and not see your friends. The D stands for *d*isputing these beliefs—which is what you must do to get out of this rut. If you do this, then E will follow—you will function more *e*ffectively.

The best way to get in touch with your irrational beliefs is to listen to what you say to yourself. The words you say to yourself and their meaning create and maintain your view of the situation. Ask yourself these questions: What's stressing me out most? What specifically am I telling myself about my infertility? What you tell yourself gives it the meaning that it has for you.

Mary Alice and her husband, Henry, are childless. When Mary Alice asks herself "What's worrying me about not having a baby?" she answers, "It means not being able to pass on my genes and my husband's for all posterity." When Henry asks himself "What's upsetting me about not having a baby?" his response is different. He says, "Without a baby I can never be a Little League coach." Such thoughts produce profound feelings of loss for these people.

As you go about your daily routine, take time out to monitor your thoughts. Stop putting yourself down for feeling jealous of your friends who have babies. Accept your humanity. Stop thinking poorly of yourself because you don't want to hold your friend's baby. Would you want to work in a pastry shop if you were dieting? The urge to steer clear of situations that would be unpleasant for you is perfectly natural. It doesn't mean you're a cruel or thoughtless person.

You can also change your thinking so that you react differently in stressful situations. You can learn to use a technique called "self-talk," which involves disputing your destructive inner dialogue. We call our version of the technique *Getting Pregnant Self-Talk*. You can choose to say, "I'm not pregnant now. But I'm hopeful that I will get pregnant. I know the odds are tough, but I prefer to think that I'll succeed. If I don't, I'll deal with that when the time comes." Viewing your dilemma from that perspective, you may be able to allow yourself to hold your friend's baby after all. Instead of thinking you are a failure, you will think about how nice it will be when your time comes—for you and your spouse.

4. WORK AS A TEAM

One of the most important aspects of living with infertility is working in concert with your spouse. Under normal circumstances, it takes two people to make a baby. For the infertile couple, the quest seems to employ a "cast of thousands." By focusing on your own emotions or the treatment you are undergoing, it's easy to forget your partner. Don't! Remember that in unity there is strength. And no matter how many doctors, nurses, technicians, friends, and family members are involved, you and your spouse—the mother and father of this desperately wanted child—are the central players.

You need teamwork to survive infertility. But sometimes it's difficult to stay united. Many couples who start with similar goals part company along the seemingly endless road. Infertility requires a reordering of priorities and a change in lifestyle. When spouses differ in their priorities, trouble looms. When treatment fails and a new course of action must be charted, conflict and disharmony may arise. These differences can strain a marriage that already may be taxed with physical discomfort, sexual deprivation, career disruption, financial woes, problems with relatives, and isolation from friends.

One of the most important tools for building a united front is developing excellent communication skills. Communication is the most important factor in determining the quality of your marriage. Therefore, the most important place to start communicating *is* in your marriage.

Like all human beings, you and your partner both live in a private world of experience, and neither of you is a mind reader. Unfortunately, couples make the mistake of believing that because they are married they ought to be able to understand one another—to know what the other is feeling or thinking, and especially to understand the reasons behind their spouse's actions. But in fact, they don't have access to the reasons, only to the actions.

Henry sees Mary Alice's sad face. He guesses she is upset because today is their anniversary and they still don't have a baby. Indeed, the anniversary has something to do with it. Mary Alice tells him that she is sad because she ruined the special anniversary cake she was baking. Henry laughs at her for getting so upset over such a trivial thing. If Henry had questioned her before jumping to conclusions, he would have understood Mary Alice better. And Mary Alice might have helped by being more specific to begin with.

Good communication involves *Active Listening* and *Leveling*. Eventually, Mary Alice explained to her husband that her sadness was about the cake but about other things as well. It was about trying to make their day special. It was about showing Henry that they had a stable, romantic marriage even though they lacked a baby. Their anniversary dinner was salvaged because they Listened and Leveled with one another.

So many aspects of infertility diagnosis can be less stressful and less emotionally devastating if you work as a team. Simple actions, such as accompanying one another to medical procedures or scheduling the receipt of test results when you can be together, can make life much more bearable. And being up front about fears concerning anesthesia, injections, and pain during necessary procedures helps you realize that you are in this together, despite your trepidations. Couples report that when they communicate with one another, using the *Getting Pregnant Active Listening/Leveling Approach* detailed in the next chapter, they feel closer and more emotionally equipped to cope with all the problems that arise from infertility.

Even after bridging communication gaps with one another, many couples find that they still have difficulty discussing their ordeal with outsiders. Bear in mind that other people can often provide additional support—which brings us to our next Pointer.

5. MANAGE YOUR SOCIAL LIFE

Rose, 28, teaches fourth grade. She's been trying to have a baby for two years. Recently, she began taking Humegon injections and undergoing intrauterine inseminations—procedures where timing is crucial. As a result, she is late to school three or four mornings a month. Rose also has gained weight and appears bloated. Fellow teachers whisper behind her back, wondering, "What's the matter with Rose?"

Martin is an attorney. Last year everyone thought that this year he would be made a partner. But this year Martin seems different. Unbeknownst to his colleagues, Martin is preoccupied with his wife Jessica's infertility treatments and test results. He's frequently on the phone, but not with clients. Everyone at work thinks something's up. Is he getting a divorce? Is he having a breakdown? Is there another woman? Whatever the problem is, his superiors surmise, Martin no longer seems to be partner material.

These stories demonstrate what can occur if you keep your fertility problems secret. Like Rose and Martin, you and your partner may have refrained from telling friends and co-workers about your problems. As a result of your new behavior or mood changes, colleagues might conclude that you're losing your edge or having a midlife crisis. Just when you need the understanding of your colleagues, family, and friends more than ever, you've alienated them.

Social psychologist Sheldon Cohen has conducted numerous studies demonstrating that social support is critical for getting through stressful situations.[12] You may feel uncomfortable discussing the intimate details with friends and co-workers, but you need not be secretive about the general problem.

Ultimately, Rose and Martin told their co-workers that they were involved in fertility treatment. Rose's principal gave her time off and assigned other teachers to fill in. The whole school seemed to rally around Rose. Now she can go to work without feeling as though she's failing as a teacher. Martin was less fortunate. He was forced to opt out of the partner track temporarily. He took the pressure off himself. His colleagues respected him for it. Martin knows that he will be able to return to a partner track once the infertility issues are resolved. But Martin is now able to be present at all of his wife's important procedures and surgeries. His main concern for now is to do everything possible to have a baby.

Disclosing the secret of your infertility frees you to interact normally with the people you care about. Psychologist Sidney Jourard, a researcher on self-disclosure,[13] suggests that distancing yourself from everyone else estranges you from yourself. On the other hand, it is inappropriate to tell anyone and everyone about your problem. Use good judgment. Think carefully about whom you should tell and under what circumstances. Maybe you will feel most comfortable telling your mother. On the other hand, you may feel better talking to a longtime friend. Whom you tell first is not important—it's the telling part that is critical. The support and encouragement you get from your confidants are often surprising. And you'll feel better, too. It's difficult at first, but you and your spouse must share what's happening, if only to unburden yourselves from feeling so isolated.

It also helps to have ready answers to embarrassing questions. Peggy took the direct approach to questions about why she had no children yet. Her answer was well rehearsed and always the same: "We want children, but we're having trouble. We're seeing the best doctor in town, and I'm hopeful all will go well. But I have trouble talking about this at happy occasions, so I hope we can change the subject." Gwen also had a pat answer, one more risqué than Peggy's: "Maybe nine months from this morning." We're not suggesting that you use either of these answers, merely that you come up with rehearsed statements that let you off the hook when you feel uncomfortable. What you tell casual acquaintances and how you talk about your infertility to people who really matter will differ drastically.

Another aspect of this Pointer concerns choosing which social occasions to attend. Bear in mind that baby-related events are difficult for most infertile women. Avoiding baby showers and baby namings or christenings protects you from directly having to experience a recent birth. Decide whether you can tolerate such events. If attending will upset you, then you are entirely justified in steering clear.

Young children's birthday parties and other family-oriented events also may be painful. Halloween, Christmas, Hanukkah, Thanksgiving, and other holidays may similarly depress you. You may decide to avoid family gatherings completely, perhaps using the occasion to get away with your partner for a few days. Or you may choose to attend the gathering only briefly and talk with individual family members prior to the event so they understand how you feel. Whatever you decide, make sure you have given these child-centered events careful consideration. Your job is to make your own life easier, not to be a dutiful daughter/sister/friend when you are not feeling strong.

6. BE A PARTNER IN TREATMENT

Arthur Greil, in *Not Yet Pregnant*,[14] makes an excellent point when he says that "infertility . . . is the process of becoming *medicalized*." He further asserts that this medicalization puts the infertile person into a "passive role" with her physician, who dominates all face-to-face interactions.

How do you view your role as the patient? Do you remain passive and let your doctor run the show? Or do you educate yourself (Pointer 1) and view yourself as a partner in your own treatment?

As a Partner in Treatment, you will feel more able to discuss the medical options, ask questions, and voice your opinions. Of course your doctor has a deeper knowledge of infertility diagnosis and treatment, but you know your own psychological responses to medication and your medical history, for example, better than anyone else. Failing to assert yourself with your doctor can make you feel frustrated and resentful of medical treatment that fails to meet your needs. Believe it or not, most doctors will welcome you as a partner.

By assertive, we certainly don't mean you should be obnoxious or constantly challenging your doctor's every word and action. Assertiveness, as one of the key aspects of this Pointer, means stating what you want and making every reasonable effort to get it. Being assertive means believing that it's your perfect right[15] to want certain things. Being assertive also means behaving in a way that is honest and relatively straightforward in terms of how you think and feel.

You are in touch with your emotional needs and your body better than anyone else ever could be. And your instincts are, more likely than not, valid. Remember that the treatment of infertility is an inexact science. Your input can influence many aspects of your treatment. Don't underestimate your intelligence just because you don't have a medical degree, and don't be intimidated by your doctors just because they do.

7. GET ORGANIZED

Making an appointment schedule, keeping tabs on where you are in your menstrual cycle, and staying on top of mounting bills and insurance payments can seem as demanding as a full-time job. And most people must maintain a full-time job in order to secure the means to pay medical bills or obtain health insurance coverage. But we have found that couples who have a system for paying bills, recording information, following up on insurance claims, and keeping a detailed appointment calendar report less stress surrounding their infertility than do couples who have no organized system.

The energy and time you spend staying organized is extremely valuable because it helps you gain control of your treatment. Women typically think they will remember the exact day of their postcoital test and its results. You probably think that you will never forget your endometrial biopsy and exactly what the doctor told you afterward. But with time, multiple treatments and doctors' reports can assimilate into a big, terrible blur. So after every treatment, we encourage you to keep a record of it—a medical one for your doctor and a psychological one for yourself.

In addition, we encourage you to keep logs of each and every menstrual cycle, master and utilize the insurance payment system we developed (only after we lost track of a few major claims of our own), and purchase and fill in an appointment calendar for all future tests, treatments, and procedures so you and your partner can better anticipate what's to come in the days and weeks ahead.

8. MAKE A PLAN

Couples battling infertility must make a myriad of decisions and judgments: what tests to have, what treatment options to explore, how many times to repeat them, how much money to spend, what doctor to select, and what procedures are most likely to bring success. Infertility decisions rank right up there with other important choices such as what college to attend and even what person to marry. While you should stay flexible to allow for medical breakthroughs, for new information about your condition, for a changing insurance policy, or even for a surprise pregnancy, it's still important to construct an overall plan so you know where you are and where you're headed at any given moment.

Forging a plan forces you to think about how much money you want to spend, how long you want to keep trying, how much physical and emotional trauma you believe you can withstand, what kinds of odds you are looking for, and other critical factors. As you make a plan, you need to ask yourself some tough questions—questions that focus on your physical, emotional, and financial wherewithal. Your inner monologue may go something like this: "I want a baby. What am I willing to do to make it happen? Am I willing to endure physical pain? Am I willing to spend my money on infertility treatments instead of a vacation? Am I willing to put my social life on hold? Can I put my career on the back burner?" Answers to these questions do not come easily. As one woman we talked to put it, "Infertility hurts my brain." What are you willing to sacrifice to achieve your goal?

Once you learn about all the available treatments and how they'll affect your life and pocketbook, you're ready to develop your plan. We recommend devising a six-month plan. By keeping things finite, you can determine your monetary and emotional limits without overwhelming yourself. If pregnancy remains elusive after six months, then reevaluate and devise another plan for the next six months. Six months is a reasonable amount of time since infertility treatment options are changing rapidly.

Once you develop your plan, stick with it unless new information warrants a change. Here's an example of a plan that was well organized and thoughtful, but not carved in stone.

Susan and Michael decided to try three in vitro procedures. If these three procedures failed, then they would begin to take steps toward adoption. Unfortunately, the three IVF procedures were unsuccessful. But then they learned about the recent great success of a procedure in which a donor gives her eggs to the couple to be fertilized with the husband's sperm, and then the embryo is transferred to the wife's uterus. Susan and Michael decided to try an egg-donor procedure before adopting. But, as they were waiting for a donor, Susan became pregnant by taking fertility drugs and having an insemination. Then Susan lost that pregnancy and became pregnant with the egg-donor procedure.

Susan and Michael are unconventional and flexible. They represent one category of planners. Many couples we talk to proceed differently. Some entertain several mini-plans simultaneously; they try a variety of treatment options in rapid succession, as well as pursue adoption at the same time. Others may tend to stay with one treatment for several years. There are many pathways through infertility. The case stories provided throughout the book can help you clarify what kind of planning style is most comfortable for you. Later in the book we provide you with a framework for decision-making and some skills and exercises that can help you make a plan that gives you the greatest degree of control.

9. MAKE DECISIONS

Making the right decisions will enable you to up the odds of getting pregnant when you thought you couldn't. Since our last edition, we have found that decision-making is central to all that we profess in this book. It is so important that we made decision-making a unique Pointer. When couples seek our help, what they want to accomplish in their sessions might be getting in touch with their feelings or changing their thinking, but in the end it's all about enabling them to make decisions about their treatment. No one would suggest that infertility counseling should not focus on thoughts and feelings—well-adjusted, thoughtful couples make the best patients. But, more importantly, people who seek our advice and read our book need to take action and make good decisions, decisions that will enable them to get what they hope for: a baby.

Often decisions are easy ones, like what month you will begin treatment, or how many months you will try Clomid before you move on to Fertinex, or who will give you shots. But, although most couples would find these decisions quite simple, we have seen countless couples who found even those decision hurdles almost insurmountable.

The McCallisters, both schoolteachers, talked for many sessions about the ideal time for treatment—summer was hard because of family commitments, September was impossible, and Christmas was no good. The Bermans focused on when they should move on to injectables. Was three Clomid cycles enough and eight too many? No amount of reading or surfing the Internet could help them decide. The Grillos almost canceled a cycle because Sam couldn't do the injections; Lilly didn't know a soul who could give the shots and the nearest hospital was forty miles away.

In some ways, these decisions were emotionally loaded—they signaled that pregnancy wasn't going to occur without assistance, that some of life is out of one's control, and that there are no absolutes about treatment. Unfortunately, the McCallisters have still not found the perfect time. They are unable to make a decision. In contrast, the Bermans, having become as educated as they could, have made a plan and, factoring in their age and their insurance coverage, have arrived at the decision to do six cycles using a pill called Clomid together with a procedure called intrauterine insemination (IUI) before moving on to injectables. The Grillos decided to bite the bullet and paid a nurse to give Lilly her injections. That decision was a good one—they are the proud parents of twin boys. Would they have become pregnant if they had decided on another choice, like Sam Grillo forcing himself to do the shots or Lilly Grillo asking her neighbor to be her injector? No one will ever know, but in fact, at this point Lilly and Sam never think about all the specifics of how they got pregnant because they are so busy with their boys.

Some decisions are infinitely more complicated and are time critical in nature. In the case of Cara and Mitch, timing isn't everything but certainly a big part of the decision. The decision to use a particular egg donor, for example, often must be made fairly quickly. Cara and Mitch have been presented with a number of donors who seemed on the surface to meet their requirements. Yet every time, Cara whines, "This is such an important life decision; what we do will determine who my child will be. We need more time and more information." They pass on each donor and then, months later, usually after they have been presented with a new profile, wish they had selected the donor presented previously. Cara and Mitch are frozen. Even though they understand that the nature of the procedure at this clinic is that they have to make fairly quick decisions, they are unwilling to go to another clinic that works differently or to recruit a donor on their own or to work with a donor broker who might be able to provide them with more detailed information. Because they can't change their thinking or get in touch with their feelings, they also can't make a decision—to accept a donor, to change clinics, or to move on to adoption. They can't put into action the decision-making techniques we've been helping them master because they really aren't ready to use an egg donor. Once they face the fact that no "perfect" donor will arrive nor will Cara's eggs rejuvenate themselves, then they will be ready to select a donor.

In contrast to Cara and Mitch, the Hollands are model decision-makers. They made choices about treatment options, clinics, insurance plans, and even whether to freeze excess embryos. The last decision they had to make was one that took them by surprise: whether or not to undergo a selective reduction from four babies to two babies when they found out that they were pregnant with quads. Probably no amount of projecting themselves into a less-than-ideal future would have prepared them for this decision—one that had to be made in less than two weeks. Using all the previous Pointers—gathering information, partnering with their doctor, talking to others who have reduced to twins and those who have delivered quads, as well as speaking to their minister and to us—the couple decided to reduce to twins. They knew that the procedure was risky and they knew that they might feel sad and depressed during the pregnancy and even after, but the Hollands made a decision quickly and definitively. The odds were on their side and, happily, they have given birth to two healthy girls.

As you read the cases in this book, we encourage you to ask yourself what you would do. In a sense, we are asking you to identify with our clients and do a rehearsal for life in your mind's eye. Some of the situations described and the choices described will ultimately be your own. Don't worry—hopefully when you arrive at these junctures, you and your partner will be armed with information and will have learned to make decisions effectively.

10. DON'T GIVE UP

Overall statistics suggest that about one out of two infertile couples will eventually produce a baby. But we believe that for some couples whose problems are not too complex or who are willing to go the limit—using repeated trials with donor eggs, donor sperm, or even both—the success rate can approach 90 percent. Of course, this 90 percent figure represents what's *medically* possible. Unfortunately, medical possibilities require economic resources. Many of the 90 percent of people whose infertility problems could be medically remedied may be unable to afford the cost of treatment. It is truly a shame that family-planning decisions are so strongly affected by finances.

Naturally, some infertility treatments are more successful than others. The "cutting-edge" treatments that offer possibilities when nothing else would ever work get the most publicity. But their odds of success are still limited. Even the top-notch programs have a take-home baby rate of about 50 percent at best with IVF and its related assisted technologies. Simpler procedures, such as artificial insemination, can also offer you reasonable success rates. Even though we encourage you to try all possible avenues optimistically, *we also encourage you to be realistic about your odds of getting pregnant.*

To appreciate fully the odds of succeeding with a single therapy, imagine that you are sitting in your doctor's office with nine other women. Each of you has dysfunctional ovaries and is about to start Pergonal therapy. At the end of six attempts, four of you will be pregnant.

No human being could sit in that waiting room and undergo treatment unless she believes she will be one of those four. Doctors encourage that optimism. Yet they walk a tightrope between encouraging you and tempering that encouragement with a realistic perspective. When a procedure fails, they urge you to try again.

And remember, technology is evolving all the time. Today's insurmountable problem may be fixable next year. For example, since we wrote the first edition of our book, the treatment of male infertility has changed radically. The technique of injecting a single sperm into an egg has allowed men who would not have been considered for IVF in the early nineties to father a biological child today. Other new and exciting techniques and medications have also improved success for other medical problems.

It is important to continue when many attempts have failed. The important key is to find ways to persevere despite these repeated failures. The temptation to give up increases if you withdraw from daily activities or let the specter of infertility color everything you do. Later in the book, we will introduce motivational (and sometimes even humorous) techniques borrowed from athletes,[16] actors,[17] artists,[18] and other successful individuals who manage to keep going in the face of adversity. The skills, modified for use with infertility, focus on helping you help yourself through all the various situations you must confront. You can choose those that work for you or adapt them to fit your circumstances. Armed with these tactics, you will be able to continue infertility treatment as long as it continues to hold out a realistic chance of success.

PUTTING IT ALL TOGETHER: HOW THE TEN POINTERS COMBINE TO HELP YOU START LIVING AGAIN

Taken individually, each Pointer probably won't seem like a major life change. But once you start putting all Ten Pointers into practice, we expect you will begin to view your infertility in a new, positive light you previously thought was impossible. Practicing the Ten Pointers can help you resume a normal, happy life even though your infertility is not yet resolved.

It's important for you to live in the present in order to make rational decisions, cope with treatment, and live a rich and rewarding life despite your infertility. It is counterproductive to regret any past actions as the real or imagined cause of your current problem. It is tempting to talk about what might have been or what you should have done. Leeanne, for example, still weeps over the abortion she had when she was eighteen, even though it seemed to be the only proper course of action at the time. "I should have had the baby," Leeanne laments. "Now my tubes are blocked and I'll never get pregnant."

Ed, meanwhile, berates himself about the vasectomy he had during his marriage to Valerie. Little did he know then that he'd one day divorce Valerie and marry another woman who wants children. "Who would have thought it? Me with new kids at my age, but it sounds nice," says Ed, whose children from his first marriage are grown.

"When Valerie suggested a vasectomy, it seemed like a good idea. But I never should have listened to her."

Leeanne and Ed are each mired in what we call "pastspeak." They dwell obsessively on their past. What they did years ago made sense at that time. They need to live in the present. You probably have some of your own should-haves and what-ifs. Everybody does. But infertile people seem to dwell on these past occurrences, perhaps to avoid the frustrations of their current dilemma. Living in the past robs you of the pleasures of today. If you live in the past, you are more likely to give up your quest to get pregnant. You must find a way to build happiness into your everyday life even as you pursue your goal of getting pregnant. Focusing on the present is more productive and healthier than dwelling on the past.

Through the Ten Pointers, Leeanne and Ed each are working to let go of their past. They are lucky to live in the twenty-first century. Their infertility problems can be treated—all with surprisingly good results. In vitro fertilization can bypass Leanne's bad tubes. And Ed has a better chance of successfully reversing his vasectomy than of reducing his alimony payments to Valerie! Our advice to you is the same as it is to Leanne and Ed: Don't look back. Plant yourself firmly in the present. Make a plan. Find a doctor who can help, and become an active, informed partner in treatment. Make decisions that take into consideration your money, your age, your need for control, and your family-building objectives.

The Ten Pointers can help you avoid another common pitfall of infertility: pining for the future. Spending all your time on "futurethought" can make your precious todays melt together. Instead of living in the here and now, infertile couples often calculate the days until ovulation, the weeks until the pregnancy test, or the months until the next IVF procedure. This hurry-up-and-wait phenomenon is one of the most difficult problems infertile people need to overcome. There is so much to wait for: the doctor, a procedure, a drug to take effect, an operation, and, of course, the pregnancy itself. Dwelling on all you have to wait for can put your life on hold. Dorothy lived her life nine months ahead. If she got pregnant in January, her baby would be born in October; if she got pregnant in February, it would be born in November. Each month she got out her astrology book and read what sign her baby would be born under if she got pregnant that month. When she wasn't pregnant that month, she'd start reading the next chapter.

Dorothy is an extreme example of somebody who was unable to live in the present. Each failure seemed to pull her farther from her immediate goals. Through the Ten Pointers, Dorothy reframed her thinking, got in touch with her feelings, developed a system to organize her bills and appointments, and made a plan. She scheduled some pleasant activities with her husband and with her friends. Dorothy is now working hard to live in the present.

We're not suggesting that it's going to be easy to live in the today world, but we believe that the wait for conception will be more tolerable if you train yourself to experience each day fully. But with all these worries on your mind, how can you possibly live in the present? The answer is to force yourself. Make a conscious effort to purge futurethought and pastspeak from your consciousness. Dispute any self-pitying or self-loathing sentiments you might harbor. To counter negative statements like "What's the use of buying a bigger house if I can't have a baby?" prepare a convincing retort, such as "My husband and I will feel more comfortable with more space." And be patient. Allow time to dig yourself out of the rut you have been in.

We provide some digging-out tools in the Getting Pregnant Workout, a set of skills described in the next chapter. The Workout, like the Ten Pointers, will help you start living again, even if your infertility seems far from being resolved.

CHAPTER 2

Helping Yourself Through Infertility: The Getting Pregnant Workout

As we went through the diagnosis and treatment of our own infertility, we felt the sort of disappointment and heartache other infertile couples tell us they feel. We learned that infertility can prevent people from living normal lives, since our own lives were incapacitated by our failures to conceive. As psychotherapists experienced in helping others cope with emotionally charged issues, we searched for ways to adapt our counseling methods to help us through our own ordeal. Our search led us to develop our Getting Pregnant Workout.

The Getting Pregnant Workout is a series of activities that puts the Ten Pointers discussed in Chapter 1 into action. The Workout blends elements used by clinical psychologists of various schools of psychotherapy—all modified to meet the unique needs of people with fertility problems. Among the traditions we draw from are cognitive and family therapy, mental imagery, communications theory, behavior modification, and Gestalt psychotherapy.

As a way to start living normally again, we began counseling infertile couples in our psychotherapy practice. These sessions provided us with new perspectives and additional psychological information, which we also incorporated into the Getting Pregnant Workout. Readers have written us letters and sent us e-mails telling us how helpful these techniques have been for them. We chose the word "workout" deliberately. We have found that you cannot cope success-fully with infertility on a casual basis. It takes psychological work to equip yourself with the tools you need to handle the tough situations that may lie ahead. With practice, healthy responses to awkward or upsetting situations will become second nature.

Linda Salzer, an infertility counselor and author of the widely acclaimed book *Surviving Infertility*,[1] tells audiences how she and her husband devised and actually rehearsed a set of signals they used to escape uneasy social encounters. At one dinner dance, she explains, Linda grew extremely anxious as several women at her table began exchanging pictures of their babies. Linda signaled her husband with a subtle hand gesture. In response, he whisked her from the table and swiftly waltzed her across the dance floor and out of the room so she could cry in private instead of embarrassing herself in front of her friends.

Like Linda, you can prepare yourself for any situation: social, med-ical, job related, or financial. The Getting Pregnant Workout is most effective when practiced for several brief periods every day. The more you practice, the better you'll get at the Getting Pregnant Workout skills: relaxation, self-talk, written self-expression, interpersonal com-munication, assertiveness training, decision-making, record-keeping, goal-setting, and using your imagination. Later in the book we'll pro-vide further details to help you cope with specific situations—such as using the decision-making technique to choose your doctor.

INFERTILITY IS STRESSFUL

The stress of infertility is inescapable. No matter what you do, you cannot entirely avoid it. Although you may be aware of your stress, you probably don't know yet how to cope with it.

For the past nine years we have asked thousands of infertile women and men to rate how stressful they found the experience of infertility. Our scale was modeled on one developed by researcher Thomas Holmes.[2] His concept was that various life events required social read-justment. For example, after a divorce one's life changes and readjust-ments must be made. Holmes and his colleagues had people rate various events in terms of the amount of readjustment they would require. He asked them to compare the amount of readjustment to the amount they thought would be required by the death of their spouse. Death of a spouse was designated 100 units. Compared with that traumatic event, Holmes research participants rated a divorce as 73 units, a jail term as 63 units, and getting fired from a job as 47 units. Our results for patients who were about to begin an in vitro fertilization procedure were remarkably stable. Time and again women rated the experience at about 60 life change units. Their husbands, on the other hand, rated the experience significantly lower (in one study as low as 47 units).

But those results were for patients in one particular clinic and for women who were about to begin an IVF procedure—a procedure that held out hope of their getting pregnant. We wanted to see how stressful infertility was for women not actively involved in treatment or for women not doing treatments as "high-tech" as IVF. To get this information, we conducted a survey on the Web site of the International Council on Infertility Information Dissemination (INCIID). More than 600 people from 47 states and 17 foreign countries responded to this survey. You can view a slide presentation of the survey results on our Web site at http://www.gettingpregnantbook.com/news_fertility.htm. And although anyone, male or female, could complete the survey, over 99.8 percent of those responding were women. These women spanned the entire range of treatment from those not currently doing anything to women undergoing the most cutting-edge treatments. What we found was that our clinic sample results were remarkably similar to the results of our Internet survey. Women who were not currently in treatment rated the stress of infertility as 60 units. Women doing relatively "low- tech" inseminations rated infertility as 68 units, and those doing the most high-tech treatments rated it as 67 units. These results confirm our view that women find the experience of infertility stressful.

The stress of infertility is both long- and short-term. Like other long-term, or chronic, stressful situations, such as poverty or cancer, there may be little you can do to change your predicament. You may feel as though you are running on a treadmill and keep failing in your attempts to jump off.

Then there are short-term, or acute stresses that last from a few minutes to a few days. Waiting for the results of a test. Receiving a medical bill you can't afford to pay. Getting invited to a baby shower. All are examples of short-term, or acute stress.

The Unique Aspects of Infertility Stress

Researchers at the University of Michigan's Institute for Social Research investigated whether men and women react differently to infertility stress than to other sources of stress.[3] They found that women do but men do not. Stress resulting from infertility or from other major life problems taxed women's marital relationships, but the infertility stress was a significantly greater contributor than stress from other life problems. Not so for men. They were not immune to the effects of stress. They too experience marital strain because of stress. The difference, however, is that fertility stress is no more disruptive than other forms of stress for men.

What about infertility was contributing to this stress?[4] The researchers found that treatment costs were an important contributor. Having to undergo numerous tests and treatments was another important source of stress. And a concern that the couple would have to use a donor rather than their own eggs or sperm was another important source of stress.

Canadian researchers Jacky Boivin and Janet Takefman[5] investigated levels of stress at various stages of an in vitro fertilization (IVF) procedure. In Chapter 7 we will describe IVF. For the purposes of this discussion we note that women undergoing this procedure go through several stages: taking fertility medications, coming in for blood monitoring and ultrasounds on an almost daily basis, having their eggs retrieved and fertilized, waiting two weeks, and getting the results of a pregnancy test. The Canadians asked women to keep a daily journal to record how much stress they experienced. They kept track of which women got pregnant and which did not. They found that neither the women who got pregnant nor their nonpregnant counterparts were particularly stressed when they were just taking the fertility medications. But the ones who did not become pregnant were significantly more stressed *even before they knew they were not pregnant* when coming in for daily monitoring and when having their eggs retrieved. Although we can offer this only as conjecture, it may be that *feeling stressed out* in some way may have lowered their chance of getting pregnant.

The Physical Effects of Stress

In times of stress, so-called fight or flight hormones kick in. It happened when your cave-dwelling ancestors confronted a lightning storm. And it happens when you confront your pregnant sister-in-law. Eventually, the fight-or-flight response can exhaust you mentally and physically. It can even make you sick or more prone to physical pain. The adrenaline flowing through your body makes you tense up during an endometrial biopsy, for example. Unlike your prehistoric ancestors, however, you can acquire the knowledge to analyze, evaluate, and even challenge erroneous assumptions about your infertility. You can learn to employ a variety of adaptive techniques that can reshape your responses, lower pain, and keep your self-esteem intact.

The following chart shows how the stress of infertility can affect your body:

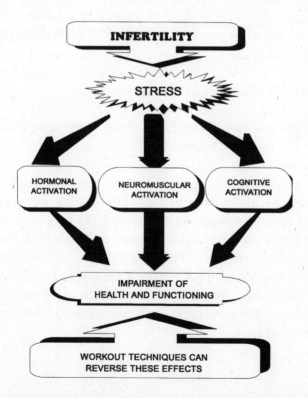

Figure 2.1 How Infertility Stress Affects Your Body

Combating Stress: Changing Your Thoughts to Take Positive Action

Look at the bottom section of the chart. It shows that the Workout techniques can reverse the negative effects of infertility stress. *How* you are affected by stress depends on how you *view* your situation. Richard Lazarus,[6] a psychologist and an eminent stress researcher, has shown that how you *appraise* a situation often determines how you are affected by it. If you view the situation as a *threat* and you believe you *lack the resources to cope* with it, you will become stressed. The critical element here is your outlook. And your outlook can be changed. If you learn to view the experience differently, you can modify how you respond to what's happening and how you behave in that situation.

Recasting your view of infertility is a key component to the Getting Pregnant Workout. The techniques we present have strong theoretical underpinnings in the field of behavioral medicine. At the core of behavioral medicine are four principles important to people confronting infertility:

- Be aware of what you are thinking;
- Change your erroneous beliefs;
- Learn various methods and techniques to assist you; and
- Carry out these skills in daily life.

You can begin by exerting some control over what happens to you. When we talk of control, we don't mean the ability to control whether you get pregnant. We mean you can develop the belief that you are not helpless and that you can take an active role in your diagnosis, treatment, and social interactions. The following model, modified from the work of two Canadians, psychiatrist Eldon Tunks and psychologist Anthony Bellissimo,[7] graphically depicts the relationship between your thoughts, your view of yourself and your capabilities, and the actions you take.

GETTING PREGNANT POINTERS

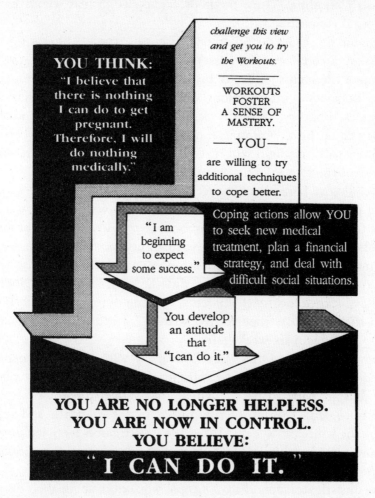

Figure 2.2 The Relationship of Your Thoughts and Your Actions

The Mind-Body Connection

Thinking optimistic thoughts won't unblock your tubes or make your husband's low sperm count suddenly become normal. Nor will reducing your stress level. But studies suggest that relaxation has many other beneficial effects. Researcher Candace Pert,[8] cancer surgeon Bernie Siegel,[9] and author Norman Cousins,[10] among many others, have all written about non-traditional, intellectual/emotional methods of healing. These methods acknowledge that we all have a body-mind connection.

Immunologist George Solomon[11] discusses studies suggesting that depression, a condition often associated with infertility, leads to suppression of the body's ability to provide immunity against certain diseases. "Behavioral interventions (such as psychotherapy, relaxation techniques, imagery, biofeedback, and hypnosis) should be able to enhance or optimize immune function," he states. And he predicts that, eventually, research will directly prove his belief. More recently, evidence of the sort Solomon was hoping for has appeared.

Psychologist James Pennebaker has been studying how the expression of thoughts and feelings, verbally or in private journal writing, affects the functioning of the immune system. He asked one group of students to write about their deepest thoughts and feelings concerning a traumatic experience for twenty minutes per day for four consecutive days. A second group of students did the same, but wrote about a superficial experience. All students consented to have their blood drawn the day before they started writing, after their last session of writing, and again six weeks later.

Immunologists at Ohio State University with whom Pennebaker worked extracted white blood cells from the samples. They placed these cells in petri dishes to which they added foreign substances called mitogens. The job of the mitogens was to attack and try to destroy the white blood cells. What the investigators were looking for was how well the white blood cells could trigger immune reactions to offer protection against the invading mitogens.

The investigators found that "people who wrote about their deepest thoughts and feelings surrounding traumatic experiences evidenced heightened immune function compared with those who wrote about superficial topics. Although this effect was most pronounced after the last day of writing, it tended to persist 6 weeks after the study."[12] Pennebaker also found that the students who wrote about their traumas showed a drop in the frequency of their visits to the Student Health Center. We will have more to say about Pennebaker's work later in this chapter and will provide you with some activities to reduce infertility stress based on his work.

First and foremost, the Getting Pregnant Workout will help you relax and feel less stressed out. We are unable to offer any scientific evidence that the Workout will combat the *physical* aspects of your infertility, but we maintain that if you do the Workout as recommended, you will be able to manage your medical treatment more effectively.

There is also some new evidence that, while not examining physiological mechanisms, is, however, suggestive that doing the sorts of activities in the Getting Pregnant Workout may actually increase the likelihood of getting pregnant. In April 2000, Alice Domar published the results of a multi-year preventative intervention trial that examined whether psychological interventions could lead to increased pregnancy rates in infertile women.[13] Three groups of women participated in the study: a cognitive-behavioral group, a support group that did not use cognitive-behavioral techniques, and a control group that received no intervention. Participants in both the cognitive-behavioral group and the support group met for ten weeks for two hours each week. In the support group, the first hour was spent updating other members about what was happening medically with each member, what was going on with family and friends, and how each participant was feeling. The second hour was devoted to exploring a particular topic in depth, including how infertility affected self-esteem, how it affected work, and how it affected relationships with their spouse or partner. In the cognitive-behavioral program participants learned many of the skills we offer you in the Getting Pregnant Workout: progressive relaxation, imagery, cognitive restructuring (i.e., Getting Pregnant Self-Talk), as well as skills at doing yoga and meditation, and nutrition and exercise counseling.

Unfortunately, a considerable number of women in all groups dropped out of the study. Of the original 184 women in the study, a total of 64 dropped out (60 percent of the control group, 26 percent of the support group, and 17 percent of the cognitive-behavioral group). But for those who remained, the exciting finding of this study was that 55 percent of the women in the cognitive-behavioral group and 54 percent of the women in the support group experienced a viable pregnancy, in comparison to only 20 percent of the women in the control group. Interestingly, of the 26 women who conceived in the cognitive-behavioral group, 11 (42 percent) conceived spontaneously in comparison to only 3 of the 26 conceptions in the support group (11 percent) that occurred spontaneously. Keep in mind that this study used very few participants, so you must exercise caution in drawing conclusions from the results. But perhaps these results are hinting that physiological changes may be taking place as a result of "workout-like" techniques. It certainly seems worthwhile to give them a try.

RELAXATION: A GOOD WAY
TO CONFRONT STRESS HEAD ON

Most of the infertile couples we counsel talk about loss, pain, and grief. They speak of feeling overwhelmed. And they worry about what infertility is doing to their marriage, their careers, and their view of themselves and others. Dawn posted this message on the INCIID emotional issues bulletin board:

"People are always saying to relax and not stress so much about getting pregnant and when you least expect it, it will happen. Anyone who can say that has not experienced the agony of infertility. How do you relax knowing that you are ovulating and this may be the only chance you have for another 28 days? How do you stop thinking about getting pregnant when your body is telling you you are ready? How do you emotionally detach yourself from wanting to get pregnant? If anyone has any ideas of how to 'relax,' please let me know."[14] To help women like Dawn, we recommend techniques such as progressive relaxation, controlled breathing, and positive imagery to break the cycle of debilitating negative emotions. By using these relaxation methods, our clients have slowly replaced their negative thoughts with a sense of peace. Gradually, they find the inner strength to take the steps necessary to increase their odds of getting pregnant.

As clinical psychologist Thomas D'Zurilla describes it, relaxation works in this way:[15]

- Relaxation *reduces emotional upheaval directly*. It helps calm you down so that you are not so overwhelmed by what you are feeling. Relaxation helps you reduce the level of your debilitating emotion.
- Practicing relaxation techniques helps you *learn to monitor your stress* and recognize the stress as it begins to occur. Mastering relaxation allows you to be on "automatic pilot," ready and able to reduce your stress as you begin to feel it.

- When you begin to achieve relaxation, you give yourself *direct access to your counterproductive thoughts* that may be keeping you from seeking treatment, preventing you from complying with your doctor's orders, or making you interact negatively with your spouse, family, or friends.

Progressive Relaxation

Progressive relaxation, pioneered in the 1930s by physiologist and psychologist Edmund Jacobson, is an effective way to relax and reduce anxiety.[16] Jacobson believed that if people could learn to relax their muscles through a precise method, mental relaxation would follow. Jacobson's technique involves tensing and relaxing various voluntary muscle groups throughout the body in an orderly sequence. According to psychologists Robert Woolfolk and Frank Richardson in their book *Stress, Sanity, and Survival*, "Despite the relative obscurity of this method, progressive relaxation is perhaps the most reliable and effective procedure of all [the different means of achieving relaxation]."[17] Since Jacobson developed and refined his techniques, people have used progressive relaxation to alleviate such diverse stress-related disorders as anxiety, ulcers, hypertension, and insomnia.

Progressive relaxation works because of the relationship between your muscle tension and your emotional tension. When you feel emotionally distraught, you automatically tense your muscles. Your muscle tension is a *cause* of the headaches and backaches of infertility, as well as a *clue* about how you are responding to your infertility.

Mastering progressive relaxation in its pure form requires extensive training and more practice than people dealing with infertility generally have time to do. Research, however, has shown that abbreviated versions of progressive relaxation can be quite effective in alleviating the effects of stress.

Five features are critical:

PLACE: Find a quiet room where you can work undisturbed.
POSITION: To learn progressive relaxation, all parts of your body must be comfortably supported. Find a bed, a couch, or a recliner.
CLOTHING: Wear loose clothing.

TIME: Designate about fifteen minutes daily. Try to schedule a fixed time every day so you won't forget to do your progressive relaxation.

FOCUS: Try to focus on the particular sensations that come from letting go of tension.

Prior to beginning your progressive relaxation routine, have someone whose voice you find pleasant tape-record the text in the box that follows. Tell that person to speak slowly and clearly, pausing to give you time to respond.

DIRECTIONS:
Turn on the tape and follow the script.

Lie or sit in a comfortable position. I'm going to ask you to tense and relax various parts of your body. When I say TENSE, I'd like you to tense that body part. When I say RELAX, I'd like you to let go of all tension. Try to focus on one body part at a time.

Get in touch with your breathing. Breathe out, breathe in. Imagine that as each body part is relaxed, all tension is gone. TENSE your toes. RELAX. TENSE your knees. RELAX. TENSE your right leg. RELAX. You should feel your whole leg relaxing and settling into the floor. TENSE your left leg. RELAX. Now TENSE your buttocks. RELAX. Press your lower back against the floor. RELAX. TENSE your stomach. RELAX. TENSE your rib cage. RELAX. Feel the tension gone in your lower body.

Push your shoulders back. RELAX. Pull your shoulders forward. RELAX. Now work on your arms. Make a fist with one hand. RELAX. TENSE that upper arm. RELAX. TENSE that whole arm. RELAX. Make a fist with the other hand. RELAX. TENSE that upper arm. RELAX. TENSE that whole arm. RELAX.

Now let's work on your face and head. Clench your jaw. RELAX. Open your mouth wide. RELAX. Grimace. RELAX. Scrunch up your whole face. RELAX. Eyes closed. RELAX. Eyes wide. RELAX. Now feel all the tension gone from everywhere in your whole body. Keep breathing. Breathe out. Breathe in. Feel completely relaxed.

Learning to Breathe

Voluntary breath control is probably the oldest known stress-reduction technique. It is a major component of yoga, the ancient Indian self-help system of health care and spiritual development; T'ai Chi, a Chinese movement art form; and the Lamaze method of natural childbirth. These and other methods share a focus on the four distinct phases of the breathing cycle: inhalation, pause, exhalation, and pause. Becoming aware of these four phases is an essential step in obtaining control of your breathing pattern. Once you gain control of your breathing in a non-stressful environment, you can more readily call up your relaxation breathing during times of stress.

Your thoughts and your internal responses are closely linked. If you think anxious thoughts, your breathing becomes shallow and rapid. Conversely, shallow, rapid breathing can make it difficult for you to think calmly and rationally. If you are caught in this vicious cycle, you can either change your thoughts or change your breathing—and the other will follow. You can use controlled breathing to implement an important Pointer: *changing how you think about your infertility.* Also, by learning to breathe properly, you can begin to feel less fatigued, less overwhelmed by your thoughts, and more able to cope with each new procedure and treatment. As you cope better, you will become more optimistic. While not a panacea, the Getting Pregnant Breathing described below is perhaps the easiest new technique you'll master.

Again, tape-record the directions in the following box. Play them back when you have a few minutes to learn to practice Getting Pregnant Breathing.

Lie on your back on a rug. Get comfortable.

Place one hand on your chest and the other on your abdomen. Without trying to change your breathing, notice which hand is rising and falling with each breath. If your belly rises as you breathe in, you are breathing from your diaphragm. If not, you are breathing from your chest.

Shift your breathing from chest to diaphragm. Inhale slowly and deeply through your nose into your abdomen to push up your hand as much as it feels comfortable. Smile slightly, inhale through your nose, and exhale through your mouth. Make a relaxed soft sound like the wind as you exhale. It should sound like "Whoosh."

Continue taking slow deep breaths. Inhale. Exhale . . . whoosh. Inhale. Exhale . . . whoosh. Think of each whoosh as a sigh of relief.

- Practice this activity for five minutes at a time once or twice a day.
- At the end of each breathing time, focus on your body and its tension. By the end of a week, you should see a noticeable difference in your tension, particularly in your neck and shoulders, and in the muscles around your jaw.
- After one week's practice, try this activity while sitting or standing.
- After one month of practicing, try this activity during a doctor's visit.

Once you've mastered controlled breathing, you can use it while driving to your doctor's office, sitting in the waiting room, or during a medical test or procedure. You can even use it while waiting to hear the results of a test. Use controlled breathing anytime you start to feel tension.

GETTING PREGNANT SELF-TALK (GPST)

Almost all infertile couples we have encountered entertain negative thoughts. One of our clients, Gloria, was trying to decide whether she should change doctors. We ask her to voice her inner thoughts. "What difference does it make," she responded. "Nobody will be able to find out what's wrong with me. I'm not pregnant with this doctor. The next one will just cost more but won't do me any good." With thoughts like these, how could Gloria ever make positive decisions? We taught her to listen to her thoughts and to say them aloud when no one was in the room. From that point, we told her to replace the negativity with positive thoughts. This self-talk method eventually motivated her to take appropriate action.

If you stop and say your inner thoughts aloud, your monologue probably sounds like this: "I'll never get pregnant. I'm sure this will go on forever. I will never be a parent." Bombarding yourself with negative thoughts like these impedes your ability to deal with the fertile world, undergo surgery, or make the first phone call to a doctor. Your negative inner statements stand in the way of what you want most.

You need to learn to use the same *cognitive* technique we taught Gloria. We call that technique Getting Pregnant Self-Talk (GPST). Implementing all Ten Pointers, GPST is the single most powerful technique in the Getting Pregnant Workout.

Self-talk is a technique used in cognitive psychotherapy, a form of counseling that focuses on how thoughts and images contribute to stress. Psychiatrist Aaron Beck, one of the country's leading cognitive therapists, discusses the importance of *automatic thoughts.*[18] Automatic thoughts are those thoughts that occur in your stream of consciousness *automatically* and are rarely questioned. They are couched with *shoulds* and *musts*, and are difficult to turn off. People erroneously treat their automatic thoughts as foregone conclusions rather than hypotheses to be questioned. Your automatic thoughts about infertility make you believe your situation is hopeless. These thoughts may prevent you from taking steps to help yourself.

Donald Meichenbaum, who developed the method of *stress inoculation*, believes that all people engage in an internal dialogue.[19] Your internal dialogue incorporates your expectations and evaluation of yourself and your behavior. The psychic pain you experience from inner statements such as "I'll never get pregnant" can paralyze you. Meichenbaum teaches his clients to use self-talk to create a productive inner dialogue that replaces these defeatist ideas.

GPST aims to boost your self-esteem and motivate you to act. GPST is *not* the vague, imprecise feelings you have regarding a situation, but rather the actual words you say to yourself in your mind's ear. Because self-talk requires that you say each word in your monologue (not just think it), we encourage you to try GPST by first writing down and then rehearsing your new inner monologue. Then, when you feel ready, use GPST during an actual situation. It may be helpful to think of GPST in the following steps:

<u>G</u>et in touch with my negative self-statements

<u>P</u>repare a counterargument

<u>S</u>ay my new statement

<u>T</u>hank myself

We'll help you get started by asking you to follow the steps and fill in the following incomplete statements. Try to be as specific as possible when writing your statements. We'll illustrate each step with responses from some of our clients.

1. Get in touch with negative statements by filling in the following blanks. We'll illustrate each step with responses from some of our clients:

   a. I don't think I can _____

   b. I'm afraid I will _____

   c. I don't want to _____

   d. I think that _____ will happen again.

   e. (Create your own phrase) _____

   Our clients said:

   a. I don't think I can *take my temperature one more time*.

   b. I'm afraid I will *never carry a baby to term*.

   c. I don't want to *get my hopes up just to have them dashed*.

   d. I think that *a miscarriage* will happen again.

   e. (Create your own phrase): *This can't be happening*.

2. Prepare a counterargument for each of these negative statements. First read how our clients prepared their counterarguments. Then prepare yours.

   Counter a: *By taking my temperature I'm upping my odds of getting pregnant*.

   Counter b: *I know I'll find an answer to this puzzle of miscarriage*.

   Counter c: *Perhaps getting my hopes up will get me through the next procedure*.

   Counter d. *I'm strong enough to deal with another disappointment.*

   Counter e: *This is not a punishment or a curse but a fact of life*.

   Now prepare *your* counterarguments.

   Counter a: _____

   Counter b: _____

   Counter c: _____

   Counter d: _____

   Counter e: _____

3. Say your counterarguments out loud in a place where no one else can hear you. Once you've said them out loud, repeat them silently to yourself several times.

4. Thank yourself for trying to cope. We'll give you the first few thank-yous; you create several more:
   a. Thanks for taking control.
   b. I like myself for helping myself.
   c. I'm proud of myself for working to change.
   d. (Your own thank-yous go here.)

Here is one more GPST memory tool to help you understand the four types of GPST statements. Examples are included with each.

Guiding yourself: *Let's figure out what this test result means.*

Psyching yourself up: *By calling the doctor I'm upping my odds.*

Soothing talk: *It's okay. This procedure will be over soon.*

Taking charge. *Come on now. Pull yourself together.*

Guiding statements help you through taxing procedures. They also assist you when you feel confused or overwhelmed. If you get a medical report that you cannot understand, don't panic. Instead, calmly guide yourself. Say, "Let's figure out what this test result means." Psyching-up statements use positive and optimistic language to motivate you. Don't let that inner voice defeat you with phrases like "What's the use of trying?" Fight back with a psyching counterargument such as "By calling the doctor, I'm upping my odds." Soothing talk is like your inner parent calming you down when you are scared. When you panic during an unpleasant procedure, use soothing words like "It'll be over soon." Finally, taking-charge statements spur you into action or shut you down if you find yourself obsessing.

MAKING YOUR PREGNANCY QUEST JOURNAL—USING EXPRESSIVE WRITING[20]

A logical extension of Getting Pregnant Self-Talk and a way to begin your Pregnancy Quest Journal is to "move outside of your head" and externalize your thoughts on paper. If you feel more comfortable dictating into a tape recorder, you can achieve the same end that way.

Your Pregnancy Quest Journal will be a series of exercises and activities to help you record your thoughts and feelings. Some activities in this journal will help you get in touch with your thoughts and feelings. Other activities ask that you probe more deeply as issues and situations are becoming difficult. Throughout the book, we present different activities to help you deal with treatment failures and successes. We also encourage you to involve your partner in participating in some of the exercises as a way to let your partner into what you are truly experiencing.

The best way to create your Pregnancy Quest Journal is to create one yourself. You will need the following materials:

- Three-inch-thick three-ring binder (to hold all your materials)
- Three-holed subject divider sheets (you will be creating lots of different sections)
- Three-hole punch (for articles you cut out or print out to include in your journal)
- Plastic pockets (for material you get at conferences, business cards, birth announcements, etc.)
- Three-holed unlined notebook paper (for drawings or diagrams you will create)
- Colored markers and highlighters (to highlight important material and to create drawings)
- Glue stick (to glue material you've cut out and to help create collages)
- Scissors
- Three-hole punched photograph holders (for your special photographs, ultrasound scans, etc.)

The activities we suggest are based on the work of psychologist James Pennebaker in his book *Opening Up: The Healing Power of Expressing Emotions.*[21] Pennebaker makes the important point that the effectiveness of writing therapy is not due to simple catharsis or to venting pent-up emotions. What is critical is how you write about your experience.

Here are your first steps:

- *Make a special writing place.* Try to find a quiet private place where you can avoid the distractions of a radio or a TV. Try to make sure that your special place affords you privacy where you don't have to worry about someone barging in and discovering what you are doing.
- *Be your own audience.* You are writing for yourself, not to impress someone else. If you find yourself thinking "I hope my mother sees this so she will know what I'm feeling," you will be writing for her and not for yourself. You will be less likely to derive therapeutic benefits from such writing. You will be writing to make an impression rather than to let go of and explore your feelings.
- *Make a journal that will become your special book.*
- *Write whatever is on your mind.* Sometimes you may find that there is a thought you keep thinking over and over again. You just can't get it out of your mind. That's a good candidate for your journal. Here is an example:

Cara couldn't get the notion that she and Ron should have started trying earlier to have a baby. She told us that she wanted to have her house all ready for her baby. Building the house and furnishing the house took much longer than she thought. Cara is thirty-four and feeling terrified. We urged her to write about this in her journal. Here is what she wrote:

We've been married for 6 years. We should have started trying when we lived in the condo. Even though there wasn't much room I bet we would have a kid by now. So what if we have a nice house. I always wanted a bay window in the baby's room. Well now I have a bay window but no baby. Why didn't I stop taking birth control pills four years ago. I'm really stupid. I'm really greedy. I can't believe I listened to my gynecologist who said it would be really easy. We made a big mistake. I'm scared now. I have a bay window but no baby.

Sometimes you might have a thought that you would love to share with others but feel too embarrassed to share. Write it down. Here is what Senovia wrote:

All my sisters all have babies. My little brothers' wives all have babies. I'm the oldest. I'm supposed to be first. In my heart I had the name Veronica, Nica, for short, for my baby. Then I find out my littlest brother's baby is going to be named Nica. They stole my name. I'm so angry. I practically raised my little brother. He knew I wanted that name and he went ahead and let his wife take it. I gave everybody everything and this is how they pay me back.

- *Write continuously.* Get it down on paper. Don't get stymied by spelling and grammar. You don't intend to publish it. You want to use it to help you feel better. If you feel blocked, write your way out of it. Write the same sentence over and over, sort of like a car getting unstuck from some mud. Write for about twenty minutes each day.
- *Don't make writing a crutch.* To everything there is a season. There is a time to write and a time to act. Don't get so caught up in writing that you use it as a substitute for taking the actions you need to help you get pregnant.
- *Be prepared for the feelings.* Research on people who use expressive writing has found that they experience powerful feelings. Sometimes they feel depressed or frightened. But studies have shown that the feelings generated by what you write subside within an hour or two or, at most, a day or so. Knowing in advance that you are likely to feel these things can be comforting when you experience them. Just use GPST to tell yourself "It's okay. The feelings will pass and I will feel better."

Now it's time to start your journal. Take out the Getting Pregnant Quiz you completed in Chapter 1. Think about each of the Pointers and how you responded to them. Now pick one of them that stimulated some thought or feeling and write about it.

LEARNING EFFECTIVE
COMMUNICATION SKILLS

Study after study has found that men and women react differently to infertility. In his thoughtful research book *Not Yet Pregnant*, sociologist Arthur Greil reports that "husbands were not only less likely than their wives to see infertility as a threat to identity, but they were also less likely to see themselves as living in a world where painful reminders of infertility were inescapable."[22] In infertility, as in other stressful situations, women tend to focus on the emotions of the situation. Even though they often are good at taking action, they also feel compelled to talk things out. Most men, on the other hand, are less comfortable dealing with feelings. They are socialized to be task-oriented. When they face a crisis, they want to do something about it rather than talk.

Our female clients, many of whom are career women, lament that their husbands have lost interest in the pregnancy quest. The women complain that their husbands don't listen to them as they did in the beginning of their crisis. Husbands are upset when they see their previously competent wives fall apart. They find it equally difficult to participate in "endless" discussions, particularly when they are not sure what their role is or should be.

Women in our society have a mandate to become mothers. Until they fulfill that mandate, everything else gets placed on hold. The only topic worthy of discussion is getting pregnant. But as Greil notes, "There is, in American society, no 'fatherhood mandate' with the same force and intensity as the 'motherhood mandate.'"[23] The bottom line, however, is that when one member of a couple has a problem, the *couple* has a problem. In order to Work as a Team, the couple must find a way to pull together.

Greil notes that despite the gender differences in motivation to have a baby, many couples report that infertility actually strengthened their marriage. Husbands and wives felt closer because of their shared experience. Admittedly, they argued more, but these intense interactions fostered greater rapport and an increased sense of empathy. Greil concludes that infertility becomes a threat to a marriage when the husband resists his wife's demands for greater communication. But if the husband accepts infertility as a problem for the marital team and is willing to talk about it with his wife, the crisis is likely to unite them.

Facing infertility as a team makes the struggle less stressful. But when stress is high, some couples have great difficulty speaking to one another productively and rationally. A few basic communication skills, mastered today and called up when communication breaks down, can help you get back on track.

Two important communication techniques are *active listening* and *leveling.* Active listening is more than just listening attentively and quietly. Active listening means trying to understand your partner's inner world. Leveling is sharing your inner world with your partner.

Listening and leveling go hand in hand. As you listen, you participate actively. As you share your reactions, you help your partner to understand your world while he is explaining his world to you. By leveling, you help your partner to listen. When you tell him about your innermost thoughts, he begins to understand you better. Also when you level, you drop your guard. Seeing that, your partner reciprocates. By leveling, you encourage him to listen; by listening, you encourage him to level. The outcome of this productive dialogue is a mutual sense of *legitimation.* Each member of the team feels that his or her partner treats his or her concerns as legitimate and valid.

The Getting Pregnant Active Listening/Leveling Approach fosters productive dialogue. The approach has three facets:

- Trying to understand your partner's world of experience;
- Conveying information about your own world of experience; and, as a by-product of the first two processes;
- Commenting on the relationship.

We've developed a checklist that can help you and your partner evaluate the nature of your communication in terms of listening and leveling:

Getting Pregnant Listening focuses on trying to understand your partner's world by:

- asking your partner for further clarification and expansion
- asking about your partner's intentions and preferences
- trying to probe for your partner's feelings about what's happening
- testing to see whether your understanding corresponds to what your partner means

In contrast, *Not* Listening communication is characterized by:

- cutting off your partner before he finishes
- telling your partner how he feels or what he wants rather than asking him
- responding literally to your partner's words instead of to the meaning of what is said

- arguing about whether your partner said something rather than whether he meant it
- treating your inferences as facts, not hypotheses to be tested

Getting Pregnant Leveling contains interactions that focus on:

- explaining your concerns
- showing how your concerns fit into your partner's concerns
- disclosing your feelings related to your partner's actions
- demonstrating how present experience relates to past experiences

In contrast, *Not* Leveling includes these interactions:

- taking action without explaining the basis for action
- not sharing information indicating whether you agree or disagree with the position your partner is taking
- not acknowledging your feelings
- not sharing the basis for your feelings
- attempting to persuade

Here are some sample conversations. Use the checklist to evaluate them. Then read our evaluation.

MARY: I just got this invitation to Beth's baby shower. I—

JOHN: I know. She should know better than to invite you to these things.

MARY: No. She is a really good friend. She's so excited about being pregnant. It's just—

JOHN: That you feel so bad that she's pregnant and you're not.

MARY: No. That's not it. I wish you'd let me say what I'm feeling instead of assuming you know how I feel. It's just that I feel so bad that I can't share her happiness. I love Beth. We're best friends. And I know she'd never want to hurt me.

Here's how we evaluated this dialogue:

Not Listening

> JOHN: cutting off his partner before she finishes
> JOHN: telling his partner how she feels or what she wants rather than asking her

> JOHN: treating his inferences as facts not hypotheses to be tested

Leveling

> MARY: explaining her concerns
> MARY: disclosing her feelings related to her partner's actions

Not Leveling

> JOHN: attempting to persuade.

How did your evaluation compare with ours? Now try this one.

DENNIS: I'm worried that I won't be able to produce a sperm sample for your insemination tomorrow.

PAULA: Don't be silly. You can do it. You're so sexy.

DENNIS: I'm not worried about my manliness. Did you think that's what was bothering me?

PAULA: Sure. You mean that's not what's really worrying you?

DENNIS: No. I'm upset because I think you'll be so disappointed in me. Here you've taken all these shots and spent all this money on medicine. And then I won't produce the samples and you won't get inseminated. I just think you'll feel angry with me. Won't you?

PAULA: No. I'd know you tried.

DENNIS: I just find that hard to believe. Wouldn't you feel let down after getting your hopes up so much?

PAULA: You're right. I would.

DENNIS: So why did you say it wouldn't bother you?

PAULA: Well, I just thought if I said I wasn't worried it would take the pressure off you.

This interaction is more complicated than the last one. Let's analyze the dialogue in greater detail.

When Dennis says, "I'm worried that I won't be able to produce a sperm sample," he is leveling by *explaining his concerns*. When Paula says, "Don't be silly. You can do it. You're so sexy," she is not leveling. She is *attempting to convince* him that he can feel sexy. She is also not listening. She *infers* that he is upset about a problem of manliness. She treats this inference as a fact rather than checking it out. Dennis levels by *explaining his concerns* when he counters, "I'm not worried about my manliness." Then he *tests his understanding* of Paula's comment by asking, "Did you think that's what was bothering me?"

Paula *asks for further clarification* when she says, "You mean that's not what's really bothering you?" Dennis responds by *showing how his concerns fit Paula's concerns* when he says, "I'm upset because I think you'll be disappointed in me." He concludes by *testing his inference* when he asks, "Won't you?"

Paula *does not acknowledge her feelings* at first. She says, "No. I'd know you tried." But Dennis finds that hard to believe. So he further probes to *test Paula's preferences.* He asks, "Wouldn't you feel let down?" Paula then *discloses her feelings in relation to Dennis's actions.* She admits, "You're right." Then Dennis *asks for further clarification* by saying, "So why did you say it wouldn't bother you?" Then Paula explains *how her concerns fit Dennis's concerns* by saying "If I said I wasn't worried it would take the pressure off you."

How did you evaluate the dialogue? Did you score it similarly? Perhaps you categorized a few statements differently than we did. That's okay. Several of the statements can be placed in more than one category. What's important here is learning to monitor your own communication to avoid making statements you'll regret. Remember:

- You and your partner are two different people with different ideas about infertility. Keep the following question foremost in your mind: *How do my partner's beliefs make sense to* him, *not to me?* No matter how silly or unreasonable his beliefs seem to you, *they make sense to him.* Your task is to investigate how they make sense to your spouse. Your partner has the same task with respect to your statements.
- Whenever your partner says something about infertility that you find unreasonable, ask him to tell you more until you get to the point where you can understand how he views the situation. And of course, he must try to understand your view.
- Try to avoid the natural tendency to think you are "more right" than the other person. Instead, tell yourself that you and your spouse are two different people with two different views about infertility.

When you feel you've mastered these communication skills, you're ready to use them in the situations described in future chapters, and in real-life ones, too.

LEARNING TO BEHAVE ASSERTIVELY

Because you are not yet pregnant, you may consider yourself deficient or unworthy because you cannot do what fertile people can do. You may believe, "I have no right to make any demands."

Such an attitude is unproductive. Often, it manifests itself in the way you behave with the medical staff during your diagnostic workup. Many of the couples whom we counsel relinquish control to the medical team. They allow the doctor or technician to call the shots. Of course doctors have a great deal of expertise, but you also have a great deal of information and experience, particularly concerning your own body. It's important to learn when and how to share this information, as well as how to ask for what you want. Only then can you Become a Partner in Your Treatment.

Start learning about assertiveness by looking at another memory device: the word ASSERT. These six statements can help you begin:

> Acknowledge your rights.
> Specify your goal (to yourself).
> State your view of the problem.
> Express and explain your feelings.
> Request what you want from the other person.
> Thank the other person for considering your needs.

First, you must believe that you have rights that deserve to be acknowledged. Then you must decide what you really want, such as a doctor's appointment or a copy of your medical records. After you have clarified your needs, you must state your desire clearly when making your request. Be ready to respond to the other person's viewpoint, as well.

Jane, one of our clients, started her infertility workup feeling particularly unassertive. She faithfully tried to master assertiveness training but never truly believed that she would need to use her new skills. Then something happened that convinced Jane of the importance of being assertive. Two weeks earlier, she had written a letter to Dr. A requesting that her records be sent to Dr. B, an infertility specialist very much in demand. His waiting list was three months long, and Jane had been placed at the end of the queue. On the day she phoned us, Jane had received a call from Dr. B's office explaining that the busy physician had a cancellation and could see her and her husband immediately.

Jane was ecstatic. She called Dr. A's office and explained that she needed her records that day. Dr. A's staff refused, stating that records were sent out in the order they had been requested and that Jane's records would not be ready for at least a month. Initially, Jane explained, "I saw red. All I wanted to do was scream. I felt like saying, 'Your patients must be exiting en masse if you're backed up six weeks,' but I took a few deep breaths, said a little GPST [Get Pregnant Self-Talk], and calmly told them that the records belonged to me, that I could come over and copy them myself, and that I was unable to accept no for an answer since I needed to see Doctor B as soon as possible."

The staff continued to balk. Even Dr. A, whom Jane asked to speak with personally (a very assertive stance in itself), called her approach highly unorthodox and refused to comply. Jane calmly stated, firmly but quietly, that she would do anything to facilitate getting her records immediately. She acknowledged that Dr. A had done the best he could and thanked him for referring her to Dr. B, but she stressed that she could not wait. Even though Dr. A had set up his practice in this rigid way and was cold and unemotional, he finally backed down and gave Jane her records. She didn't get a smile, but Jane knew that friendly behavior was not critical to her getting pregnant.

Jane got her meeting with Dr. B and was excited by what she learned. She told us, "Dr. B said that a new procedure might help us. We can do it next month, and maybe then I'll get pregnant. Thanks for helping me learn to ask for what I want. I always felt I deserved things but never knew how to ask."

Like Jane, you may find it difficult to ask for what you want. Yet your diagnosis and treatment has short- and long-term implications for your body and your life. Express your opinions. Clarify what you want. Make demands. Don't be afraid to make simple requests such as asking for a sheet in a cold examining room or an appointment at

9 A.M. instead of at 3:30 P.M. Your comfort and convenience are important. And be bold when asking for more complicated and critical considerations, even if a doctor implies that your opinions are not important. You're paying for your treatment, not asking for a handout. Insist on the best possible treatment. But be diplomatic. Avoid being obnoxious or overly aggressive in making these requests.

DECISION-MAKING

More often than not, the clients we see have no plan for their treatment. They have fallen into what writer Kassie Schwan has called "the infertility maze."[24] They flounder here and there with no clear direction. Having no plan makes you feel helpless, and helplessness fosters feelings of depression, so common in infertility. The way out of the infertility maze is to formulate a plan and take responsibility for making important decisions. You will have to decide whether to see an infertility specialist or an OB-GYN who does not specialize in infertility. You may have to decide how best to spend the money you have on treatment—whether to try many repeated cycles of a less-expensive low-tech treatment or to go with fewer but more expensive high-tech treatments. The volume of information you must consider when drafting your plan of action can be daunting.

There is no simple way to make these choices. But there is a method that can help. The method we present is based on one model of decision-making discussed by psychologist Ward Edwards[25] and on another model of choice discussed by psychologists Amos Tversky and Daniel Kahneman.[26]

First, a scenario: Your mother is planning a visit during the Christmas vacation. You can't decide whether to pursue treatment while she visits or take a month's rest.

Begin your decision-making process by gathering information about the factors you must weigh. You talk to friends and acquaintances who have experienced a similar dilemma. You read books and magazine articles that discuss the problem. You post your quandary in a discussion group on the Internet. And then you and your spouse develop a list of those factors. At the end of this phase, you prioritize.

A list (which we have deliberately simplified for illustrative purposes) includes these factors:

- Preventing stress to your body
- Getting closer to your goal of having a baby
- Avoiding family friction

These are just a few of the many considerations you would list. Your next step is assigning a "grade" to each factor. The grade, which is a number from 1 (worst) to 10 (best), indicates the effect of each choice on that factor. So you might assign the following grades:

FACTOR	CHOOSING TREATMENT	CHOOSING REST
1. How much will this choice prevent stress to my body?	2	8
2. How much closer will this choice bring me to my goal of having a baby?	7	1
3. How much will this choice prevent friction in the family?	1	10

Next, assign a weight from 1 (least) to 10 (most) to the importance of each factor. You need to weigh the benefit of treatment at a distant clinic against the cost of family friction that would result if your travel prevented you from spending relaxed time with your mother during her visit. You then multiply the weight by the rating to get a factor score. Finally, you add the total factor scores for each choice. Here's what your chart might look like:

FACTOR	WEIGHT FOR THIS FACTOR	GRADE FOR TREATMENT	FACTOR SCORE FOR TREATMENT (WEIGHT × GRADE)	GRADE FOR RESTING	FACTOR SCORE FOR RESTING (WEIGHT × GRADE)
Prevent stress to body	2	2	4	8	16
Closeness to goal	10	7	70	1	10
Avoid family friction	9	1	9	10	90
TOTAL SCORE			83		116

Looking at the table, you can see that your best choice would be to rest for the month. In later chapters, we will apply this technique to other important decisions, such as choosing a doctor, freezing embryos or doing a fresh cycle, or selecting an egg donor. When we do, we will guide you through a more thorough examination of the various factors to take into account.

RECORD-KEEPING

Once your diagnosis begins, you'll be swamped with papers: receipts, test results, insurance forms—the sheer volume is enough to make you stuff it all into a drawer and forget about it or, worse yet, leave the materials scattered around the house. Instead of becoming preoccupied with how difficult getting pregnant is, channel some of your energy into getting and staying organized. Put copies of your medical records, as well as your own logs of monthly cycles, in a convenient file or loose-leaf notebook. Getting Organized is probably the most effective way to reduce your feelings of being overwhelmed. Following the organization Pointer also can help you develop your Getting Pregnant Plan.

The Cycle Log

The first section of your Getting Pregnant Journal will be the information section. Use this section as the place to keep your Cycle Log, which will help you chart your menstrual cycle. Sometimes as you record information in your journal, you feel powerful emotions that you can write about in the expressive writing section of your journal. For example, on the day you ovulate and have intercourse, you may feel very optimistic and want to write about your feelings of hope.

On the next page, you will find a Cycle Log form to photocopy and put into your portfolio. A copy of the Cycle Log can also be found on our Web site at http://www.gettingpregnantbook.com. This log can help you record every aspect of your cycle: how you feel, what medications you took, what your blood levels were, or what tests were done on any given day. Although you may think you'll remember that you had unusual cramps on Day 21 or that your temperature fell on Day 25, you probably won't. Daily events, even those that seem momentous at the time, often blend together or fade from memory. Detailed records of each cycle allow you and your doctor to compare one treatment or one cycle to another or begin to see patterns suggesting why you are not getting pregnant.

CYCLE LOG

Directions: Use this log to enter important information about your cycle. The days of the cycles are listed at the left of the page. Next to the day of the cycle, write the date. Then record essential information under the heading "Notes." In your notes keep track of the following (and anything else that may be important to you):

- Symptoms: Any important symptoms you experienced
- Estradiol information (E2)
- Progesterone levels (P)
- Sonogram results (number of follicle size for Left (L) and Right (R) ovaries)
- Medication taken (meds)
- Questions to ask your doctor (Qs)

Day of Cycle	Date	Symptoms or Comments	E2	P	Left Ovary: Size of Each Follicle	Right Ovary: Size of Each Follicle	Medications Taken: Lupron (L); Progesterone (PR); Pergonal (PG); Fertinex (F); hCG (H); Other (O)						Questions?
							L	PR	PG	F	H	O	
1													
2													
3													
4													
5													
6													
7													

Day of Cycle	Date	Symptoms or Comments	E2	P	Left Ovary: Size of Each Follicle	Right Ovary: Size of Each Follicle	Medications Taken: Lupron (L); Progesterone (PR); Pergonal (PG); Fertinex (F); hCG (H); Other (O)						Questions?
							L	PR	PG	F	H	O	
8													
9													
10													
11													
12													
13													
14													
15													
16													
17													
18													
19													
20													
21													
22													
23													
24													
25													
26													
27													
28													

GOAL-SETTING

Coping with infertility is like coping with any chronic illness. Our clients often feel that their condition is entirely out of their control. While they cannot control whether they get pregnant, they *can* choose their physician, their treatment, and how long they will remain in treatment. Goal-Setting is a skill that can help you enact many of the Getting Pregnant Pointers: Getting Organized, Making a Plan, Managing Your Social Life, Making Effective Decisions, and Being a Partner in Treatment. In setting your Getting Pregnant Goals, follow these *dos* and *don'ts*:

- *Do set realistic goals.* When you set goals, consider time, travel, work and family commitments, financial resources, and all the other real-life situations that can get in the way of accomplishing these goals.
- *Do make specific concrete goals.* Think in terms of both short- and long-range objectives. A long-range objective might be to undergo all the tests your doctor recommends by a particular date. That particular long-range objective can require short-range objectives such as having one test during each cycle.
- *Do divide the goals into discrete, manageable steps.* These steps are what you actually have to do to meet your goal, such as checking your temperature, making a doctor's appointment, or arranging time off from work.
- *Do set verifiable milestones to check your progress toward your goals.* Write—and follow—reminders such as these on your calendar: when to call for test results or fill a prescription. You are your own best monitor, so don't cheat.

And also remember the *don'ts*:

- *Don't set yourself up for failure.* Sometimes when you are pessimistic, you expect failure before you even start. Then you might set unrealistic goals that you can never accomplish and say, "See, I knew it was impossible."
- *Don't retreat into passivity.* By becoming passive, you ensure that

nothing good happens and thus confirm your prediction that "nothing good will happen."

- *Don't become exhausted.* Pace yourself. Budget your energy.
- *Don't catastrophize.* See the situation for what it really is and hold on to hope.

The Getting Pregnant Monthly Plan

On the next page you will see a model of the Getting Pregnant Monthly Plan. Photocopy it, punch holes in it, and insert it into the second section of your notebook. You can also find a copy of a Getting Pregnant Monthly Plan form on our Web site. Together with your spouse, set a short-term goal, one you can envision reaching this month. Do not make your goal, "I will get pregnant this month." Make your goal, "This month, I will schedule and undergo the diagnostic test."

The monthly plan on the next page suggests a number of possible goals for the coming month. Your first step is to decide upon your goal. Once you've established what your goal is, write it on the form.

Next, use GPST (Getting Pregnant Self-Talk) to psych yourself up to accomplish your goal. Make a GPST statement that you find particularly motivating. For example, if you hate calling doctors, try psyching yourself up by saying, "By calling the doctor, I'm upping my odds." Keep your GPST statement in mind if you find yourself procrastinating.

Now you are ready to formulate an action plan. The action plan is critical and easy to put off. Make your spouse your consultant. Ask him to review the plan and add any important steps you might have omitted. Your task for this month is to put your plan into action. At the end of this month, assess how your plan worked out. If your plan worked, congratulate yourself. If it didn't, figure out why and modify the plan for the next month.

THE GETTING PREGNANT MONTHLY PLAN

MAKE THIS MONTH COUNT. Now is the time to make sure you accomplish something important this month.

Directions: Even if you will not be able to try to conceive during this month, you must view this cycle as a chance to get closer to your goal. It's important to think of a month during which only tests occur as providing you with information that confirms or rules out causes for infertility. Cycles that fail also can provide new knowledge. You can't control whether you get pregnant this month. But you *can* do something to up the odds. This planning sheet will help you do so.

First list your goal for this month. Make it something manageable—something you can definitely accomplish. This month you can:

- Find out new information
- Get the results of an important test
- Strengthen your body and your mind
- Try a treatment
- Do something else (Supply your own goal)

_____

MY GOAL FOR THIS MONTH IS:

_____

Now you must psych yourself up to accomplish this goal. Do this by making a *motivating GPST.* For example, a person who hates having tests might say, "By having the test, I may learn what's wrong." Write your motivating GPST below.

_____

MY MOTIVATING GPST STATEMENT FOR THIS MONTH IS:

_____

Now that you have a goal and you've psyched yourself up, it's time to formulate your action steps. For example, suppose you set the goal of finding out whether your tubes are blocked. You might formulate the following plan:

1. I'll contact my doctor to set up the test.
2. I'll read the section in the diagnosis chapter describing the test.
3. To work as a team, I'll ask my partner to read about the test and discuss it with me.
4. I'll mentally rehearse experiencing the test so I'm ready for it.
5. As a partner in treatment, I'll call the doctor to clear up any questions I might have.
6. I'll ask my partner to take time off from work to accompany me to the test.
7. I'll get the insurance material ready in advance.

MY ACTION PLAN FOR THIS MONTH IS:

In the next part of this form, write down how it worked out.

HERE IS HOW MY PLAN WORKED OUT:

Now that you took the steps to carry out your plan, congratulate yourself for taking a positive action.

CONGRATULATE YOURSELF!

USING YOUR IMAGINATION

When we tell our clients that we are going to ask them to use their imagination in helping them through their infertility, they initially reject the idea. They mistakenly fear that we're going to have them imagine that they are pregnant, and they find that thought too painful. Or, worse yet, they think that we're going to ask them to imagine a sperm fertilizing an egg, and they find this scenario too weird or off-putting. Unfortunately, most of the infertile couples we see have lost so many dreams that their imagination is dulled. They are almost ready to give up. They fear entertaining any new dreams. Yet once they have learned to use imagery techniques and incorporate them into real-life situations, couples report that they feel much more able to cope with their experiences. And some even tell us that they also allow themselves to dream again.

Before you begin your imagery work, we want to clarify that we are *not* introducing imagery as a way for you to explore your complex unconscious mind. Such personal introspection takes intensive one-on-one work with a qualified therapist. What we want you to do is to gain access to your inner world of ideas, modify those images that hinder you, and expand and detail those images that help you—all for the purpose of harnessing the power of your mind to help you through infertility.

For this imagery section of the Workout, we've collected a wide range of imagery procedures, modified them, and tested them with infertile couples. The result is a series of techniques that possess amazing power. These are not mystical exercises, but straightforward techniques and scenarios that help relax, inspire, motivate, and prepare you for what you must do to enhance your chances of getting pregnant.

What Are Mental Images?

Mental images are those pictures that you see in your mind's eye when the object is no longer present or the situation is in the past. Your mental image may be visual, olfactory, auditory, gustatory (recorded through tasting), tactile, or kinesthetic (recorded through moving).

Your images may be spontaneous, like a daydream, or they may need some prodding and shaping.

In the Workout, we focus on developing your ability to imagine procedures and interactions that you've yet to experience. You will use these images together with breathing or progressive relaxation to reduce your stress. And you will employ these images in conjunction with GPST to help you reframe unproductive experiences and to assist you in cultivating a sense of optimism.

Mental Rehearsal

Experts believe that having a mental picture of an upcoming event can help you cope better when it happens. For example, having a mental picture of how to react in an awkward social situation—the words you'll say or the things you'll do—can be very reassuring. Likewise, the more familiar a medical procedure is, the less likely you are to panic or experience extreme discomfort during the procedure. In subsequent chapters, we describe many of the tests and treatments used to help infertile couples. If you use these descriptions to help you form a "movie in your mind" and then rehearse what will occur, you can prepare yourself for what will happen.

Once you develop a clear and detailed picture in your mind's eye, add some GPST. For example, while imagining that you are having one of the tests many find unpleasant you might add a soothing statement to your mental rehearsal like, "This test is almost over. I've passed the worst." Just as we encourage you actually to imagine yourself experiencing the test step-by-step, we also encourage you to hear yourself saying your GPSTs.

Rehearsing for a Diagnostic Test or a Medical Treatment

Medical researcher Jennifer Wilson-Barnett has investigated the stress of diagnostic testing. She states that "one of the most common fears expressed by those scheduled for tests is the 'fear of the unknown.' For those experiencing a procedure for the first time, in particular, anticipation may be tainted by various fantasies."[27]

To overcome that fear, follow these steps:

- Read the description of the procedure with your spouse.[28] Together, use the information to write a brief script of the procedure, which includes all of the relevant details. (A sample script follows).
- Sit in a comfortable position. Close your eyes.
- Have your spouse actually read the script to you or tape-record it for playback at a later time. Make sure your spouse gives you sufficient time to really picture the scene. You may have to coach him to read or record at a slow enough pace.
- Mentally rehearse the scene in as much detail as possible. Allow yourself to feel the anxiety. Also picture yourself coping with the worst-case scenario, knowing that once you've dealt with your ultimate fears, you are ready for anything.

I'm going to read you a description of the _____ (name of test). I want you to see yourself coping with your anxiety by using the deep breathing technique you've been practicing. I'm going to help. I'll be your coach and cheerleader. Whenever you feel anxious, just raise your little finger. I'll help you relax. Take slow deep breaths. INHALE. EXHALE . . . WHOOSH. GOOD. Again. INHALE. EXHALE . . . WHOOSH. Okay, here we go. I'm with you, so you don't have to be afraid. C'mon. You can do it! Good. You're doing it. As you see yourself exhaling, get in touch with the feeling of relaxation and control the air you are bringing forth. GREAT. Add your GPST. Tell yourself, "I can do it! I've done tougher things before." GOOD. Keep breathing slowly and deeply. GREAT. Now stop that image and relax. GOOD WORK!

Following is an example of a script, based on the model above, that you and your spouse might write to mentally visualize and rehearse yourself going through a hysterosalpingogram (HSG) procedure. (You can find a detailed description of this procedure in Chapter 4.)

> *You've arrived at the radiologist's suite. You are signing in. The receptionist is giving you a consent slip to read and sign. It says that you will release the doctors from any responsibility for any problem that might happen as a result of the procedure. Now you're signing it. Now you're going into a dressing room, taking off your clothes and putting on a dressing gown. The nurse is escorting you to the examination room. You are lying on the table. It feels cold. You look around and see an X-ray camera and an X-ray screen. The room is dark. Here comes the radiologist. She's putting a tube into your uterus. Now she's squeezing dye into the tube. Now you can feel the dye traveling through your tubes. You feel pressure and maybe some pain. The doctor is going behind a screen. Now she's telling you to turn to the right so she can get a picture of that side. Now she's telling you to turn to the left. Now she's finished. She's telling you to get dressed.*

Mental imagery also can help you prepare for difficult or awkward situations that can arise socially or on the job. In her pamphlet *Getting Around the Boulder in the Road: Using Imagery to Cope with Fertility Problems,* psychologist Aline P. Zoldbrod encourages readers to "try working with your imagery during demanding periods in your treatment regimen, when your life feels out of control, or when you feel distant from your spouse . . . to make you feel more comfortable during social situations, or to control pain during surgical procedures."[29]

Guided Fantasies

An entirely different approach to mental imagery is called creative visualizations or guided fantasies. These activities, which deal almost exclusively with your sense of sight, focus on using images to help you relax, get motivated, or even inspire you to develop a more upbeat attitude toward fighting infertility. An important benefit of guided fantasies is that they often are accompanied by physiological changes, such as relaxation.

Guided fantasies, or "mind journeys" as they are sometimes called, are a set of guiding phrases, read or tape-recorded. While in a relaxed state, you are encouraged to visualize the picture or experience suggested by the reader. Generally, infertility guided fantasies require that you, the listener, experience the journey firsthand, with such sentences as "Together we are going to develop a circle of friends who are your supporters," which is the beginning of a guided fantasy called "Circle of Friends" that appears in Chapter 6. There are just a few simple rules to remember:

- Find a calm and quiet place to practice your imagery.
- Set a regular time each day to do imagery activities. Just like physical activity, you need to practice mental activity on a regular basis.
- Sit in a chair or lie on the floor—whatever position seems to be easier.
- Start with controlled breathing, as described earlier in this chapter.
- Try to direct your focus inward, instead of on the chaos around you.
- At the beginning of each exercise, always state your goal to yourself, using GPST.
- For the time you are imaging, allow yourself to go with the images.

ONE FINAL THOUGHT

In the first chapter, we gave you Ten Pointers that can help you get pregnant when you thought you couldn't. In this chapter, we have given you a set of skills that will allow you to enact the Pointers. Some skills, such as GPST, are so useful that they can help with all of the Pointers. Other skills, such as controlled breathing, are more limited in what they can do for you. In each of the succeeding chapters, we will describe pitfalls and obstacles to getting pregnant. Then we will show you how to apply the skills learned from the Getting Pregnant Workout to help you avoid them.

Practice the Getting Pregnant Workout on a regular basis. The Workout could very well contain the tools you need to help you get pregnant when you thought you couldn't.

CHAPTER 3

The Miracle of Life

GETTING PREGNANT WHEN THINGS WORK RIGHT

or many who have been trying for a long time to have a baby, the thought of actually conceiving a new life seems like a miracle. And in truth, conception itself—even for the most fertile people—is surely miraculous. A myriad of events must occur at exactly the right time and in the proper place for pregnancy to happen.

Broadly speaking, there are four milestones to conception, some involving both partners, others involving the woman only. The first milestone is production of a *gamete*, or reproductive cell: the man's sperm and the woman's egg. Next, the *sperm meets the egg and fertilizes it* to produce an embryo. Third, the *embryo implants* itself in the uterus. Finally, the *implanted embryo divides, flourishes, and fully develops.* Each milestone is controlled by a cascade of chemical and hormonal reactions. Through "feedback mechanisms," hormone production is turned on and off, just as a thermostat senses temperature changes in your house to control whether your furnace turns on or off.

Gamete Production in the Woman

A female is born with all the eggs she will ever produce—about 1 to 2 million.[1] As she gets older, her supply of eggs decreases. From the onset of puberty, when she has about 400,000 eggs, until menopause, a woman normally has a menstrual cycle culminating in the release of one or more of those eggs. This menstrual cycle is spawned at the base of the brain, right above the pituitary gland, in an area called the hypothalamus. The hypothalamus produces a hormone called *gonadotropin releasing hormone* (GnRH). About every ninety minutes, for about one minute, the hypothalamus pumps out a small dose of GnRH.[2] This periodic pumping is necessary to set things in motion for ovulation to occur. If the hypothalamus pumps out a steady stream of GnRH, for example, the entire pregnancy process will be pushed off balance.

When the hypothalamus works properly, the GnRH stimulates the pituitary gland to release two more hormones: *follicle-stimulating hormone* (FSH) and *luteinizing hormone* (LH). As its name implies, FSH stimulates the ovaries to start developing one of many *potential* follicles that are available. A follicle is a sac that will contain an egg. Why a particular follicle is selected over another one is a mystery. Some follicles contain healthy eggs; others contain poor-quality eggs that are unable to develop into an embryo. Ideally, FSH stimulates the follicle to grow large enough to be "ovulated," or ejected.

As the sac grows, the egg is being genetically prepared to become susceptible to fertilization. Again, timing and hormone levels are critical. FSH production must start and stop at the proper times. The ovary must secrete increasing amounts of estradiol, a form of the female hormone, *estrogen,* which performs many functions. It's important to note that most women rotate ovulation: They ovulate one month from the left ovary and the next month from the right.[3] Other women ovulate almost consistently from only one ovary. When one ovary is surgically removed, the other generally takes over the monthly job.

The estrogen first stimulates the development of the lining in the uterus. The lining, or *endometrium*, must grow thick enough to allow an embryo to implant and grow. Secondly, the estrogen rise increases the quantity and consistency of cervical mucus. You may notice this extra mucus midway through your menstrual cycle. The mucus serves as a vehicle for sperm as it journeys to the egg.

Thirdly, high levels of estrogen in the bloodstream enlarge the opening of the cervix. Estrogen's fourth function is to signal the pituitary gland to stop producing FSH and to send a tremendous surge of LH instead. The LH surge signals the ovary to ovulate an egg.

In addition to stimulating ovulation, meanwhile, the LH surge also initiates a series of genetic events inside the egg. Like every cell in the human body, the egg cell contains forty-six chromosomes—strands of genetic material. When an egg gets fertilized, it combines with a sperm, which has twenty-three chromosomes of its own. (Sperm shed their other twenty-three chromosomes sometime prior to ejaculation.) If the fertilized egg retains all forty-six female chromosomes as well as the male chromosomes, the resulting cell could not grow into a healthy baby. So the LH surge prepares the egg cell to expel half of its chromosomes.

After the egg is ovulated, the leftover sac develops into a yellow structure called the *corpus luteum* (literally "yellow body"). The corpus luteum produces a second important hormone called progesterone. For most women there is a sharp increase in progesterone secretion at the beginning of the second half of the menstrual cycle. This part of the cycle is known as the *luteal phase.* As estrogen makes the uterine lining grow thick, progesterone makes the lining soft and spongy—a good environment for embryo implantation. If a pregnancy occurs, progesterone will continue to be secreted throughout the pregnancy. However, if there is no pregnancy, progesterone secretion stops at the end of the luteal phase. The decrease in progesterone and estrogen levels sends a signal to the hypothalamus to trigger a new stream of FSH. Then the ovulation cycle begins anew.

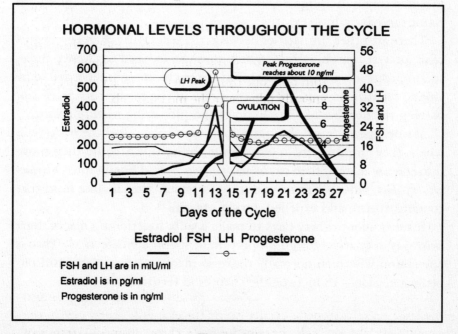

Figure 3.1

Gamete Production in the Man

Unlike women, men are not born with all the sperm cells they will ever have. Sperm are born, grow, mature, and eventually die (save for the ones that ultimately fertilize eggs).

Men are like women in that they also have a GnRH "pump" that pulses periodically, stimulating the production of FSH and LH. In men, however, LH causes the production of *testosterone,* not estrogen. Testosterone is the male hormone that increases sex drive and stimulates the development of secondary sex characteristics, such as beard growth, at puberty. FSH, on the other hand, regulates the production of immature or primitive sperm cells known as *sperm precursors.* These precursors are *not* the same as the mature sperm used to fertilize an egg. As with females, there is a feedback mechanism in males that regulates FSH and LH levels. When testosterone levels increase, LH production decreases, and vice versa. Likewise, when sperm precursor levels are low, FSH levels rise to increase their production.

It's important to keep in mind that so-called manliness is not related to the ability to make sperm. A high sex drive can be present in a man totally lacking in sperm, just as a man with a very high sperm count can have a low sex drive.

There are other similarities between the sexes. Just as an egg begins with forty-six chromosomes, which must be reduced to twenty-three, sperm precursors have twice the number of chromosomes needed to be able to fertilize an egg. FSH plays a role in triggering this process of halving the number of chromosomes and producing mature sperm.

Mature sperm travel through a long, thin tube called the *epididymis,* where they improve their swimming ability. Eventually, they move into the *vas deferens,* then to the *seminal vesicle,* and finally into the *ejaculatory duct,* where they are mixed with semen, the alkaline fluid that contains sperm, and expelled during orgasm.

It takes about ninety days to make a fully functioning sperm. Surprisingly, a relatively high proportion of sperm are defective.[4] That is one reason why men normally make so many sperm—many millions per ejaculation—to increase the chances of fertilization.

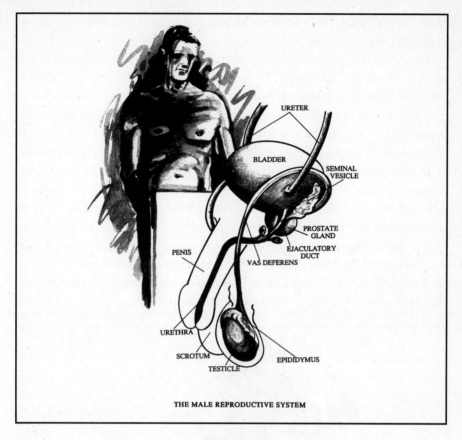

URETER

BLADDER

SEMINAL
VESICLE

PROSTATE
GLAND

EJACULATORY
DUCT

PENIS

VAS DEFERENS

URETHRA

SCROTUM

TESTICLE

EPIDIDYMUS

THE MALE REPRODUCTIVE SYSTEM

Figure 3.2

Journey and Rendezvous: Sperm and Egg Meet

Again, timing is crucial during this stage. First, the sperm must travel from the penis and through the vagina, cervix, uterus, and fallopian tubes to get to an egg. To optimize the chance of pregnancy occurring, intercourse should occur just before ovulation. One reason is because the life of the egg is very short; estimates run from twelve to twenty-four hours. If intercourse does not take place at the right time (around the time of the LH surge), the sperm can travel to the right site but fail to meet its target. If the sperm does encounter the egg, it must be able to penetrate and fertilize the egg. As you are beginning to see, both the egg and the sperm must survive an arduous journey before getting a chance at conception.

As the sperm prepares for the journey, the ovaries are getting ready to ovulate an egg or eggs. The ovaries lie just outside the end of the *fallopian tubes.* The fallopian tubes are extremely narrow, the narrowest part having an outer diameter about as wide as angel hair pasta at the point where it hooks up with the uterus. Inside the tube is a canal lined with millions of tiny hairs called *cilia.* It also contains special cells that secrete a fluid that plays a critical role in fertilization. The narrow portion of the tube that joins the uterus is called the *isthmus.* The isthmus is barely wide enough to allow a fertilized egg to pass through. However, as you proceed down the tube, the tube widens into a bell-shaped structure called the *ampulla.* At the end of the ampulla are fingerlike structures called *fimbria*, which contain little petals of tissue. The ampulla is "hinged" to the ovary in such a way that it is able to swing over to catch the ovulated egg.

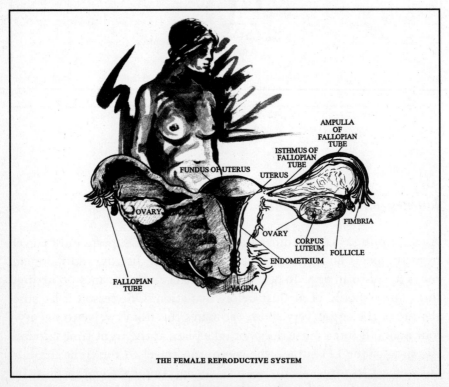

THE FEMALE REPRODUCTIVE SYSTEM

Figure 3.3

Just before the egg is ovulated, the fimbria are positioned above the dominant egg follicle. When it leaves its follicle, the egg is covered with a sticky substance that helps it adhere to a petal of the fimbria and get trapped. Once the egg is trapped, the cilia on the lining of the fimbria beat rapidly and push the sticky egg mass into the crevices of the lining of the ampulla. Here, the fluid of the lining dissolves the sticky coating and nourishes the egg. As the fluid dissolves the egg's coating, it also softens the egg's shell so that the egg will be more susceptible to penetration by a sperm.

Assuming that the man and woman have just engaged in intercourse, the man will ejaculate semen into the woman's vagina. The semen is an alkaline fluid, which protects the sperm from the vagina's acidic environment. Typically, an ejaculate contains many millions of sperm. The first portion of the ejaculate has the highest concentration of sperm, most of which are spewed forth during the first ejaculatory pulse. A significant percentage of these sperm are poor swimmers. *Fewer than 1 percent of the sperm ejaculated will make it to the site of fertilization.* Some sperm, however, can live up to three or four days in the cervical mucus.

Once sperm reach the cervix, they encounter the cervical mucus, which, under the influence of estrogen, has built up during the first half of the woman's cycle. The estrogen has created an abundance of thin, stretchy mucus that, under normal conditions, serves as an ideal sperm-transport system. The cervical mucus creates a reservoir of sperm in the cervical canal, releasing only a few at a time.

The heads of the sperm are covered by a cap, which is altered just prior to egg penetration. With this change, each sperm secretes an enzyme called *acrosin,* which further softens the outer covering of the egg. Like battering rams, these top-of-the-line sperm butt up against the *zona pellucida*, the hardest part of the egg's outer covering, with their heads. Fertilization is a precisely organized cascade of events. If this complex multistep process is not properly orchestrated, fertilization will not take place. As soon as the sperm enters the egg, a chemical reaction occurs to prevent any other sperm from coming in. In a precisely timed series of events, the sperm and egg cells combine their chromosomes. The now-fertilized egg, called a *zygote*—the first stage in embryo development—is ready to begin the final leg of its journey to the uterus, where it will attempt to implant and grow.

Womb with a View

The cilia beat rapidly, propelling the fertilized egg down the fallopian tube. At the same time, the muscles of the tube contract to further aid the embryo's travel. The embryo remains in the tube for about three to five days, until the uterine lining is ready to receive it.

When it enters the uterus, the cells of the embryo have divided many times but remain enclosed in the zona pellucida. It is now called a blastocyst. Signals are sent from the embryo to the uterus and from the uterus to the embryo in an attempt to locate an optimal site for implantation. The blastocyst "hatches" and implants in the endometrium, which, as you recall, has thickened under the influence of estrogen and softened under the influence of progesterone. The embryonic cells secrete yet another hormone, called *hCG*, which stimulates the corpus luteum (vacated egg sac) to continue secreting progesterone. In this favorable environment, the implanted embryo grows and develops over the next nine months.

NOT GETTING PREGNANT WHEN YOU THOUGHT YOU COULD

Given the complexities of conception, it is no wonder that perfectly fertile couples have only a one-in-five chance of conceiving during any given month. Yet even with those odds, 90 percent of couples without fertility problems will achieve pregnancy within one year.

If you are not one of those lucky ones, you may be tempted to believe simply that the odds have worked against you. But it is that line of reasoning that might work against you if you delay seeking a medical evaluation at this point. Postponing diagnosis can waste precious time, especially if your problem is easily correctable. It's our belief that the sooner you find out what, if anything, is wrong, the sooner you can cradle your baby in your arms.

Here, we examine what can go wrong at each stage of the process. Later in the book we will discuss the various procedures and drugs available to correct many of these problems.

The Woman Fails to Ovulate

As we pointed out previously, you enter puberty with a store of about 400,000 eggs (on average) and will produce no more. Each month, numerous follicles start to develop, of which one will become the dominant one. The remaining follicles will wither and die.

One reason older women have trouble conceiving is that they simply have used up their supply of eggs or the few remaining ones are of very poor quality. A blood test conducted on the second or third day of your cycle can provide an indication of your "follicle store." For younger women, the failure to ovulate probably lies elsewhere.

The ovulation process is controlled by numerous hormones whose levels must attain a proper balance. If your hormonal levels are off balance, you will not ovulate, or you will ovulate before the eggs are ripened. Other problems that can affect ovulation include polycystic ovaries, high prolactin levels, and other less common conditions, which are discussed in Chapters 4 and 5.

The Man Fails to Produce Sperm

Just as with ovulation, hormones regulate sperm production. Therefore, indirect evidence of whether a man is producing sperm can be gathered through hormonal testing. As we noted earlier, FSH controls the production of sperm *precursors* (immature sperm). If a blood test shows an adequate FSH level, it means the man is making these precursors. However, in order to have sperm that can fertilize eggs, these sperm cells must mature and lose half their chromosomes. Cases where this does not happen are exceedingly rare.

By obtaining a semen sample, a laboratory technician can check the number of sperm, their shape, and their ability to swim. All three factors give doctors enough data to diagnose whether or not the man has a problem.

The Egg Does Not Get Fertilized

If the woman is ovulating and the man is making sperm, infertility may result from a problem in the rendezvous stage. These problems may involve *travel*, *timing*, or *penetration*.

- **Travel:** The sperm that is ejaculated must travel from the vagina to the fallopian tubes, where they can attempt to penetrate the egg. Sperm can be blocked, lost, or killed before they reach their destination. The acid in the vagina may kill all the sperm. The cervical mucus may be too thick to allow penetration, or the mucus may contain antibodies that are lethal to sperm. Ironically, the sperm itself may have antibodies that cause it to self-destruct. Also, sperm may be poor swimmers. Instead of swimming straight to the tube, they may swim off course or in circles and never reach their destination. Or they may be straight swimmers but too weak to buck the tide in the female's reproductive tract.

  Like the sperm, the egg also can encounter travel problems. Although a fine egg may have developed and been ejected from the ovary, it may never be "caught" by the fimbria. To catch the egg, the tube must have rotated into the proper position. But adhesions or scar tissue might have interfered with the structure's ability to move and turn. If this is the case, the egg gets lost in the abdomen instead of making its way down the tube.

- **Timing:** Mature eggs can live in the body for only twelve to twenty-four hours. If sperm aren't available during this "window of opportunity," fertilization cannot occur. Sperm can live in the woman's body longer than eggs, up to four days in some cases, in fact. A supply of sperm must be released to get to the tube several hours before the egg's arrival. The goal is to have a constant supply of sperm at the site of fertilization awaiting ovulation.

- **Penetration:** The third main cause for a lack of fertilization stems from a sperm's inability to penetrate the egg. The egg's covering is hard. It needs to be softened by enzymes secreted in the fallopian tube and by the sperm. Nearby sperm actually help to break the egg's barriers and assist the chosen sperm to penetrate.

Fertilized Egg Fails to Implant

Generally, three types of problems can thwart success during the implantation stage. These involve *travel, roadblocks,* and *lodging.*

- **Travel:** The fertilized egg must be swept through the fallopian tube on a current of fluid. It must pass through a narrow opening linking the tube and the uterus. Then it must land upon a soft, spongy endometrium, where it takes up residence. Problems with the fallopian tube muscles or the cilia may impair movement of the fertilized egg.
- **Roadblocks:** The narrow passage leading from the tube to the uterus may be blocked by inflammation, thereby preventing the fertilized egg from leaving the fallopian tube. If this happens, the fertilized egg can die or, worse, it can implant and begin to grow in the tube. This so-called *ectopic,* or tubal, pregnancy can be life-threatening if not treated promptly.
- **Lodging:** Finally, if the fertilized egg enters the uterus, it must land on the soft, spongy endometrium and implant there. Throughout the early stages of pregnancy, the endometrium is nourished by a constant supply of progesterone. This lushness will not occur if there is insufficient progesterone being produced either naturally or through drug therapy. Scar tissue, adhesions, or fibroid tumors inside the uterus can also prevent implantation.

The Implanted Embryo Divides for a Time but Fails to Flourish

If things have gone well at each of the previous stages, a pregnancy test will be positive. From this point on, the embryo must continue to be nourished or it will die and miscarriage will occur, sometimes before the woman even realizes she was pregnant. Researchers estimate that a large percentage of pregnancies end this way.[5] Since infertile couples tend to take pregnancy tests at the earliest possible moment, they are often painfully aware of early miscarriages. Even when an embryo begins to grow, many problems—both with the developing fetus and with the mother—can contribute to a miscarriage.

Nature has a way of fostering preservation. Some embryos were not meant to develop because the resulting fetus would be deformed. Some eggs, particularly very old ones, are genetically nonviable. Even if they are fertilized, they may contain genes that could contribute to a genetically defective baby. To prevent these defects, nature causes a spontaneous abortion—a miscarriage.

THE DISORDERS OF FERTILITY

Various factors—male, female, or unexplained—can prevent you from getting pregnant. Male problems almost always are associated with sperm production, sperm transport, or the health of the sperm itself. The root of female problems, on the other hand, can lie in the ovaries, fallopian tubes, uterus, cervix, or any combination thereof. As you see from Figure 3.4 showing the distribution of infertility causes for patients undergoing assisted reproductive technology (ART) in the United States,[6] doctors are unable to pinpoint the cause of infertility in about 9 percent of cases.

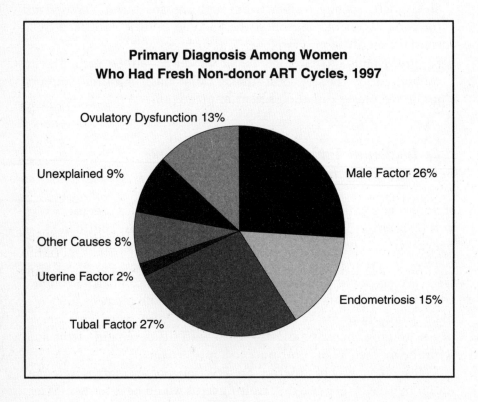

**Primary Diagnosis Among Women
Who Had Fresh Non-donor ART Cycles, 1997**

Ovulatory Dysfunction 13%

Unexplained 9%

Male Factor 26%

Other Causes 8%

Uterine Factor 2%

Endometriosis 15%

Tubal Factor 27%

Figure 3.4

Ovulatory Disturbances

Ovulation is the key to conception. More than one-quarter of all infertile couples have ovulatory disturbances. Some disturbances are:

- A woman may not ovulate.
- A woman may fail to ovulate consistently.
- A woman may produce eggs that are too ripe.
- A woman may produce many tiny egg follicles that fail to ovulate.

For ovulation to occur, a woman's body must produce various hormones in proper sequence in the right amount and at the right time. Chapter 4 covers ways to detect whether you have an ovulatory problem.

Tubal Problems

Blockages or adhesions involving the fallopian tubes are another major cause of infertility. A common cause of blockages and adhesions is pelvic inflammatory disease (PID), which can result from sexually transmitted infections such as gonorrhea or chlamydia. Many women who have had PID have no symptoms and are surprised when they learn, during a routine infertility workup, that they have blocked tubes.

Some women are born with abnormal fallopian tubes. A major cause of this damage is the fetus's exposure to diethylstilbestrol (DES), a drug prescribed to pregnant women to prevent miscarriages starting in the 1940s and ending in the early sixties.

Damaged fallopian tubes also can result from an ectopic, or tubal, pregnancy. Damaged tubes may be unable to transport the embryo into the uterus, increasing the risk of another ectopic pregnancy. Chapter 4 covers the tests doctors use to discover these problems, some of which can be corrected surgically.

Endometriosis

Endometriosis is a condition where the lining of the uterus, the endometrium, grows outside the uterus, causing scarring, pain, and heavy bleeding each month. It affects an estimated 10 to 15 percent of the female population. A leading theory or the cause of endometriosis involves the concept of "retrograde menstruation"—a backflow of blood tissue from the uterus into the pelvis during menstruation. A second theory is that the surface of the pelvis is lined by cells that can be changed to endometrial cells. Whatever the cause, endometriosis sufferers often describe pain—during menstruation or at other times in the cycle—as the primary symptom. Pain may or may not signal endometriosis, however. Even women with severe endometriosis may not necessarily have pain. Endometriosis can mimic many other disorders, including colitis and PID. Moreover, the severity of the symptoms often does not match the severity of the disorder. Very few disorders associated with infertility have so many unanswered questions as does endometriosis. And doctors aren't always sure exactly how endometriosis prevents pregnancy.

Cervical Problems

Cervical problems can involve the mucus in the cervix or the structure of the cervix itself. Mucus problems usually hinder conception, while structural deformities can make staying pregnant difficult. Mucus can be too scant, too thick, too acidic, or otherwise hostile to sperm. Mucus problems can shorten the life of the sperm or prevent it from swimming to the egg. The primary cause of abnormal cervical mucus is lower estrogen levels resulting from altered follicle development.

In addition to hostile mucus, bacteria in the cervix can kill sperm. The responsible microorganism, which is sometimes hard to identify, is studied by means of a cervical culture test. When the cervix is infected by one of these microorganisms, it becomes inflamed. Inflammation of the cervix is referred to as *cervicitis*.

Uterine Problems

Three types of uterine disorders can impair fertility and sometimes be corrected surgically. Women can have congenital uterine abnormalities such as a uterine "septum," a fibroid band of tissue that divides the uterus. There are also a host of other minor birth defects that can alter the structure of the uterus, but, unfortunately, they are very difficult or even impossible to correct surgically. While structural abnormalities don't necessarily prevent conception, they can be a source of repeated miscarriages.

A second uterine disorder is fibroid tissues. Fibroid tissues are benign tissue growths within the smooth muscle of the uterus. Fibroids do not always cause infertility, but when they do, they usually result in a miscarriage rather than in a failure to conceive. A fibroid is most likely to interfere with conception if it grows near the entrance to the tubes, obstructing the embryo's way into the uterus. The effect of a fibroid on fertility and possible pregnancy loss depends on the size and position of the fibroid.

A final type of uterine disorder involves scarring of the uterine lining. One cause of scarring is infection, which can result from a dilation and curettage (D&C) and can cause Asherman's syndrome—scar tissue between the opposing walls of the uterus and destruction of the endometrial cavity.

Egg Problems

Since the publication of the first edition of *Getting Pregnant When You Thought You Couldn't,* much greater attention has been given to the role of poor-quality eggs in the inability to become pregnant and/or stay pregnant. Many of the problems that ten years ago were classified as "unexplained infertility" are now recognized to be the result of poor-quality eggs. Some women have hormonal levels that suggest that their egg supply is diminished. Surprisingly, some of these women are relatively young. Currently, the only treatment for this problem is to use an egg donor. However, on the horizon is a treatment that will allow some of these women to use their own eggs once they have been "specially treated."

Male Problems

By all accounts, a significant proportion of infertility problems is attributable to a "male factor," such as:

- Making no sperm, called *nonobstructive azoospermia*
- Making sperm that fail to reach the ejaculate (because of a blocked duct, for example)
- A low sperm count, called *oligospermia*
- Ejaculating enough sperm, but some aspect (their ability to move or their shape, for example) prohibits them from fertilizing the egg

Rapid weight gain, weight loss, or malnourishment also can hurt sperm quality or quantity. DES exposure in the womb is another factor that can create fertility problems in males.

Radiation treatment or chemotherapy also can cause sperm problems. Also, chronic alcoholism can create impotence and contribute to male infertility. Exposure to high heat from Jacuzzis, long-distance driving, excessive bicycling, too much jogging, or the wearing of tight underwear also can contribute to male infertility, as can infection of the genital-urinary tract. The primary diagnostic tool for detecting male fertility problems is a *semen analysis*, discussed in detail in the next chapter.

YOUR ROAD TO PREGNANCY

Once you have become pregnant, you can look back at this chapter and marvel at the miracle of conception. For now, though, we urge you to Educate Yourself About Infertility, our first Pointer. Educating yourself is critical to becoming a Partner in Your Treatment, another Pointer. Consider the knowledge you gained through this chapter your first step toward getting pregnant when you thought you couldn't.

CHAPTER 4

Diagnostic Testing: Finding Out What Is Wrong

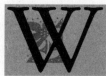hen you are having trouble getting pregnant, time is a precious commodity. Each month that passes without a pregnancy is likely to increase your level of stress. Therefore, it is in your best interest to find the source of the problem and correct it as quickly as possible. Having accurate information about your menstrual cycle helps your gynecologist determine which diagnostic tests to order or whether you need to see a specialist.

In this book we provide you with the information you will need to help you "up the odds" of getting pregnant. We can also help you by pointing out resources on the Internet that contain valuable information. One of the most useful starting places for this information is the Web site of the International Council on Infertility Information Dissemination (INCIID). You can find it at http://www.inciid.org. The INCIID Web site contains a fact sheet called "Basic Fertility Testing Information." Consult that fact sheet for another perspective on the basic testing process.

Begin by trying to get pregnant on your own for a specific amount of time. If you are younger than thirty-five years old, try for twelve months on your own. If you are older than thirty-five, try on your own a maximum of six months. If you are forty or older, you should probably try on your own for no more than three months.

Here is how to try on your own. First you must determine when you are ovulating. To find out when you are ovulating, measure your basal body temperature and use ovulation predictor kits (as described on page 88) so that you will know when you are most fertile. You can do other things to help increase the likelihood of getting pregnant on your own. There is a large amount of literature on "home remedies" that couples claim have helped them get pregnant. Examples include drinking several tablespoons of Robitussin to improve cervical mucus and having your husband change from jockey to boxer shorts. Can these techniques help? We don't know. But they may help you feel that you can exercise a measure of control over a fertility problem that seems beyond your control.[1]

Diagnostic tests help figure out why you are not yet pregnant. Physicians perform most of these tests. However, you can also collect information on your own that can save time and be very helpful in aiding your diagnosis. We begin with what you can do on your own to Become a Partner in Your Treatment.

DETECTING OVULATION

Infertility problems can be detected either directly or indirectly. The only *direct* evidence of ovulation is pregnancy. Indirect evidence can be provided through an endometrial biopsy, through an analysis of your hormonal levels during specific days of your menstrual cycle, through a cervical mucus check, basal body temperature charts, and home ovulation-predictor kits. These charts and tests look at clues that arise from the hormonal events associated with ovulation. Try to keep your information *organized* so that you can readily share it with your doctor. Keep this in the information section of your Pregnancy Quest Journal.

Cervical Mucus

As your estrogen levels change, so does the quantity and quality of the cervical mucus. Just before and around the time of ovulation, mucus production increases, and the mucus becomes clear and stretchy, almost like raw egg white. One test you can do yourself is to examine your cervical mucus during your cycle. Try to discern when it changes from scant to copious and from thickish to thin and stretchy. Immediately after ovulation, it changes again from the consistency of egg whites back to a small amount of thick mucus.

Basal Body Temperature

Another hormonal event you can monitor indirectly is the level of progesterone in your bloodstream. At the beginning of the cycle, the progesterone level is low and your body temperature is correspondingly low. Just before ovulating, there is an LH surge, sometimes associated with a slight drop in basal body temperature. Following the surge, the egg is ovulated from the follicle, and the remaining sac becomes the corpus luteum, which secretes progesterone. When this happens, body temperature jumps one-half a degree to a whole degree.

You can chart these temperature changes using a basal body temperature (BBT) thermometer. Most basal body thermometers come with temperature charts. Pharmaceutical companies also produce these charts. Your doctor should have an ample supply of temperature charts to give you. All charts contain spaces where you date each day of your cycle. *The first day of your menstrual period is Day 1.* In addition to showing graphically any temperature changes, the chart also helps you determine exactly how long your cycle is and how regular you are. Keep your BBT chart in one of the plastic pockets you have purchased for your Pregnancy Quest Journal. You will then have it easily available to share with your doctor.

For charting to be of value, you *must* heed the following precautions:

- Take your temperature *as soon as you wake up, before you get out of bed.*
- Do *not* move around before taking your temperature.
- Record the temperature on the chart right after you take it. Do not rely on your memory.
- Record your temperature every morning.

Your BBT changes constantly, according to activity levels and time of day. Readings taken any time other than the moment you wake up are useless. Keep your thermometer, the chart, and a pencil at your bedside. Shake the thermometer down immediately after recording your temperature so it is ready for the next morning's reading.

Keeping track of your temperature can be nerve-wracking. A reading that is not what you hoped for may tempt you to fudge or to take a second reading. Resist this temptation, because inaccurate data can mislead a doctor into thinking you are ovulating when you really aren't. If you would like to use your computer to keep your BBT chart in the form of an Excel spreadsheet, you can download one that has been created as a template for you at http://www.fertilityplus.org/faq/bbt/bbt.html. If you use this spreadsheet, you should print out a paper copy to place in your journal and have available to share with your doctor.

Ovulation-Predictor Kits (OPKs)

In addition to monitoring your BBT and cervical mucus, you also can test your urine for an LH surge, which generally starts twenty-four to forty hours before ovulation, the time of peak fertility.[2] There are some ten brands of ovulation-predictor kits on the market, and all are available without a prescription. They vary in complexity as well as in price (the average is about $23 for a five-day supply of testers). The kits cannot be reused. All of the kits require that you either collect your urine and mix it with chemicals or put the urine in contact with a chemically treated surface. A color indicator will tell you whether you are having an LH surge. You may wonder why you need to spend so much money on an ovulation-predictor kit when you can find out when you ovulate using a thermometer, at no cost. The reason for spending the extra money is that the OPKs tell you twenty-four to thirty-six hours *ahead* of time when you are about to ovulate. The BBT, on the other hand, only lets you know that you most probably have *already* ovulated.

Most kit manufacturers claim that ovulation will occur twenty-four to forty hours after the change in color on the indicator stick.[3] The tests are reliable if used correctly. Test your urine for three or four consecutive days, beginning about four days before the time you usually ovulate as shown by previous BBT charts. For most women (those with cycles that last from 26 to 30 days), this will be between Days 9 and 13 of their cycle. If your cycle is very short (21 or 22 days), you should begin testing on Day 5. For cycles between 31 and 42 days in length, add one day to 13 for each day over 30. Thus a woman with a 31-day cycle should begin testing on Day 14 and a woman with a 42-day cycle should begin testing on Day 25.

Kits can sometimes give a "false negative" reading if your urine is diluted as a result of drinking too much water. Kits can also sometimes give a "false positive" reading if you have polycystic ovary syndrome (PCOS) or if you have taken Clomid within the previous two days.

Once you have a positive test, stop testing and be sure to have intercourse within the window of time recommended on the kit's instruction leaflet. Note on your BBT chart when the LH surge occurred.

When you first run a series of ovulation-predictor tests, you may feel like a mad chemist. But rest assured, you soon will be able to perform the tests in a more matter-of-fact way once you get accustomed to the procedure. Knowing when to time intercourse is a definite help in getting pregnant.

You can find some valuable information about ovulation-predictor kits on the Internet at http://www.fertilityplus.org/faq/opk.html. This site, compiled by Rebecca Smith Waddell as a resource for several Internet infertility discussion groups, lists information about ten different kits ranging in price from a low of $13.87[4] (Answer Ovulation Test Kit) to a high of $50 to $70 (OvuQuick). Ms. Smith has monitored Internet discussions about ovulation-predictor kits and notes that patients talk most about Clearplan and OvuQuick. Patients indicate that these two kits are easiest to find.

COLLECTING MEDICAL HISTORY INFORMATION

Another way to aid your gynecologist is to gather critical medical history in a systematic and organized way. To help, we provide you with separate forms for both you and your partner to photocopy, fill out, and give, along with your temperature charts and a list of questions, to your gynecologist during your consultation.

WOMAN'S MEDICAL HISTORY FORM

Name:

Age: ___ Years married: ___   1st marriage ___ 2nd marriage ___

Height ___   Weight ___

Menstrual History Information:

Age at first period:

Characteristics of early periods:

___ cramps   ___ light flow   ___ heavy flow   ___ erratic period

How long did it take for your periods to become regular?

Do you remember anything unusual about your early menstrual history?

Current Menstrual Information:

When was your last period?

How long is your typical menstrual cycle (from the beginning of one period to the beginning of the next period?)

How many days do you bleed?

Do you have:

___ cramps   ___ clotting   ___ heavy flow

___ light flow   ___ irregular flow

Do you experience pain during intercourse?

Is your period usually regular?

Have you had any missed periods lately?

Do you take pain medications (e.g., Tylenol/Motrin) when you have periods?

Can you tell when you are ovulating?

What are the signs:

___ pain in your ovaries   ___ pain in your lower back

___ heavy watery cervical mucus   ___ other

History of Birth Control

Have you ever used birth control?
Have you used:

___ birth control pills   name ___   date of use ___   duration

___ diaphragm   date of use ___   duration

___ IUD   kind ___   date of use ___   duration

___ condom

___ sponge/foam

___ rhythm method

___ coitus interruptus

If you used an IUD or birth control pills, describe your cycles while using either of them.

What were your cycles like after you stopped using them?

How long has it been since you stopped using birth control?

Pregnancy History:

Have you ever been pregnant?

PREGNANCY HISTORY

Year	Spontaneous abortion? Yes/No	Karyotype: Normal Male Normal Female Abnormal Male Abnormal Female	Therapeutic abortion? Yes/No	Ectopic pregnancy? Yes/No	Any infertility treatment for this pregnancy?	How much time did it take to conceive?	Did this pregnancy result in a live baby?	Was the current husband the father?

Past Gynecological History:

What was the age of first intercourse?

Have you had any sexually transmitted diseases?

___ gonorrhea ___ syphilis ___ chlamydia

___ venereal warts ___ herpes ___ pelvic inflammatory disease

___ other

When did you have them?

How were they discovered and treated?

Have you ever had:

irregular periods ___ previous colposcopy ___

abnormal Pap smear ___ previous laser surgery (cervix) ___

previous cryosurgery ___ history of fibroids ___

history of endometriosis ___ history of uterine cancer ___

history of ovarian cysts ___ history of breast disease ___

history of ovarian cancer ___ previous uterine surgery to correct uterine

previous breast surgery ___ septum ___

Did your mother take the drug DES while she was pregnant with you?

   If yes, how did you find out?

   Has any doctor commented on your DES exposure?

Family Pregnancy History

Mother's number of pregnancies ___ number of live births ___

Age of mother at her first conception ___ last conception ___

Number of mother's miscarriages ___

Age at menopause ___

Sister's number of pregnancies ___ number of live births ___

Age of sister at her first conception ___ last conception ___

Number of sister's miscarriages ___

General Medical History:

Have you ever had the following immunizations?   DATE

MMR   _____

Tetanus   _____

Hepatitis B   _____

Influenza   _____

Chicken Pox   _____

Physical Conditions:

Skin

Acne ___   Eczema ___   Rashes ___

Hairiness

Face ___
Chest ___
Abdomen ___

Have you had any surgeries or illnesses that required hospitalization?

Name of illness or surgical procedure	Date	Reason for hospitalization	Findings	Complications

Have you had any chronic illness now or in childhood?
Have you ever been on medication for a long time?
Are you taking any medication now?
Are there any chronic diseases or conditions in your family?

Lifestyle History:

Name of exercise	How often do you do this exercise?	How much time do you spend on this exercise?

Are you a vegetarian? ___

Does your weight fluctuate much? ___

Do you diet? ___

Have you ever had an eating disorder? ___

Do you drink alcohol? ___

   How often? ___

Do you smoke cigarettes? ___

   How often? ___

Are you frequently exposed to the sun? ___

Are you exposed to any chemicals or radiation on your job? ___

Do you consider yourself to be under a lot of stress at home or at work? ___

History of Infertility:

How long have you been trying to get pregnant? ___

When did you discontinue contraceptives? ___

Intercourse:

Frequency (times/wk)	Position	Lubricant? Yes/No	Douche? Yes/No	Pain? Yes/No

MEDICAL HISTORY: MALE

Name:

Age: ___ Years married: ___   1st marriage ___ 2nd marriage ___

Height ___   Weight ___

Childhood Information:

Were you an: ___ only child   ___ middle child   ___ last child

Were you born prematurely?   ___ yes   ___ no

Were you circumcised?   ___ yes   ___ no

Did you ever have mumps?   ___ yes   ___ no   At what age? ___

Did you ever have surgery for a hernia? ___ yes   ___ no   At what age? ___

Sexual Information:

What was the age of first intercourse?

Have you ever fathered a child?   ___ yes ___ no

Have you ever had gonorrhea?   ___ yes ___ no

Have you ever had syphilis?   ___ yes ___ no

Is intercourse painful?   ___ yes ___ no

Do you have trouble maintaining an erection?   ___ yes ___ no

On a scale from 1 (low) to 5 (high), how would you characterize your current sex
    drive? ___

Do you ejaculate in the vagina without difficulty?   ___ yes ___ no

Genital/Urinary Information:

Have you ever been treated for an infection of the testicles?   ___ yes ___ no

Is urination painful?   ___ yes ___ no

Did you ever have undescended testes?   ___ yes ___ no

Was the problem corrected?   ___ yes ___ no

Did you ever have any injury to your testes?   ___ yes ___ no

Have you ever had a vasectomy?   ___ yes ___ no

Have you ever had varicocele surgery?   ___ yes ___ no

Other Information:

Do you use hot tubs regularly?	___ yes ___ no
Are you exposed to high temperatures at work?	___ yes ___ no
Are you exposed to radiation at work?	___ yes ___ no
Were you ever exposed to Agent Orange in the military?	___ yes ___ no
What type of underwear do you use?	___ boxer shorts ___ jockey shorts
Do you drive long distances on a regular basis?	___ yes ___ no
Do you bicycle-ride excessively?	___ yes ___ no
Do you jog excessively?	___ yes ___ no

Have you had any surgeries or illnesses that required hospitalization?

Name of illness or surgical procedure	Date	Reason for hospitalization	Findings	Complications

Have you had any chronic illness now or in childhood? _____

Have you ever been on medication for a long time? _____

Are you taking any medication now? _____

Are you taking any herbal medicines? _____

Do you use recreational drugs now? _____

Have you ever in the past used recreational drugs? _____

Are there any chronic diseases or conditions in your family? _____

Lifestyle History:

Name of exercise	How often do you do this exercise?	How much time do you spend on this exercise?

Does your weight fluctuate much? ___

Do you diet? ___

Have you ever had an eating disorder? ___

Do you drink alcohol? ___

    How often? ___

    How much? ___

Do you smoke cigarettes? ___

    How often? ___

    How much? ___

This information probably will have to be supplemented with information gathered through laboratory tests and medical examinations. Knowledge of the tests and procedures described in this chapter should prepare you for whatever your diagnosis might be. Finding out that you have a problem is discouraging news. But remember that many fertility problems can be fixed or circumvented and that advances in this area of medicine are happening all the time.

BEGINNING THE PARTNERSHIP

Prior to testing, your doctor will probably request a consultation session with you. Try to have your partner accompany you to this visit to help you Work as a Team. During this initial visit, your doctor will review your medical histories and probably schedule some diagnostic tests, technically known as an "infertility workup." Be on alert that this workup is physically taxing, emotionally draining, and can deplete your finances quickly if you have no health insurance. The diagnostic process may span many months.

Life during diagnosis is extremely stressful. You may feel bombarded by disturbing and possibly conflicting thoughts. It's quite normal to want several things at the same time. You want to learn what the problem is. You want to hear there is no problem. You want to know whether the problem is fixable. The bottom line is that you want to know whether you will ever be pregnant.

If you are feeling scared or overwhelmed at this point, realize that just knowing the names of the tests, what problems they might uncover, and what you can expect to happen during your workup will provide some relief and give you a sense of control.[5]

When you schedule your doctor's appointment, make sure you tell the nurse or secretary the purpose of the visit: to begin diagnosing why you are not yet pregnant. When you see the doctor, request that you have a Pap smear, cultures of your cervix, and some basic hormonal tests and blood work. These tests are the building blocks of your basic workup.

Many of the hormonal tests must be conducted on a particular day of your cycle, for example Day 3 for FSH. So try to schedule your visit to correspond with the early days or the midpoint of your cycle. Don't worry if your cycle is irregular. You can have your entire physical one day and then return on Day 3 of your next cycle to have blood drawn.

This initial visit is your first opportunity to Become a Partner in Your Treatment. As a partner, you should take the responsibility of setting an agenda for the visit. The agenda should be:

- What do we know?
- What do we need to find out?
- What do we do next?

When talking to your gynecologist, explain clearly that you have been trying to get pregnant for X months and would like to begin testing as soon as possible. When you leave the office, you should have a clear-cut plan for the next several months, fulfilling yet another Pointer.

PLANNING A COST-EFFECTIVE WORKUP FOR INFERTILITY

In this chapter we will discuss numerous tests to rule out various problems that may be preventing you from getting pregnant. But not all tests need to be done to arrive at a proper diagnosis and develop an effective treatment plan. What is needed is a cost-effective workup. Fortunately, Dr. Annette Lee, a reproductive endocrinologist, has developed a strategy for a cost-effective workup. Here is what Dr. Lee suggests.

Step 1: Determine Your Insurance Benefits

You want to make sure that, if you have insurance that will cover treatment and/or diagnosis, you are doing what you need to do and avoiding any missteps that will disqualify you from receiving benefits. To do this properly:

- Call the insurance company to verify what benefits you are entitled to. State specifically that you wish to verify what, if any, infertility benefits you have.
- Document this contact and then determine whether you will need any preauthorization.

Step 2: Participate in a Directed History and Physical with Your Physician

The physician will do a physical exam and take your medical history and your partner's history. The information you have gathered with the medical-history forms in this chapter will be very useful. Make sure to bring them to this meeting. In taking the history, the physician will ask about such things as your cycle length, how regular the cycle is, whether you have PMS, Mittelschmerz (pain around the time of ovulation), and dysmenhorrhea (painful menstrual periods). The physician will inquire about coital frequency, timing, and your use of lubricants. Believe it or not, some lubricants, such as petroleum jelly, can reduce your chances of getting pregnant. He or she will ask your partner whether he has ever created a pregnancy, about any exposure to health hazards at work, and lifestyle factors that may have a bearing on his fertility. In your physical, the physician will be looking for hirsutism (hairiness) that may suggest polycystic ovary syndrome, fat distribution, and estrogen status. The physician will also conduct a breast and pelvic exam.

Step 3: A Non-Invasive and Cost-Effective Workup

Physicians and insurance companies use different approaches to determine how to conduct a workup. While physicians typically use an approach based on their experience diagnosing a large number of patients sharing common characteristics, insurance companies turn to a computerized analysis of statistical predictions of treatment outcomes. This difference in approach may explain why sometimes your insurance company will refuse to pay for diagnostic procedures your doctor has ordered.

Your doctor will probably take the following steps:

1. *Rule out anovulation (Price range: $7–$75).* If you want to get pregnant you must release eggs, so you need to know whether you are ovulating. According to the latest available CDC national statistics, approximately 12 percent of the women who underwent assisted reproductive technology (ART) procedures had a primary diagnosis of ovulatory dysfunction. Of all the infertile women who have failed to conceive after engaging in unprotected intercourse for twelve months, 40 percent are diagnosed with an ovulatory disorder. So it is important that you rule out this possibility. The inexpensive way to do this is to use a basal body temperature thermometer for three months, at a cost of about $7. A more expensive way to diagnose this problem is by

measuring your blood progesterone level during the luteal phase of your cycle. This will cost about $75.

2. *Rule out a male factor problem ($60–$125).* Approximately 35 percent of couples who have not conceived after one year of trying on their own are diagnosed with a male factor problem (25 percent who are trying ART have this diagnosis). The diagnosis requires collecting a semen sample from the male partner and conducting an analysis using the Kruger strict criteria system. Ideally, your partner should abstain from ejaculating for two to five days before producing the sample to be used for the analysis. The cost of the analysis and report is about $125.

3. *Evaluate the status of the fallopian tubes and the uterine cavity ($250 physician fee and about $1,000 for radiology fee).* More than 30 percent of the patients doing ART are diagnosed with either a tubal or a uterine problem. You can get information about your tubes and uterine cavity by having either a hysterosalpingogram (HSG), which is an X-ray procedure, or a sonohysterogram, which is an ultrasound procedure.

4. *Rule out a cervical factor problem ($125).* Fewer than 10 percent of infertile women have a cervical problem. You can diagnose this problem using a postcoital test (PCT) that is timed using an ovulation-predictor kit.[6]

5. *Evaluate your ovarian reserve ($150–$360).* The importance of this evaluation increases as you get older. Dr. Lee estimates that less than 10 percent of women under age thirty who experience unexplained infertility have an inadequate ovarian reserve. For women between ages thirty and thirty-five, perhaps as many as 30 percent may have diminished ovarian reserve. This figure increases to 40 percent in women between the ages of thirty-five and forty and rises to 50 percent for women who are over the age of forty.

Dr. Annette Lee suggests that there are certain tests you should avoid. She believes that you don't need to have a routine TSH and prolactin screening (saving you $100) if you have very regular cycles. You can also avoid a routine endometrial biopsy, which costs about $300, unless you have symptoms suggesting that you have a luteal phase disorder. She also cautions you to avoid having several cycles of Clomid therapy without any other monitoring if you already know that you are ovulating and making a sufficient number of follicles. Finally, if you do not have insurance that covers a diagnostic laparoscopy, you may decide to pursue treatment for three to six months before undergoing a diagnostic laparoscopy, unless there is a strong suspicion that you have endometriosis or your HSG shows that you have tubal disease. On the other hand, if your insurance carrier will cover a laparoscopy for a patient with your diagnosis, you may decide to have a laparoscopy before beginning treatment.

Dealing with Experts Other Than Your Primary-Care Physician

Unfortunately, the key to getting the diagnosis and treatment you want can mean seeing a battalion of specialists. Many of the tests described in this chapter can and should only be done by experts who perform them regularly. Although your gynecologist can orchestrate the general plan of action, you most likely will also require the services of radiologists, laboratory technicians, and urologists who specialize in male infertility.

Unlike your own doctor, who is familiar with your personality and probably has a good bedside manner, doctors in these specialties may see patients only once or for short periods of time. They may seem gruff or cold. Their relationship is not with you but with your personal physician, to whom they will submit the results of your test. Prepare yourself for this detachment by realizing that the doctor's expertise and competence—not charm—are the only important factors. You want to get pregnant, not find a new friend, so seek emotional support outside the specialist's office.

HORMONAL TESTS FOR WOMEN

The simplest tests are generally performed first, either in your doctor's office or in a laboratory.

Even if your basal body temperature (BBT) thermometer shows the appropriate rise and fall in temperature and your LH surge kit reveals a color change, your doctor may order a hormonal analysis to confirm that your ovaries are functioning normally. These tests are almost always covered by health insurance. You need only have a few vials of blood drawn, a relatively painless procedure. Having the test done does not prohibit you from trying to get pregnant during that month, although you may experience some stress awaiting the test results.

Follicle-Stimulating Hormone/Estradiol Levels

The brain, the pituitary gland, and the ovaries work together through feedback mechanisms. When the brain wants the ovary to begin to mature a follicle, it sends a signal to the pituitary gland to release follicle-stimulating hormone, called FSH for short. As the follicle grows, the level of FSH decreases. When the follicle is mature, the brain communicates that it is now time to decrease the level of FSH. If you look at the chart of hormonal levels in figure 3.1, you will see that between Days 3 and 10 the level of FSH decreases. After Day 10, it increases until just about the time of ovulation, after which it declines until progesterone levels start to fall in the last week of the cycle. This increase and decrease in FSH level that is coordinated with the development of the egg in a normal cycle reflects a state of good "communication" between the ovaries and the brain. The key "players" in this process are the egg and the cells surrounding the egg. If the quality of your eggs is poor, this state of affairs will be manifested by poor communication between the ovaries and the brain. And the clues about whether communication is likely to be poor can be found when your doctor measures your FSH level early in your cycle.

Therefore, perhaps the most important hormonal level that your doctor will be determining is your "Day 3 FSH" (which can actually be measured on Days 2 or 3, or even Day 4). More than any other hormonal level, your Day 3 FSH level (in conjunction with your Day 3 estradiol level) will determine the nature of your ovarian reserve and your potential for conceiving, either on your own or with assistance.

When a woman enters menopause, she is essentially running out of eggs (follicles) in her ovaries. A woman can be forty with exceptionally good-quality eggs and still be fertile or she can be twenty-four with poor-quality eggs and be infertile. More typically, a woman's egg quality tends to decline in her late thirties and declines even more quickly in her early forties.

When the brain senses that eggs are not being produced, in part from the low estrogen level and in part due to the hormone inhibin (a female feedback hormone made in the ovary to regulate FSH production by the pituitary gland), it orders up more FSH in an attempt to compensate and maintain ovulation. As the ovarian reserve declines more and more, the pituitary produces more and more FSH to help the ovaries produce a follicle, but the ovaries cannot respond. At some point, no matter how loud the brain and the pituitary gland shout, there are just too few follicles remaining in the ovaries to maintain normal functioning. This leads to a state of low estrogen and high FSH levels in the blood.

So if the hormonal level tests show that on Day 3 the FSH is high and the estrogen is low, it is an indication that the ovarian reserve is declining. But several other factors complicate the reading of these levels. For example, the estrogen level can be high on Day 3, and the Day 3 FSH can be low. If you are young and this is your result, the high estrogen can mean that you have a residual cyst (an unovulated egg from a previous cycle) or that the estrogen level in your system is high (because you are young), and this result is good. If you are older and have these results, the test could be showing that the high estrogen is driving down the FSH level and affecting the hormonal balance. Since the estradiol level is elevated, it may be artificially suppressing the FSH level into the normal range but not really representing what is happening in your body.

The final complicating aspect of this test is that labs use different scales. In the United States there are several different assays (ways of measuring hormonal levels); the two most common are Leeco and Becton Dickinson.[7] These assays use different solutions and therefore give different results for the exact same sample. A value of 25 IU/L on the Leeco assay corresponds to approximately 10 IU/L on the Becton Dickinson assay. The Leeco assay has a normal range of 5 to 20 IU/L. The Becton Dickinson assay has a normal range of 1.5 to 8.6 IU/L.

While an abnormal result can indicate poor egg quality, a normal result does not necessarily mean that the egg quality is good. If you have an elevated Day 3 FSH level, you may still become pregnant on your own even though you would not be considered a good candidate for stimulation using injectable medications.

There is another method of assessing how good your FSH level is. Recall that in a normal cycle the FSH level is expected to decrease between Day 3 and Day 10. If your eggs are good, they will maintain this decreased level even when they are "put to the test." The way doctors put them to the test is to challenge them with a dose of clomiphene citrate in a test called the Clomid challenge test. A clomiphene challenge test is a dynamic type of test that can discover some cases of poor ovarian reserve in women having a normal Day 3 FSH. Therefore, this test is sometimes administered *in addition to* the Day 3 FSH test, especially if the doctor suspects that a woman has problems with her ovarian reserve or if she is older than thirty-five.

The test works as follows. On Day 2 or 3, a blood sample will be taken to ascertain your FSH and E2 levels. On Day 5 of your cycle you will take two Clomid pills (100 mg. each) and continue taking them until Day 9. (You will have taken a total of ten pills.) On Day 10 you come to the doctor's office and have another blood sample taken to evaluate your FSH level and your E2 level. The doctor will be looking to see whether you have a high FSH level on Day 10. If your egg reserve is poor, the FSH level will rise in response to the stimulation by Clomid. But if the reserve is good, it will resist this challenge and remain low.

A high Day 10 FSH level is as bad a signal as a high Day 3 FSH level. Sometimes the Day 3 level can be low because your FSH level is actually fluctuating from day to day. If only the Day 3 level is measured, the doctor may incorrectly assume that everything is okay if that level is low. By obtaining two pieces of data—the Day 3 level and the Day 10 level in response to a challenge by Clomid—the doctor has a much more accurate picture of your ovarian reserve. As you can see, the Clomid challenge test is more accurate in detecting decreased ovarian reserve than is a Day 3 FSH test alone.

Other Hormonal Levels

LH (luteinizing hormone) level is monitored when Day 3 FSH is taken and again around mid-cycle. LH is a hormone that stimulates the release of an egg. A normal base level is between 2 and 20 mIU/ml. During the mid-cycle peak, the level is many times higher than the base level value. Often the ratio of LH/FSH is considered in the diagnosis of PCOS (polycystic ovary syndrome) and may help in designing a stimulation protocol.

Estradiol level, the amount of estrogen in your blood, is monitored at various times. On cycle Day 3, it can normally range between 25 and 75 pg./ml. During the mid-cycle peak it can range between 200 and 600 pg./ml., and during the luteal phase it will be between 50 and 300 pg./ml. As discussed above, estradiol levels are usually considered in conjunction with the results of other hormonal tests.

The level of progesterone, the hormone secreted by the corpus luteum of the ovary after ovulation has occurred, can be monitored at mid-cycle and after ovulation. The level at mid-cycle is typically under 2 ng./ml. before the LH surge and rises to between 10 and 40 a week after ovulation.

The level of prolactin, too much of which can inhibit ovulation, is best measured in the morning after you have been fasting in the early follicular phase of your cycle. The level is normally less than 20 to 25 ng./ml. If the level is elevated, an additional test for thyroid function (TSH) should be performed.

SEMEN ANALYSIS FOR MEN

While a woman undergoes ovulation tests, her partner's sperm quality and quantity can be analyzed through a test known as a *semen analysis.*[8] To obtain a semen sample, the man must ejaculate through masturbation into a sterile cup. Lab technicians have told us that some couples have brought in samples in Tupperware saltshakers or other unusual containers. For best results, obtain a sterile specimen cup from your doctor or pharmacist.

The sample can be collected at home, in a doctor's locked examination room, or in a lab that has a private room for this purpose. (If religious practices conflict with masturbation, other methods of obtaining semen can be used. Consult a clergyperson.)

If the specimen is to be obtained at home, be sure to keep the semen at room or body temperature en route to the lab. The sample should be provided 2 to 5 days after the man last ejaculated and should be brought to the lab within one to two hours of leaving the man's body. Try to keep the sample warm while transporting it. If someone else is driving keep the sample under your armpit to keep it warm. The test is usually repeated at least once to increase reliability.

It is important to remember that "normal" has a wide variety of meanings. What's normal for getting pregnant on your own is different from normal for someone about to embark on an IVF procedure that utilizes intracytoplasmic sperm injection (ICSI). So when comparing your husband's results to those given below, you must keep in mind what procedure they will be used for.

A standard for assessing sperm adequacy was developed by the World Health Organization (WHO). The WHO procedure provides normal values for a routine semen analysis.

Specifically, the lab technician will measure:

- *Semen volume:* How much liquid is produced? Normal value is 2 to 6 ml.
- *Semen density:* How many sperm per milliliter of semen? (At least 20 million sperm per milliliter is considered sufficient to conceive.)
- *Total sperm count:* Greater than 40 million per ejaculate.
- *pH:* Acidity or alkalinity (7 to 8).
- *Sperm morphology:* Shape of the sperm. (At least 30 percent should be of normal, oval shape.)
- *Sperm motility:* Swimming ability. Graded on five-point scale:
  0: sperm are not moving
  1: staying in place and vibrating
  2: moving slowly
  3: moving forward in a straight line at a good pace
  4: racing forward in a straight line
  If 50 percent are grade 3 or better or if 25 percent are grade 4, the sample is adequate.
- *Semen viscosity and liquefaction:* How thick or watery. (Good semen is not too thick. It liquefies within one hour.)
- *Sperm agglutination:* How much do the individual sperm stick to each other? (Good semen has no significant clumping.)

Your physician may also use a different scale for further morphological analysis called the *Kruger strict criteria test.* The Kruger test is more time consuming because detailed measurements of the sperm are taken by the technician viewing them under the microscope, but the results of this assessment may correlate better with fertilization during

IVF cycles. The method employing strict criteria for normal shapes has a normal range of greater than 14 percent normally shaped sperm.

Results are usually available on the same day the test is performed. The lab sends results to the referring physician, who will pass the information along to you. While many times routine semen analysis can allow a definitive diagnosis of infertility, such as in a man with azoospermia—the absence of sperm in the ejaculate—in many cases there remains a question of the impact of more minor semen abnormalities on your chances of becoming pregnant naturally with your husband's sperm.

While there are no ill effects associated with providing a semen sample for analysis, there could be some emotional upheaval should the specimen prove to be less than ideal. It is important to emphasize to your husband that the quality of a man's sperm has nothing to do with his masculinity or sexual attractiveness. If the semen analysis reveals a problem, the doctor may order one or more of these additional tests: a *fructose test,* a *testicular biopsy,* and *hormonal analyses.*

Fructose Test

This test is done *only* if the semen analysis reveals a complete absence of sperm. Its purpose is to determine whether an obstruction is preventing sperm from getting into the ejaculate.

Sperm cells and the seminal fluid are produced in separate areas of the testes. They flow through separate tubes, which merge into a single tube, the vas deferens, which carries the semen out of the penis during ejaculation. The seminal fluid contains a sugar called fructose. If no fructose is detected in the semen, the doctor knows there must be a blockage somewhere before the epididymis, causing the sperm to be trapped in the testicle. If fructose is present but *no* sperm are seen, it usually indicates that the testes are producing few, if any, sperm. Results should be available within one week.

Hormonal Analysis for Men

Analyzing the levels of hormones in the man's blood is another method of finding out possible causes of a low sperm count. The pituitary gland may not be secreting enough FSH to stimulate the testes to make sperm, or there may be testicular failure indicated by an elevated FSH level. The three hormones usually tested are LH, FSH, and testosterone.

Testicular Biopsy

If a fructose test reveals no sugar, the doctor may order a testicular biopsy to determine whether the man is making sperm. The value of a biopsy is limited if FSH levels are high. The biopsy examines the entire sperm "production line"—the area where sperm precursors are made, whether precursor sperm cells are changing into mature sperm, and whether sperm tails are being formed. It seems remarkable that so much information can be gathered by examining a tiny snip of tissue, but it helps to remember that all these things happen on a microscopic level.

The biopsy is taken under local anesthesia, usually in the doctor's office. The doctor, preferably a urologist, makes a one-quarter-inch incision in the scrotum and snips a small piece of tissue from the testes. The tissue is sent to a lab and examined under a microscope. The actual removal of tissue takes about ten minutes, and results are available in a week or two. Taking Tylenol prior to the test can reduce pain.

While physical discomfort is minimal and temporary, most men who undergo a testicular biopsy experience anxiety. They are concerned about both their masculinity and their potential inability to father a child. Again, it is important to be emotionally supportive of your husband as he waits for the results of this test. In some cases, sperm that is extracted during the biopsy can be frozen for possible use in assisted reproduction.

DOES THE COUPLE HAVE A PROBLEM?

Once the doctor has established that the woman is making eggs and the man is producing sperm, the next logical question is, Can the sperm get to the eggs to try to fertilize them? There are several barriers that can keep this from happening.

During the initial consultation, the physician should determine whether the couple is using a proper intercourse technique. Although there is no special technique or position that will assure a pregnancy, there are some improper techniques that can prevent sperm and eggs from meeting. If the doctor discovers that you are using one of these, he will advise you of an appropriate change. For example, during one of our sessions with a couple who had been trying unsuccessfully for almost a year to become pregnant, the wife mentioned to us, in a fairly offhand way, that they had been having intercourse using petroleum jelly as a lubricant. We explained that the only lubricants that were conducive to baby making were olive oil and saliva because neither of these lubricants kill sperm. The couple stopped using petroleum jelly and became pregnant the next month. The lesson to be learned: Provide as much information as possible to your doctor. Sometimes a piece of seemingly innocuous information may hold the key to unlock the door to a successful pregnancy.

Postcoital Test (PCT)

In perhaps 2 percent of infertile women, the cervical mucus is "hostile" to sperm and kills them long before they can swim to the egg. Hostile mucus can be diagnosed through a *postcoital test,* or PCT. This test is also known as the Sims-Huhner test, and it is performed two to twelve hours after intercourse.[9] However, there is no need to feel pressured to rush in immediately for this test.

A PCT also can be performed twenty-four hours after intercourse to determine the sperm's long-term survival in the vagina. A negative finding may stem from poor timing, poor-quality mucus, acidity, inadequate sperm, lack of estrogen, or from sperm-killing antibodies in the woman's vagina. It is not always clear which is to blame.

Prior to the PCT, you will use your basal-body temperature chart and LH test kit to determine when you are ovulating. Just before ovulation, you will be instructed to have intercourse. When you arrive at the doctor's office, the gynecologist extracts a small sample of cervical mucus and examines it under a microscope to see how many sperm are alive and swimming. The procedure takes a few minutes, and some doctors allow you to view the sample under the microscope. While the

PCT is relatively painless, it can cause emotional upset due to "sex on demand" pressures.

Testing for Bacterial Infections

One of the earliest tests that should be done is a genital-tract culture to look for bacterial infections. Many different strains of bacteria can live in the male and female genital tracts and can cause a variety of problems at many different stages of the pregnancy process. Some of these bacteria are transmitted in "Ping-Pong" fashion from one partner to the other during sexual intercourse. Certain bacteria may create problems that interfere with ovulation. Bacteria may contribute to a low sperm count or to sluggish sperm swimming. Bacteria also can advance the formation of scar tissue, which can block sperm transmission or damage sperm-production apparatus in the testes.

For women, certain bacterial infections can be a factor in pelvic inflammatory disease. These bacteria include chlamydia, mycoplasma, streptococcus, and enterococcus, among others. The cervical mucus and the semen should be tested for the presence of a bacterial infection. These infections are, in most cases, easily treatable with antibiotics.

As benign as this testing seems, it can spur emotional upset because a chlamydia infection can bring up discussions of past and present sexual activity.

Immunobead Test for Antisperm Antibodies

The body has an immune system designed to prevent attack by foreign bodies. The husband's sperm cells normally are treated as "friendly foreigners" by a woman's body, but some women's bodies mistakenly treat sperm as an enemy and send antibodies to destroy it. The woman can have antibodies that attack the head, the tail, or the midpiece of the sperm. Antibodies to the head can make the sperm incapable of penetrating the egg. Antibodies to the tail can impair the sperm's ability to swim properly.

Sometimes, too, a man can produce antibodies that actually attack his own sperm. This is a serious problem. Fortunately, the incidence of so-called antisperm antibodies is low for both the male and female populations.

To find out whether either or both members of the couple are producing antibodies, the doctor orders an *immunobead test.* A blood sample is drawn and a mucus sample obtained from the female and blood and semen samples are obtained from the male. Results, available in a few weeks, are given in terms of percentage of antibodies attacking the head, midpiece, or tail of the sperm.

The doctor will discuss the specific proportions of the various types of antibodies found. In instances where significant immunological problems are encountered, the doctor may discuss using one of the assisted reproductive techniques described in Chapter 7.

DOES THE WOMAN HAVE A PROBLEM THAT IS PREVENTING FERTILIZATION?

If the tests for ovulation suggest that you are ovulating, the doctor needs to find out whether the ovulated egg is getting into the fallopian tube. Some women have "adhesions," or scar tissue, which impede the ability of the tube to rotate into position to catch the egg. Even if the tube is in position, the egg may not be picked up because the fimbria at the upper end of the tube may be damaged.

If the egg does get into the tube, it may get stuck in one spot, unable to travel to the location of the sperm. The tube itself may contain internal adhesions or fibroids, which act like roadblocks preventing movement of an egg.

There are several diagnostic procedures that provide information about the internal and the external condition of the fallopian tubes. These tests differ in terms of their cost, physical discomfort, risks, and the amount of information they provide. Understanding these tests can give you an idea of which ones should be done before others and whether the costs and risks are worth it.

The Hysterosalpingogram (HSG)

Useful information about the internal condition of the fallopian tubes is provided by a *hysterosalpingogram,* or HSG. The HSG does *not* allow the doctor to see the actual inside of the tube *directly.* Instead, it shows only the *outlines* of the inside of your tube. Only a procedure called falloposcopy allows the doctor to observe the inside of the tube *directly.* Not only can he see it, he can also perform minor surgery to correct some problems.

A hysterosalpingogram is an X-ray showing the shape of the uterus and the fallopian tubes and whether the tubes are open. The amount of radiation exposure is minimal. It also provides information about abnormalities of the uterine cavity such as adhesions, polyps, fibroids, or congenital abnormalities. The X-ray also can reveal scarring in the reproductive tract. An HSG is a test that is done by a physician other than your own doctor. Your reproductive endocrinologist may or may not accompany you to this test.

To obtain the X-ray, a tube is inserted into your uterus and dye injected into the tube. As soon as the dye begins to travel through your tubes, you will feel mild to moderate pain. Performed in a radiologist's office or hospital, the procedure takes about fifteen to thirty minutes and is done early in the menstrual cycle prior to ovulation so as not to disrupt a potential pregnancy.

It is not unusual to feel emotionally distraught over the HSG procedure. You may be worried, and rightly so, that the test will reveal blocked tubes. You may be upset about having to sign a waiver releasing the doctor from responsibility should anything go wrong. You may feel uncomfortable about having to be undressed in front of an unfamiliar doctor. And finally, since your doctor may have prescribed antibiotics, you may be worried about a bacterial infection resulting from the procedure. To cope, we recommend that you:

- *Work as a Team.* Have your partner read the description of this procedure and write a script to help you mentally rehearse it. Also have your partner accompany you to the test.
- *Make a Plan.* Use the Getting Pregnant Workout techniques to rehearse the procedure, and relax using controlled breathing

before and during the HSG. Part of your plan should be taking three or four ibuprofen tablets (400 to 800 mg.) several hours before the test to reduce discomfort. Your doctor also may prescribe antibiotics prior to the test to minimize the possibility of infection.

Sonohysterogram (SonoHSG)

A SonoHSG is a good alternative to evaluate the inside of the uterus. The SonoHSG is an ultrasound monitored procedure. It may be a safer alternative than an HSG because it does not involve any exposure to radiation.

In contrast to an HSG, which is usually performed in a radiology department, a SonoHSG can be performed in a doctor's office. The physician places a speculum into the vagina and inserts a catheter into the uterus. Through the catheter, he injects a saline solution into the uterine cavity and performs a transvaginal ultrasound. Although you may experience discomfort with this procedure, it may be less uncomfortable than an HSG because the saline solution is less irritating than the iodine used in an HSG. The salt solution separates the two sides of the endometrium and helps the doctor see whether you have any polyps, adhesions, or fibroids.

Dr. Michael Applebaum, a physician with a great deal of experience doing SonoHSGs, advises that if you are looking for more information about the fallopian tubes than whether they are blocked, you may be better off using an HSG than a SonoHSG. You should ask your physician about the relative merits of each of these alternatives to provide the best information in your situation. If you are contemplating a choice between these two procedures, use the Decision-Making Pointer discussed earlier in this book.

Hysteroscopy

The HSG or SonoHSG does not allow a doctor to examine the uterus directly. The hysteroscopy looks for problems such as adhesions, polyps, fibroids, or the formation of a wall in the uterus called a septum. It takes thirty minutes to two hours and is generally done early in the cycle. Under some circumstances, a hysteroscopy can be performed in a doctor's office using a combination of local anesthesia and a sedative. More commonly, the hysteroscopy is performed on an outpatient basis in a hospital operating room under local or general anesthesia. Sometimes the hysteroscopy can be combined with a diagnostic laparoscopy. It is generally performed by an OB-GYN, who may also be your infertility specialist.

Before the procedure, you must disrobe, put on a hospital gown, and lie on an operating table, which may feel cold and uncomfortable. During the procedure, the uterine cavity is inflated with carbon dioxide or a sterile water solution. The doctor inserts a telescopic instrument called a hysteroscope through the cervix. Using a scalpel or a laser attached to the end of the hysteroscope, the doctor can cut away adhesions or polyps he might see. While the doctor is examining the inside of the uterus, he can also obtain tissue for an endometrial biopsy.

The operation itself is not very painful, but you may feel nauseous afterward from the anesthesia. Some patients vomit and many are groggy after the procedure. Patients sometimes feel a temporary pain in the shoulders and neck from carbon dioxide bubbles rising from the abdominal cavity. Do not be alarmed by these symptoms. The body will absorb the bubbles within the next twenty-four hours, and the pain will disappear. Lying down prevents the bubbles from rising and also relieves pain.

To cope with the anxiety over the surgery, use the same Pointers described for the HSG, and in addition Make a Plan. Ask your doctor if he plans to do a laparoscopy or endometrial biopsy, and if so, discuss with him the pros and cons of scheduling the two procedures simultaneously.

Falloposcopy

Falloposcopy is a procedure that allows your doctor to visualize the inside of your fallopian tubes.[10] As of this writing, the procedure is still considered experimental. The optics used on the instrument are less than optimal, and better medical instruments for use with this procedure need to be created. For this reason, the procedure is not widely used at the moment. However, medical technology changes rapidly and by the time this book is published, falloposcopy may be more widely used. We therefore describe the technique briefly.

The doctor inserts a tiny flexible catheter through the cervical canal and uterine cavity into the fallopian tube. Then he threads a tiny flexible fiberoptic endoscope through the catheter into the fallopian tube. He is then able to look at the inside of the tube on a TV monitor. Looking at this TV image, he can see obstructions, scar formation, and any other abnormalities. The procedure takes between one-half hour and forty-five minutes. The procedure is performed under local anesthesia or IV sedation. You can resume normal activities the day after the procedure.

Diagnostic Laparoscopy

While the hysteroscopy concentrates on the inside of the uterus, the *laparoscopy* provides much valuable information about the *outside* of the tube as well as what's going on in the abdominal cavity. Laparoscopy is usually recommended for women who used IUDs in the past, have had a previous tubal pregnancy or painful periods, have had previous pelvic surgery or previous pelvic infections, or have failed to become pregnant after a year of trying. In some cases a diagnostic laparoscopy may be the next step before using injectable medications or turning to assisted reproductive technology.

A laparoscopy is performed in a hospital or outpatient operating room under general anesthesia. Be aware that you will be wearing a hospital gown and be wheeled into the operating room while you are still conscious. After you are unconscious, a needle will be inserted through your belly button. An incision of about 10 mm. (½ inch) will be made just below the belly button and a laparoscope inserted. Carbon dioxide gas will be introduced to inflate the abdominal cavity and make it easier for the surgeon to view the internal organs.

Through the laparoscope, the surgeon inspects the uterus, tubes, and ovaries for evidence of adhesions, endometriosis (uterine lining tissue present outside the uterus), or other problems and fixes what can be corrected. Usually, another instrument is inserted through an incision elsewhere in the patient's abdomen. After the operation is completed, the incision or incisions are closed with one or two stitches and covered with a Band-Aid. The patient is taken to the recovery room. A few hours later, she is discharged.

The surgery takes a minimum of thirty minutes and a maximum of several hours if the surgeon needs to correct many problems. It is advisable to have a surgeon who specializes in this procedure and in the treatment of infertility perform the laparoscopy. Although the surgery is quite safe, complications such as perforated blood vessels, bowels, or stomach have occurred in a small minority of cases. In addition, if your OB-GYN does not specialize in laparoscopic procedures, he or she may be unable to correct problems encountered and you would then need to undergo a second procedure. Reproductive endocrinologist Dr. Samuel Thatcher recommends that most laparoscopies for evaluation of infertility should include an hysteroscopy, which is performed at the same time.

The side effects, both physical and emotional, are similar to those of the hysteroscopy.

To cope:

- *Work as a Team.* Have your partner read the description of this procedure and write a script to help you rehearse it mentally. Also, have him accompany you to the operation.
- *Be a Partner in Your Treatment.* Assertively discuss your concerns about anesthesia with the anesthesiologist and insist on a protocol that will minimize the likelihood of discomfort.

CAN THE SPERM FERTILIZE THE EGG?

Once the aforementioned tests and surgeries confirm that the man is making sperm and that there are no blockages in the woman's reproductive tract, the next logical question is, Are the man's sperm capable of fertilizing the woman's eggs?

The ultimate test to answer this question is *in vitro fertilization.* When the doctor retrieves a woman's eggs and places them together with her husband's sperm in a petri dish, the doctor can actually see whether the sperm successfully penetrates and fertilizes the egg. Short of that, there is no direct measure.

Hamster Penetration Test

Since there is no easily obtained measure of fertilizing ability, some doctors have tried to get an indirect indicator of the sperm's ability to fertilize an egg using a *hamster penetration test.* The idea is that if a man's sperm can penetrate a hamster's egg, then it probably can penetrate a human egg as well. There is controversy, however, regarding the value of this test. Some doctors believe the information gleaned from this test is useful. Others believe that the conditions of the test are so unlike those in nature that the test does not provide valuable information.

DOES THE FERTILIZED EGG IMPLANT IN THE ENDOMETRIUM?

The next step is ensuring that the embryo can implant successfully in the endometrium, the lining that grows inside the uterus and is shed each month during menstruation when pregnancy does not occur. When the endometrium is too thin or not soft enough due to a lack of estrogen or progesterone, respectively, successful embryo implantation is less likely. When things work properly, the LH surge ovulates an egg and the leftover corpus luteum secretes progesterone, which makes the endometrium soft and lush. If the woman has a so-called *luteal phase defect,* the endometrium is not ready to receive the embryo when it arrives in the uterus.

Endometrial Biopsy

To determine the receptivity of the endometrium, the doctor performs an *endometrial biopsy,* a procedure in which a tiny piece of lining is extracted and examined. The biopsy is performed in the doctor's office before the expected onset of the next menses. By studying the tissue sample, it is possible to "date" the age of the endometrial tissue. Endometrial tissue is dated on the basis of an idealized twenty-eight-day menstrual cycle. Careful laboratory investigations of endometrial development have revealed how endometrial tissue should look at different "ages." Using these standards, the age of the biopsied tissue is determined.

The observed age is interpreted relative to the *start* of the menstrual period *following* the biopsy. Then the doctor counts backwards from the first new cycle day until he reaches the day on which the biopsy was performed. So if the biopsy was performed three days before the onset of the next menses, the laboratory tissue analysis should look like tissue that is three days prior to menstruation. If the "histological" (tissue) date is three or more days out of sync with the date determined by counting backwards from menstruation, then a luteal phase defect is said to exist. The endometrium is not ready for the egg and may have difficulty allowing for implantation.

Extraction of the tissue sample takes about ten minutes. The biopsy is done around Day 26 or 27. You may actually be pregnant at this time. But be assured that the risk of a miscarriage due to a biopsy is less than one in one thousand. Nonetheless, you may wish to have a pregnancy test before the procedure. During the procedure, the woman lies on the table just as she would during a pelvic examination. The doctor inserts a speculum into the vagina and examines the cervix. He cleans the vagina and then grasps the cervix with a clamp. That causes a sudden cramp, and the patient may react with a startle. A good physician will alert the woman ahead of time and talk her through this phase in a calm manner. Then the doctor inserts a metal instrument called a curette into the uterus and scrapes off a bit of the lining. The effect of this action produces a sensation similar to a menstrual cramp. The woman will feel discomfort for several minutes following the procedure. Some women bleed and should use a sanitary napkin. To reduce cramping, take Advil one-half hour before the procedure.

To lessen the pain of a biopsy, doctors have recently investigated the use of topical intrauterine lidocaine and found that it provides safe and effective anesthesia during endometrial biopsies.[11] Women who were given a placebo had pain scores of 9.9 compared to a score of 4.7 for women using lidocaine. The study concluded that using lidocaine added only a few minutes to the length of the procedure and did not affect the overall cost. If you are scheduled for a biopsy, ask your doctor about using lidocaine.

Women typically are frightened by the endometrial biopsy, but that fear can be lessened by the realization that the information gained through the procedure may be helpful in getting them pregnant.

To cope:

- *Work as a Team.* Have your partner read the description of this procedure and write a script to help you rehearse it mentally. Also have him accompany you to the test.
- *Make a Plan.* Use the Getting Pregnant Workout techniques to relax. Use GPST. Tell yourself, "It's going to be easy; the pain is minor and will subside shortly." Before the procedure, take a mild pain medication such as Motrin (800 mg.).
- *Be a Partner in Treatment.* Ask your doctor to prescribe Valium, which you can also take before the biopsy. A half-tablet can help you relax during the procedure. The more relaxed you are, the less discomfort you will experience. Also, remember to ask your doctor whether lidocaine can be used.

BEYOND IMPLANTATION

Once implantation takes place, the concern becomes making sure that the embryo continues to grow and develop into a healthy baby. For information on those stages of pregnancy, we refer you to Dr. Jonathan Scher's excellent book titled *Preventing Miscarriage.*[12]

Diagnosing the reason or reasons for infertility takes good detective work and skilled craftsmanship. As with any job you contract for, you want to use only highly skilled professionals. Some doctors are "jacks-of-all-trades." They do both the detective work and the repairs. As a consumer of medical care, it is your responsibility to make sure that the doctors you are working with are experienced. And remember, the doctor who is a skilled technician may not necessarily be a skilled diagnostician. In Chapter 6 we include a Doctor Interview Guide, which has important questions for you to ask when selecting the infertility specialist who is best for you.

Also keep in mind that *the ability to make an accurate diagnosis does not require the skills to perform the test.* That means your gynecologist may diagnose you solely by reading the laboratory and surgical reports. That also means that you can logically deduce that some tests are inappropriate or redundant for your case, given what you already know. For that reason, it is essential that you Assert Yourself in discussing your case with your doctor, another of our Pointers.

CHAPTER 5

The Treatments of Infertility

s in diagnostic testing, infertility treatment runs the gamut from the simplest and cheapest to the more complicated and costly. "Simple" and "cheap" are relative terms, however. As you have already read in Chapter 3, reproduction is a complicated business. The ways of correcting fertility problems are therefore, by definition, complicated. But don't let the strange-sounding names or procedures intimidate you. None of these concepts are beyond your comprehension, especially if you try to remain objective. Once you know what to expect, you can anticipate how various procedures may affect your body, your mind, and your pocketbook.

This chapter focuses on the relatively simple, or "low-tech," treatments to correct your fertility problems. These treatments include drug therapy, artificial insemination, and surgery. (Artificial insemination with donor sperm also is a low-tech treatment, but we address that topic along with other third-party pregnancy approaches in Chapter 11.) Once you have Educated Yourself about these low-tech ways of getting pregnant, you can go on to Chapter 6, which addresses the emotional and psychological aspects of the issues covered in this chapter.

After obtaining diagnosis from your physician—even if the diagnosis is unexplained infertility—it's time to begin Making a Treatment Plan in earnest. Depending on your doctor and your case, you may be advised to pursue one of two conflicting strategies. One strategy suggests that you go directly to the "high-tech" assisted reproductive technologies, which have higher success rates and potentially a shorter time to success. The other strategy explores less-invasive, less-costly, low-tech treatments first. Couples pursuing this strategy may try a low-tech treatment for several cycles. If that treatment fails, the couple "graduates" to a more aggressive low-tech treatment (from pills to injectable medications, for example) for the next several cycles. Only when they've exhausted all the appropriate low-tech treatments do they consider moving on to the high-tech area.

Regardless of what your doctor recommends, the ultimate choice is yours. The path you choose will reflect your finances, your timetable, the advice of your physician, and a host of other individual considerations, not the least of which is your psychological well-being.

We believe you owe it to yourself at least to consider low-tech treatments before trying high-tech measures such as in vitro fertilization. Last week, for example, five women at IVF New Jersey, where we counsel couples, learned that they were pregnant, not through in vitro, but as a result of taking drugs to stimulate egg production followed by intrauterine insemination—the mainstay of low-tech treatment.

DRUGS OF INFERTILITY TREATMENT

Most people, when they are trying to conceive a child, stop taking all drugs—even aspirin and alcohol. So it's ironic that for many infertile couples their only chance of becoming pregnant is by using drugs—fertility drugs, that is. Listen to the conversations between people combating infertility and the topic is almost always centered on medications: dosage, administration, costs, effectiveness, and side effects.

Here are the pros and cons, costs and side effects of the pharmaceutical arsenal available at this writing.[1,2] Since the time when we wrote the first edition, many new fertility medications have been developed. Perhaps because of resulting competition, the price of many of these drugs has decreased. We urge you to ask your doctor whether newer, better drugs have hit the market. We will also keep you informed of changes in available medications and research concerning these medications on our Web site, http://www.gettingpregnantbook.com.

Clomiphene Citrate

The most commonly prescribed drug to correct ovulation problems is clomiphene citrate, sold under the brand names Clomid and Serophene. By manipulating hormonal output, this oral medication stimulates the ovaries to produce one or more eggs in women who do not otherwise ovulate or have irregular cycles or infrequent periods. Clomiphene may also be prescribed to induce "superovulation" in women who have unexplained infertility "empirically," that is without clear scientific proof, on the chance that there may be subtle abnormalities in ovarian function that can be helped by clomiphene therapy.

Clomiphene, priced at about three to five dollars a tablet,[3] is generally taken for five consecutive days beginning on Day 3 to Day 5 after the onset of menstruation. The standard dosage is one tablet (50 milligrams) a day. If your body responds properly to the drug, you should ovulate about a week after you have taken the last tablet. If ovulation or pregnancy does not result, the doctor may increase the dosage to two or three tablets a day with the next cycle. The doctor also may prescribe the drug for more than five days. Most women need 150 milligrams a day or less to ovulate.

While on clomiphene, be sure to record your BBT carefully each morning and perform ovulation-predictor (LH surge) tests beginning on Day 10 of your menstrual cycle (see Chapter 4). Unless you will be artificially inseminated, your doctor will likely advise you to have intercourse every other day (to maximize sperm count) for at least one week starting about four days after you've taken the last tablet.

Following these guidelines, about 70 percent of women treated with clomiphene will ovulate, and 30 percent will get pregnant within six cycles.[4] Those women who do conceive have about a 5 to 10 percent chance of giving birth to twins.

Caution: Clomiphene therapy often lengthens a woman's cycle by two, three, or even more days, which can give her a false sense of being pregnant.

Researchers have found that if clomiphene treatment has not led to a pregnancy after six cycles, however, it is unlikely that it ever will.[5] If you have not gotten pregnant after six clomiphene cycles, therefore, it is time to Make a New Plan.

Clomiphene creates some undesirable physical and emotional side effects in some women. The most common physical side effect is a reduction of cervical mucus and a thinning of the uterine lining. There have been some reports that this "anti-estrogen" effect can be partially counteracted by taking supplemental estrogen. Other women report bloating, weight gain, hair loss, vision changes, and headaches while on clomiphene therapy. Many patients we counsel report fairly substantial emotional side effects from clomiphene as well. To investigate this phenomenon, we placed an inquiry in the national RESOLVE Inc. newsletter. Within several weeks, we received about thirty letters stating that clomiphene produced an array of negative emotional effects. Norma, a social worker, described profound depression, which caught her off guard since she generally was an upbeat person. Abby called Clomid's emotional impact "devastating." Phyllis said she was so depressed that she would sit and cry for hours. Others reported that they would suddenly burst into tears without provocation. Nanette described apparitions that haunted her. (Clomiphene sometimes changes pressure in the eye, which can cause what seem like ghostly flashes of light.)

In contrast, some women wrote that they had no significant emotional side effects. Although our survey was informal, it is clear that the response varies substantially from person to person. So if you're feeling sad and "cry at every Hallmark card" commercial like Jean told us, or have dramatic mood swings during a clomiphene cycle, you are not going crazy; you're just having intense responses to the drug, particularly because of its "anti-estrogen" characteristics.

Dr. Melvin Taymor, clinical professor emeritus at Harvard Medical School, calls clomiphene "one of the most widely used medications in gynecology; unfortunately, it is also one of the most misused.

"Most infertility specialists will have had the experience of seeing many patients who at the very first interview have already been on clomiphene—sometimes for up to one year or more," Dr. Taymor continues. "Many of these patients have not had a simple basal body temperature chart followed to see whether or not they are ovulating. In addition, many have had no infertility workup. This misuse has probably been fostered by the fact that clomiphene citrate has been called a 'fertility drug.'

"The fact is that if a patient is ovulating normally on her own, there is little likelihood that clomiphene will further increase the quality of that ovulation. The administration of clomiphene without a workup will, in most instances, only delay the resolution of the problem. In addition, clomiphene may have inhibiting effects upon fertility"[6] such as diminishing the quality of the cervical mucus.

Dr. Taymor's warnings are worth heeding. To avoid misuse of clomiphene or any fertility drug, you must Be a Partner in Treatment. Be sure your doctor has completed an adequate workup before determining whether clomiphene treatment is appropriate in your situation. If it is not, you should move on to another treatment that is right for you.

Clomiphene also can be used in men in an effort to improve sperm count. A typical male regimen is taking 25 milligrams of clomiphene daily, with interspersed five-day rest periods. The therapy is generally continued for up to nine months.

Clomiphene is also used in a diagnostic test called the Clomid challenge test (CCT), as described in Chapter 4.

Human Menopausal Gonadotropin (hMG) Medications

Human menopausal gonadotropins (hMG) are much more powerful than clomiphene. When we wrote the first edition of this book, we included only two drugs, Pergonal and Metrodin, in this class of medication. Serono, Inc. manufactured both of these medications. Since that time, the variety of hMG medications has increased considerably. Now, in addition to a group of natural hMG medications, several pharmaceutical companies are producing recombinant (i.e., created through genetic-engineering processes) forms of these drugs. These follicle-stimulating hormones include medications known by the following names: Pergonal, Fertinex, Humegon (manufactured by Organon), Follistim, Repronex (manufactured by Ferring), and Gonal-F. Unlike clomiphene, these medications are administered by injection only—some with intramuscular needles (the larger ones) and some with subcutaneous needles (the littler needles)—and require much more intensive monitoring, as well as an additional drug, human chorionic gonadotropin (hCG), to trigger ovulation.

Pergonal, the original injectable infertility medication, contains equal parts of the hormones FSH and LH, which are extracted from the urine of postmenopausal women, purified, and freeze-dried in glass ampules (small glass containers that keep the medicine fresh and sterile). Before injection, the white powder must be reconstituted with sterilized water. The FSH and LH in Pergonal have a direct impact on the ovaries, causing them to produce several eggs during one cycle, giving sperm more targets.

Humegon and Repronex are similar to Pergonal in their composition. They all consist of a combination of FSH and LH. Similarly, each of these medications requires mixing, intramuscular injections, and monitoring (regular blood work and ultrasound scans). Repronex is considered a generic equivalent of Pergonal and its cost is considerably less than that of Pergonal or Humegon.

In 1993 Serono introduced a new form of a medication, Metrodin, that was widely used up until 1999. The new medication, called Metrodin HP, is a highly purified version of Metrodin containing more than 95 percent pure FSH. Serono claims that one of the benefits of the purity of Metrodin HP is that it is less likely to cause skin irritation or allergic reactions such as little red bumps. But the more important benefit of creating a highly purified version of Metrodin is that it can be injected subcutaneously (under the skin) with a very small needle rather than requiring an intramuscular injection, although it still must be mixed and its levels monitored. The medication that is known as Metrodin HP in some countries is more often known as Fertinex in the United States. Fertinex is not often used, however, if the woman is overweight. Physicians have reported a lower success rate with the subcutaneously administered Fertinex for women who are moderately to severely overweight. It may be that this higher body mass index interferes with optimal absorption of the medication.

In 1997, the pharmaceutical company Organon, Inc. received FDA approval to market a recombinant DNA follicle-stimulating hormone called Follistim. Unlike Pergonal, Humegon, or Repronex, Follistim is not extracted from the urine of postmenopausal women. Researchers at Organon isolated the genes responsible for producing human FSH. After isolating the human FSH genes, they merged them with host-cell DNA, and this enabled the cells to produce human FSH. Because the manufacturer does not have to obtain large quantities of postmenopausal urine to create this medication, Organon is able to create a larger supply of the medication. Like Fertinex, Follistim is injected subcutaneously. Gonal-F is just like Follistim but a different pharmaceutical firm, Serono, manufactures it.

According to research studies, about nine out of ten women treated with follicle-stimulating hormones will ovulate. Most women begin their injections on Day 2 to Day 4 of their cycle. Typically, patients are injected with one, two, or three ampules (75 units per ampule) of medication daily for seven to twelve days. On average, patients given recombinant medications require about one less day of stimulation than those using nonrecombinant medications. Also, the estrogen level may rise more slowly in the beginning of the cycle for patients using recombinant medications. In general, however, overall success rates with each of these medications are comparable. Your physician will consider the specific data in your case and determine which medication or combination of medications is best for you.

Follicle-stimulating hormone injections should be administered around the same time each day. Many doctors prefer evening doses, between 7 P.M. and 9 P.M.; however some instruct patients to have medications in both the morning and the evening. For most women, the schedule means that they or their partners (not the doctor, whose office has closed for the day) must give the injections. At the end of this chapter is a detailed guide to help both of you through the rigors of hMG therapy.

The number of days for administering follicle-stimulating hormones is based on results of ongoing blood tests and ultrasound scans of the ovaries. The blood tests measure estradiol levels, and the scans enable the doctor to measure the growing egg follicles and the size of the ovaries themselves. While inconvenient, this intensive monitoring is vital to avoid overstimulating the ovaries, a condition that can lead to discomfort or pain.

Most doctors order the first blood tests and scans on Day 3, before your first injection. This initial monitoring is to ensure that you have no residual ovarian cysts or follicles left over from previous cycles. The next monitoring is generally done on Day 6, then every day or every other day, depending on the individual. When the follicles grow big enough, you will stop taking follicle-stimulating medication and get an injection of hCG (human chorionic gonadotropin), which will cause your eggs to ovulate.

Since you will produce several eggs with fertility medications, the risk of having multiple births becomes higher than average, about 38 percent compared with 2.7 percent for the general population not using ART treatments.[7] There is no direct evidence that fertility medications cause birth defects. On the other hand, a multiple-birth pregnancy is associated with more problems than a singleton pregnancy. These problems include higher cesarean-section rates among mothers, premature births, low birth weights, and developmental disabilities among infants born prematurely.

hMG therapy can be used in conjunction with intercourse, artificial insemination to the cervix (intracervical insemination), or artificial insemination directly into the uterus (intrauterine insemination, or IUI). Some doctors use a combined dose of hMG and clomiphene with or without insemination.

Physical side effects of hMG medications may include breast tenderness, swelling or rash at the injection site, abdominal pain and bloating, and enlarged ovaries. Emotional side effects may include mood swings and depression. However, some women, rather than feeling depressed, experience a sense of elation, known as a "Pergonal high." Interestingly, our inquiry about Pergonal side effects in the RESOLVE Inc. newsletter solicited only one letter and one phone call describing emotional problems. This was in marked contrast to a large number of complaints about clomiphene.

One side effect from hMG, albeit a rare one thanks to the advent of sophisticated monitoring, is hyperstimulation syndrome, a condition in which the ovaries grow abnormally large. The typical treatment for hyperstimulation is bed rest, pain medication, and observation by your doctor. In rare extreme cases the condition may require hospitalization, during which a catheter may be placed in the abdomen to drain excess fluids that build up. Even more rarely, hyperstimulation may cause the ovaries to become "twisted," a condition that requires surgery. Contrary to popular belief, Pergonal does not make ovaries "explode."

Perhaps the most painful aspect of a fertility medication is its damage to your pocketbook. Depending on where you live, the drug can be expensive. In the summer of 1999 the cost of these medications was: Pergonal: $55 per ampule; Fertinex: $51 per ampule; Gonal-F: $58 per ampule; Humegon: $33 per ampule; Follistim: $57 per ampule; and Repronex: $33 per ampule. If your insurance does not cover pharmaceuticals, you may find yourself canceling a vacation or forgoing that new stereo in order to pursue your pregnancy quest. Syringes, by the way, should not cost more than $2 apiece and some pharmacies include them free of charge when you purchase fertility medications.

Lupron

Lupron (leuprolide acetate) is a medication that has several uses in the treatment of infertility. Lupron is available in two different forms, each used to treat a different problem. One, Lupron Depot, is administered once per month primarily for the treatment of endometriosis. Lupron Depot is administered intramuscularly. The second form is a daily dose taken for approximately twenty-one days when used in conjunction with ovulation induction. This form of Lupron is injected subcutaneously. Usually, Lupron is not used in "low-tech" treatments such as insemination in conjunction with injectable medications. It is, however, a mainstay of the drug regimen used in in vitro fertilization.

Lupron blocks the release of gonadotropins (hormones capable of stimulating the testicles or ovaries to produce a sperm or an egg) from the pituitary gland. It helps reduce the secretion of FSH and LH by your pituitary gland. Instead of getting your FSH and LH from your own body, you get these hormones from the FSH/LH medications you inject. Before Lupron was used as part of the "high-tech" regimen, some women would have an unwanted LH surge and possibly ovulate prematurely. But by including Lupron in the protocol, the doctor determines when the eggs are ripe enough to ovulate. Then he instructs you to stop taking Lupron and inject hCG to trigger ovulation. Thirty-four to thirty-six hours later, he retrieves your eggs in an in vitro fertilization procedure.

Lupron is also used to treat endometriosis. Endometriosis is a condition where the tissue lining the uterus grows outside the uterus. When Lupron is administered, ovarian follicles stop growing, a woman stops having her period (temporarily), and, as a result, she stops making estrogen. This decrease in estrogen is the goal of Lupron treatment for endometriosis. Sometimes Lupron is used without surgery. When used without surgery, treatment may last up to six months. About six to eight weeks after the Lupron is discontinued in the treatment of endometriosis, periods resume. Average cost of Lupron: $245 for a 2.8-milliliter vial, which can last for approximately one month, depending on the specific daily dose.

The side effects of Lupron mimic those of menopause. They included hot flashes, night sweats, headaches, vaginal dryness, and reduced sexual drive. During longer-term therapy (six months for endometriosis), the drugs deplete calcium in a woman's bones and reduce bone density. Bone density returns when treatment is completed.

Why Should I Take One Medication and Not Another?

Since publication of our first edition, drugs that are subcutaneously injected have been developed and seem to have come into favor. Many women (IUI, IVF, and egg donors) find it difficult to give themselves an injection in the hip. They find it easier to administer subcutaneous injections to themselves. Doctors, too, often prefer to have their patients use subcutaneous injections because the medication itself is of a more purified nature than the medications that are injected intramuscularly. Also, theoretically, women with polycystic ovary syndrome are more suitably treated with one of the newer FSH only drugs, although evidence supporting this claim is not currently available. There is still a place, however, for the original intramuscularly injected medications consisting of both FSH and LH. For example, some individuals respond better to these drugs than to pure FSH drugs. Also, a small amount of LH may be desirable for individuals who do not already have high LH levels. Sometimes patients are started on FSH and then the medication protocol is changed to an LH/FSH combination to improve the later stages of follicle development. Also, women who are overweight may respond better to the original FSH/LH combination medications. The chart that follows should help you make your way through the menu of fertility medications available to you. We expect that in the near future additional medications, including a recombinant LH medication, will be added to this list.

Buyer Beware:
Buying Drugs on the Internet

Before you buy infertility medications on the Internet, make sure that you are dealing with a reputable pharmacy. We also suggest that you not buy medications from a person who advertises on the Internet unless you know that person or have a mutual acquaintance. Internet discussion forums try to remove postings in which people offer to sell drugs. Yet during your participation in a discussion group, one of your "chat" buddies may offer to sell you her excess drugs. Because the price seems so much less than in your local drugstore, you may be tempted to buy. Don't do it. You have no idea what you are buying. One reproductive endocrinologist told us that he had a patient who sent a cashier's check to someone selling medications on the Internet. She received only vials of water. She had no more money to purchase medications and her cycle had to be canceled. Please don't let this happen to you. *Caveat emptor!* (Buyer beware!)

Synarel

Like Lupron, Synarel (nafarelin acetate) is used to combat endometriosis. Instead of being injected into the body, however, Synarel is a nasal spray. Some practices use Synarel instead of Lupron for IVF. Potential side effects of Lupron and Synarel are some symptoms of menopausal women, including hot flashes, vaginal dryness, headaches, insomnia, diminished sex drive, depression, and breast tenderness.

Zoladex

Like Lupron and Synarel, Zoladex (goserelin acetate) is sometimes used for the treatment of endometriosis. It works by suppressing estrogen and reducing estrogen to a postmenopausal level. Its side effects are similar to those reported for Synarel.

Many women with endometriosis who have taken medications such as Lupron, Synarel, or Zoladex report that the side effects of these medications are almost as painful as the discomfort they experience from endometriosis. Furthermore, the medications are approved only for a six-month course, and the recurrence of endometriosis after taking

GUIDE TO INJECTABLE MEDICATIONS

Brand Name	Generic Name	Manufacturer	Type	Uses	Composition	How Injected?	Side Effects	Same As
Pergonal	Human Menopausal Gonadotropin (hMG)	Serono	Natural—obtained from purified urine of postmenopausal women	Stimulate development of follicles	FSH & LH	Intramuscular	Abdominal pain, bloating, nausea, irritation at the site of injection	Humegon, Repronex
Repronex		Ferring			FSH & LH	Intramuscular		Pergonal, Humegon
Humegon		Organon			FSH & LH	Intramuscular		Pergonal, Repronex
Fertinex	Urofollitropin	Serono	Natural—made from urine of post-menopausal women	Ovulation induction in women who have a high blood level of LH (such as women with PCOS)	FSH (highly purified FSH)	Subcutaneous	Abdominal pain, bloating, nausea, irritation at the site of injection	Metrodin HP
Follistim	follitropin beta	Organon	Synthetic—produced through recombinant DNA technology	Ovulation induction in women who have a high blood level of LH (such as women with PCOS)	FSH	Subcutaneous	Abdominal pain, bloating, nausea, irritation at the site of injection	Gonal-F
Gonal-F	follitropin alpha	Serono			FSH	Subcutaneous		Follistim
Pregnyl	Chorionic gonadotropin	Organon	Urinary Hormone	Trigger ovulation in women; treatment for decreased level of testosterone in men	Hormone produced by the human placenta; made from purified urine of pregnant women	Intramuscular	No severe side effects	A.P.L., Profasi
A.P.L.	Chorionic gonadotropin	Wyeth-Ayerst	Urinary Hormone			Intramuscular		Pregnyl, Profasi
Profasi	Chorionic gonadotropin	Serono	Urinary Hormone			Intramuscular		Pregnyl, A.P.L.
Lupron	Leuprolide	TAP	Gonadotropin releas-ing hormone (GnRH) agonist	Prevent the pituitary gland from releasing an LH surge at an inopportune time	Synthetic analogue of naturally occurring GnRH	Subcutaneous	Mimics the effects of menopause, including hot flashes, headache, night sweats, and reduced sex drive	

these medications is high. Additionally, these medications have not proven to be effective for treating infertility associated with minimal levels of endometriosis.

Cetrorelix and Antagon

Lupron, Synarel, and Zoladex belong to a group of drugs known as GnRH agonists. By injecting these medications daily during the time you are also taking ovulation-induction medications, you can prevent a premature LH surge that can decrease the quality of your eggs or release your eggs too soon, resulting in the cancellation of your cycle. But GnRH agonists are expensive and have to be injected daily. Currently researchers are experimenting with another class of medications called GnRH antagonists that can also prevent a premature LH surge. One such drug that received FDA approval in 2000 is Antagon (made by Organon). A second medication, still in the experimental stage, is called Cetrorelix (made by ASTA Medica). These medications need to be injected less often than Lupron. They need to be injected only during the time period when an LH surge is likely to occur. As we write, doctors are currently experimenting with two different protocols with Cetrorelix. In the German protocol, the medication is injected starting on Day 7, when a premature surge becomes possible, and is continued daily until the eggs are ready to be ovulated.[8] In the French protocol, 3 mg. of Cetrorelix is injected on Day 9. If the patient is not ready to ovulate by ninety-six hours after this injection (Day 13), she takes 0.25 milligram injections until she is ready to ovulate. Both the German and the French protocols seem to prevent premature ovulation adequately. Cetrorelix and Antagon seem to offer the promise of several advantages over Lupron: Fewer injections are required so that you spend less money on medication. Another benefit reported by researchers is that patients do not experience the sorts of menopausal side effects they have with Lupron.

Danazol

Danazol (danocrine) is a synthetic derivative of the hormone testosterone. Since endometriosis is the result of excess estrogen, Danazol is designed to reduce estrogen levels. The standard dose of Danazol is two 200-milligram tablets twice a day, or a total of 800 milligrams a day. The treatment is continued for six months. While Danazol does not *cure* endometriosis, it prevents its growth temporarily. Once a patient stops taking the medication, the endometriosis can return. While doctors advise against trying to get pregnant while on Danazol, there is a six-to-twelve month window of opportunity to conceive after stopping the drug and before endometriosis potentially builds up to where it was before treatment.

Unfortunately, Danazol has a number of undesirable side effects. A deepening of the voice, a decrease in breast size, weight gain, hair growth in various parts of the body, and acne occur in some patients, particularly when high doses are used. Lower doses reduce the side effects but also reduce the drug's ability to fight moderate or severe cases of endometriosis. Since the FDA approved Lupron and Synarel in the early 1990s, Danazol is not prescribed as often, primarily because of its side effects.

hCG/Profasi/Pregnyl

Human chorionic gonadotropin (hCG) is a clear liquid that is injected into the buttocks to trigger the release of the eggs after blood tests or ultrasound scans indicate that the eggs are mature. hCG is frequently given during ovulation-induction cycles, as well as during clomiphene cycles. In addition, hCG also is used to improve the quality of a man's sperm. Marketed as Profasi or Pregnyl, hCG is obtained from the urine of pregnant women, refined, and purified. (At press time, pharmaceutical firms report that they are working on the development of a recombinant form of hCG.) The medication costs about $32 per ampule for 10,000 IU (international units). Physical side effects of hCG may include abdominal distention, abdominal pain, and headache. Emotional side effects may include irritability, restlessness, depression, and fatigue.

Parlodel

Parlodel (bromocriptine mesylate) is prescribed for women whose pituitary gland produces too much prolactin (called hyperprolactinemia), which can cause a milky discharge from the breasts (called galactorrhea), menstrual irregularity, lack of ovulation, and infertility. Parlodel can also be used in the treatment of polycystic ovary disease, but it cannot be recommended *solely* for this purpose. It is taken in tablet form one to three times daily until blood tests indicate that prolactin levels are normal.

There is a fairly high incidence of mild adverse reactions to Parlodel, including nausea, vomiting, headaches, dizziness, fatigue, lightheadedness, abdominal cramps, nasal congestion, and drowsiness. These adverse effects usually disappear after one to two weeks of use. Some women are able to avoid the nausea and cramps by taking bromocriptine via vaginal suppositories. Parlodel's cost: $1.50 to $2.50 per dose.

Dostinex

Dostinex (manufactured by Pharmacia & Upjohn) is another medication used to treat hyperprolactinemia (too much prolactin). In contrast to the multiple daily doses required by Parlodel, Dostinex requires only two doses per week. A study cited by Pharmacia & Upjohn claims that it is more successful than Parlodel in reducing excessive milky discharge. The most common side effect of Dostinex is nausea.

Progesterone

Progesterone prepares the lining of the uterus for implantation by an embryo. Progesterone is used to treat patients having a luteal phase inadequacy. The value of such treatment as luteal phase support is somewhat controversial, because some studies have shown a benefit and others have not. Progesterone is also given to women after they are artificially inseminated to help support a possible pregnancy. Under normal circumstances, progesterone is produced by the ovary in slight amounts just before ovulation and in increasingly greater amounts by the corpus luteum during the luteal phase. Progesterone also is produced in large quantities by the placenta during pregnancy.

When patients undergo IVF, the follicle aspiration procedure may reduce the body's capability to produce its own progesterone during a pregnancy resulting from that cycle. When the woman fails to produce enough progesterone, the hormone can be taken in injections, vaginal suppositories, pills, or a vaginal gel.

In the past, intramuscular (IM) injection was the preferred method of administration by most physicians. Unfortunately, IM injections, lasting for up to twelve weeks of gestation, can be painful and difficult to administer. Both the pain and the difficulty in administration are attributable to the oil in which the progesterone is dissolved. Another form of progesterone administration is a vaginal suppository. On the positive side, there is no pain associated with suppositories. On the other hand, they can be messy, irritating to the vaginal tissue, and provide inconsistent absorption. Progesterone pills are easy to take but can cause gastric and bowel discomfort. They also do not provide consistent absorption.

The newest and most widely used form of progesterone administration involves the use of a vaginal gel. The gel is known as Crinone and is applied in a manner similar to inserting a tampon. Several well-designed studies have found that Crinone is as effective as IM injections of progesterone. Cost of Crinone is $175 for eighteen applications (3 grams each). The side effects for all forms of progesterone may include mild acne, oily skin, oily hair, and increased hair growth.

It is important to realize that the progesterone supplement you are taking is *natural* progesterone, which does not cause birth defects. There also are *synthetic* forms of progesterone known as progestins, which can harm a fetus and therefore should be avoided when you are trying to get pregnant.

Immune Globulin (IVIg)

IVIg is used primarily in the treatment of congenital immunodeficiencies. IVIg is not a medication used in low-tech procedures. We include it here because it is one of the drugs sometimes used for infertility treatment. In reproductive medicine, IVIg is used *experimentally* to prevent recurrent pregnancy loss and repeated IVF failure.

IVIg consists of antibodies purified from pooled serum provided by blood donors. Since IVIg is derived from donor blood, contracting blood-borne diseases from treatment is a remote possibility. IVIg treatment is administered intravenously in a number of different protocols. Many of these protocols are very expensive and time consuming, but physicians who believe in this approach encourage their patients to undergo IVIg treatment. A few studies performed to date have had conflicting results in terms of IVIg's effectiveness. To date, physicians have reached no consensus on its value for IVF. The American Society for Reproductive Medicine (ASRM) has cautioned that IVIg be used *only* in research settings.

Side effects include injection-site reactions, malaise, fever, chills, headache, nausea, vomiting, chest tightness, difficulty in breathing, and pain.

Antibiotics

Antibiotics are used to treat bacterial infections and to prevent the possibility of infections that can impair fertilization or embryo implantation. A frequently prescribed medication for treating or preventing such infections is the antibiotic doxycycline. A typical regimen is two 100-milligram tablets daily for fourteen days. Side effects may include upset stomach and sensitivity to the sun. Antibiotics are sometimes prescribed as a preventative measure for both members of the couple in conjunction with a high-tech treatment such as IVF.

Aspirin

Aspirin is used to treat pain and inflammation as well as to reduce the risk of heart attack and stroke. In assisted reproduction, aspirin is used alone or in combination with other medications to reduce the risk of recurrent spontaneous pregnancy loss associated with high levels of autoimmune antibodies. Most frequently, low-dose aspirin is given in conjunction with heparin, a powerful anticoagulant.

Recent research on the effects of aspirin on the reproductive system examines whether or not the anticoagulative properties of aspirin will lead to an increased supply of blood to the ovaries and to the uterus. If there is an increased blood supply to these areas the ovaries could be more productive and the uterine lining could become thicker and more well developed. Consequently, low-dose aspirin could be beneficial in some way to all infertility patients.

At IVF New Jersey, where we consult, all patients who are egg recipients are asked to take one tablet of baby aspirin daily when their donor begins taking fertility medication. We urge you to ask your physician whether taking aspirin is right for you.

Fertility Medications and the Risk of Ovarian Cancer

In 1992 Alice Whittemore of Stanford University and her colleagues in the Collaborative Ovarian Cancer Group created a great stir and considerable consternation for infertile women when they suggested that fertility drug use may cause increased rates of ovarian cancer. The Whittemore study was widely reported by the popular media. Reporters wondered whether the study's results predicted a looming cancer epidemic. Not surprisingly, pharmaceutical companies and academic scientists quickly responded with criticism of the study's design and execution. They suggested that Whittemore's conclusions were premature and they published studies that concluded that there was no real risk.

Since the publication of the 1992 study, numerous other studies on this topic have been published. Although physicians feel comfortable that they are not putting women at risk when they tell their patients to use fertility medications, we still do not really know whether the medications may have an adverse effect.

Let's examine the Whittemore study more closely to understand how it was done and why others believe that there were flaws in its design and conclusions.

The Whittemore study examined the fate of more than 1,700 women who, in their past, recalled using some type of fertility medication. It included 622 women who developed ovarian cancer and 1,101 who did not. The authors concluded that women who had used fertility drugs had nearly three times the lifetime risk of ovarian cancer compared with women with no history of infertility. They also characterized the cancer risk by whether or not a woman who used fertility drugs became pregnant. Note carefully what they found: If a woman became pregnant after using fertility drugs, she had no increased risk of ovarian cancer. On the other hand, if she did not become pregnant, her risk was approximately twenty-seven times higher than that of a woman who became pregnant.

How did the authors reach these conclusions? First, you must realize that the conclusions are based on a very small number of cases. The overall study was large, but the twenty-seven-fold higher risk figure is based on only twelve women who used fertility drugs, did not become pregnant, and developed ovarian cancer. You should also be aware that the study relied on the recall of the women studied. Ovarian cancer is a disease that typically occurs late in life. In fact, the median birth date of women in the study was 1924. So imagine that you are an elderly woman and you are asked to recall whether perhaps twenty years ago you used a fertility medication. Remember that the era when these women may have used a fertility medication preceded the time when injectable medications were available. If the recall of some of the elderly women was flawed, the results would be unreliable. If even just a few of the women who did not get cancer forgot that they used fertility medications, the conclusions would be invalid. But even if their recall was accurate, we do not know what medication they considered a fertility medication. Moreover, whatever medication they may have taken certainly could not have included drugs such as Pergonal or Humegon or Gonal-F or Lupron or any of the medications you may be taking. Clomid wasn't marketed in the United States until 1961, Pergonal until 1970, and the others much later. The only possible medication the study may have included that is still used today is Clomid, and those born in 1924 or earlier would have been in their late thirties when they first got a chance to try it.

The study certainly doesn't prove a link between fertility-drug use and ovarian cancer. Sadly, the fear it caused may have been unnecessary. Four other studies—one in China, one in Italy, one in Israel, and one in Denmark—failed to find any connection between fertility drugs and ovarian cancer, although each of them was too small to rule out the threefold increase in risk cited by Whittemore. On the whole, the medical community discounted the risk and recommended no changes in ovarian stimulation as part of assisted reproduction.

We mention the Whittemore study because many of our clients have told us they are concerned about the risk of getting ovarian cancer after taking fertility medications. The decision about whether to use these medications in light of the possible risks is an important one. We believe that the possible gains far outweigh the risks. We ourselves were willing to take this risk. Helane subjected herself to numerous cycles of Pergonal injections. Like us, our donor was also given the information about possible cancer risks and she too was willing to take that chance. Thanks to this risk taking, we are now able to enjoy the incomparable experience of parenting our twins, Nathaniel and Allegra.

INSEMINATION AS A TREATMENT FOR INFERTILITY

Artificial insemination is a procedure that separates reproduction from sexual intercourse. The procedure involves placing the husband's sperm into the wife's vagina, cervix, or uterus, so that she can become pregnant. Initially, many couples view insemination as "unnatural." But after they have time to think about the procedure, they usually welcome it as a means to assist them in their pregnancy quest. Some even welcome insemination as a break from "sex on demand." Doctors are often pleased to use insemination as a way to help couples feel that they are "doing something" to remedy their problem.

Intracervical Insemination

Intracervical insemination is the least invasive form of artificial insemination. Although this procedure was once widely used, nowadays it is used almost exclusively for insemination with donor sperm. The goal is to get the sperm, which may be poor swimmers, as close as possible to the cervical mucus so that they avoid the treacherous journey through the vagina. The cervical mucus acts as a reservoir for the sperm, releasing a few at a time during the next twenty-four to forty-eight hours. In this way, the chances are very good that some sperm will arrive in the fallopian tubes at the time when the ovulated egg gets there.

Since you may be artificially inseminated with sperm from your husband or from a donor, doctors draw a distinction between the two for clarity. This chapter addresses only artificial insemination by husband (AIH). AIH is performed in the doctor's office, usually the day after you first detect an LH surge. Your husband provides a semen sample (after having abstained from any form of ejaculation for two to five days to increase his sperm count). Some clinics, however, ask you to have intercourse the night before the procedure. The doctor draws the semen up into a syringe. You will lie on the examining table with your feet in stirrups. The doctor first inserts a speculum and then puts the syringe into the opening of your cervix and squeezes out the semen. The whole procedure takes less than a minute. In some cases, the doctor then inserts a cap, similar to a diaphragm, over your cervix to help keep the sperm pooled in the area. You remove the cap using your fingers about twelve hours later. Cost of the insemination runs about $150.

Success rates for intracervical insemination vary depending on the nature of your fertility problem, what, if any, fertility drugs you are taking, and how many inseminations you have attempted. The pregnancy rate is higher (26 percent to 56 percent) when the problem is a low sperm count compared to a cervical problem, when the pregnancy rate is only 17.5 percent.[9] If after six trials of AIH you are not pregnant, it's probably time to try another technique or conduct more diagnostic tests.

Intrauterine Insemination

Intrauterine insemination (IUI) consists of introducing sperm that have been separated from semen in a procedure called "washing" through the cervix and directly into the uterus. (Unwashed semen can cause uterine cramping.) IUI is recommended to counter a variety of male factor problems, such as low sperm count or high semen viscosity (clumpiness). IUI is also recommended in cases where the woman's cervical mucus is hostile to sperm, is not plentiful enough, or is too dense. People with unexplained infertility also may benefit from IUI. The goal of IUI is to introduce the sperm directly into the uterus and bypass the cervix, thus enabling more sperm to travel a shorter distance to the fallopian tubes and the waiting egg.

IUI may be done with or without clomiphene or hMG therapy. The advantage of combining IUI with fertility drugs is that you are increasing the number of targets for the sperm to reach. Superovulation, and the monitoring and hCG injection that go along with it, also help the doctor to time the IUI more precisely to coincide with when your eggs are most likely to ovulate.

IUI is similar to intracervical insemination in that the husband produces a semen sample into a sterile cup. It differs, however, in that a nurse or technician "washes" the sample to remove prostaglandins (hormone-like substances) that would otherwise cause cramping in the uterus. The washing procedure involves using a solution called Percoll in a filtering process to rid the sample of non-motile sperm and malformed sperm. Then the technician places the sperm in a tube containing culture media. This tube is then placed into a centrifuge, which spins the sperm so that they are separated from the semen. The sperm sink to the bottom of the tube and the other material is removed. The "dirty" culture media (fluid) is then replaced with fresh culture media.

At this time, the strongest swimming sperm swim up into the media. This procedure is referred to as "swim up," which allows the doctor to use the best sperm for the insemination. It takes one to two hours to prepare a sperm sample in this manner. If your husband's sperm have poor motility, it might take a bit longer to give slower-swimming sperm more time to reach the top.

Be aware that the "swim up" procedure is not appropriate in some situations. Your doctor will know what techniques take best advantage of your husband's sample. Many women worry that the sperm will die unless the insemination takes place immediately after the sample has been prepared. Be assured that this is not the case. Once the sample is ready, it is placed in an incubating device until the time of the insemination.

When the IUI is about to begin, you will lie on an examining table. The doctor will insert a speculum into your vagina and introduce the washed sperm directly into your uterus with his choice of several possible types of catheters. Catheters vary in their rigidity, and doctors differ in how high in the uterus and how close to the tube they introduce the sample. You may feel some cramping during the insemination, but it should pass in a few minutes. We encourage you to relax and/or use mental imagery (see "Circle of Friends" in Chapter 6) to get you into a relaxed and peaceful state of mind. After the insemination, you will probably be told to remain lying down for about ten minutes. There is no need for a cervical cap with IUI. IUI fees run about $250 each for sperm preparation and insemination.

The reported success rate of IUI varies depending upon the nature of the problem. Dr. Nancy Allen and her colleagues,[10] researchers at the Vanderbilt Medical Center, reviewed published studies about the use of artificial insemination for various problems. Success was reported as the percentage of couples who became pregnant after several attempts. When the major problem was male factor, the average success rate was 25 percent. When the problem stemmed from cervical factors, the average success rate was 60 percent, since IUI enables the sperm to bypass the cervix completely. And when the problem was immunological, success, on average, was 22 percent. More than a decade has elapsed since Dr. Allen's study. In reviewing the literature, we were unable to locate a more recent review as comprehensive as hers. One recent large-scale study of 811 cycles was conducted in Finland.[11] The authors of that study reviewed other reports and indicated that pregnancy rates typically tend to vary between 8 and 22 percent. The least successful study found reported a rate of 4 percent, and the most successful study reported 40 percent success. The large-scale Finnish study reported an overall pregnancy rate of 12.6 percent per cycle and a multiple pregnancy rate of 13.7 percent. Additionally, the authors found that 23.5 percent of the more than 800 cycles studied resulted in a miscarriage. The authors conclude that IUI is a useful treatment for women younger than forty years old who do not have endometriosis and have been trying to get pregnant for less than six years.

When you think about your own attempts to become pregnant, you probably do not think about your success rate after *many* cycles; rather, you focus on your chance of success for *that* cycle. For studies reporting success *per* cycle, the percentage is about 9 percent.

But we believe that the per-cycle success rate can be made considerably higher than 9 percent. What's needed to improve the success rate is careful timing. And while doctors all agree that timing is crucial, they disagree about how long after hCG the insemination should take place. It is our *personal* belief that inseminations are most likely to succeed when they are performed thirty-six to forty-two hours after hCG. This belief is bolstered by the results of a study done at Duke University. In the Duke protocol, IUIs were performed thirty-eight to forty hours after hCG. Doctors at Duke report a take-home baby rate of 14 percent *per cycle*.[12] And physicians at the University of Miami report that a single IUI timed at thirty-six to forty-eight hours after hCG administration was as effective as two separate IUIs administered at eighteen to twenty-four hours and thirty-six to forty-eight hours after hCG.[13]

SURGERY

In addition to drugs and insemination, surgery is also used to remedy certain infertility problems. Sometimes it is used by itself and sometimes it is combined with drugs to optimize success.

Endometriosis Surgery

Surgery can enhance fertility rates for patients experiencing endometriosis only when their endometriosis is moderate or severe. On the other hand, if you are experiencing significant pain because of endometriosis, you should consider surgery to relieve the pain. The operation's objective is to remove the migrated uterine lining, which can cause tremendous pain and impair fertility. Once done with scalpels, endometriosis surgery now employs lasers to vaporize the endometriosis and adhesions. Laser surgery has reduced the complications and pain associated with nonlaser surgery for endometriosis. Doctors charge up to $5,000 to perform laser surgery, and that excludes anesthesiologist's and hospital charges. The good news is that often insurance covers this surgery.

Surgery for Other Female Disorders

There are countless conditions for which surgery is indicated. New surgical techniques have created possibilities to repair problems that twenty years ago could not be remedied. Here are just a few of the many conditions that can be surgically corrected: Uterine polyps and fibroids, which can prevent embryo implantation, can be removed surgically. A uterine septum can be similarly removed or reconstructed. Tubal blockages can be repaired through microsurgery.

Surgery to Correct Male Infertility

A similar situation exists in terms of surgery for male infertility. One type of male fertility surgery is a *varicocelectomy*, which is used to correct a varicocele. A varicocele is a varicose vein in the scrotum, usually on the left side, which causes the temperature in the testis to be abnormally high. Optimally, sperm need a relatively cool environment, several points below core body temperature.

The varicocelectomy involves tying off the impaired vein and redirecting the blood flow. Doctors are divided in their opinion about whether this procedure is advisable. Just as many doctors strongly advocate performing a varicocelectomy, others have cautioned against having this operation performed. Many couples feel that despite this controversy they are willing to undergo the pain, cost, and discomfort involved just to have a chance at success. Doctors charge about $2,300 for a varicocelectomy on one side, $4,550 for both sides.

Another type of surgery involves clearing a blocked duct. Through microsurgery, surgeons may be able to clear blockages in the tiny ducts of the vas or epididymis. Because the success rate is relatively low, men with duct blockages often use other procedures to retrieve the sperm.

Another type of male fertility surgery is the vasectomy reversal. Dr. Sherman Silber, a prominent urologist, describes the reversal procedure in detail in his book *How to Get Pregnant with the New Technology.*[14] Briefly, the procedure consists of reconnecting the severed vas deferens so sperm can again be present in the ejaculate. Just as in the previously described procedures, this operation does not guarantee that fertility will be restored. Moreover, if the reversal is performed more than five years after the vasectomy was done, there is a good chance the man has developed antibodies against his own sperm, which can destroy his ability to impregnate his wife. Despite this condition, doctors can aspirate sperm from the testes and use these successfully to create an IVF pregnancy.

MEASURES OF INFERTILITY

Infertility treatment requires that you interpret a myriad of numbers. Mostly, these numbers represent various levels of hormones in your blood. Doctors monitor the progression of your treatment cycle so they know how well you are responding to the drugs. It's important for you to know what they are talking about and to record the information in your Cycle Log. By doing so, you Become a Partner in Your Treatment. Here is a rundown of what some of these numbers mean.

Estradiol Level

Estradiol is a measure of the estrogen produced by the developing follicle or follicles. This level rises daily throughout the cycle. In natural cycles when no fertility drugs are used, the estradiol level reflects the size of the follicle. But when drugs are used and multiple follicles develop, the estradiol level by itself is not a good predictor of the size of the follicles. Generally speaking, though, doctors want to see a level of 100 to 200 pg. of E2 for each mature follicle. So if you have eight mature follicles, expect levels between 800 and 1,600. Such levels indicate that at least some follicles have matured and that it is time for an hCG injection to cause the eggs to ovulate.

Day 3 FSH Level

The Day 3 FSH level is an indicator of ovarian reserve—that is, the number and quality of eggs available to be fertilized. Studies have shown that using one particular assay, the Leeco assay, a level greater than 25 milli-international units (mIU) predicts a very low likelihood of getting pregnant.[15] Ideally, patients respond best to infertility treatment when FSH levels are below 20 mIU on Day 3. Using the Becton Dickinson assay, this value would be between 8 and 12.

Progesterone Level

The progesterone level is another important indicator of ovulation and pregnancy. In a basal body temperature chart, the average temperature during the luteal phase of the cycle is between 0.3 and 1.0 degrees higher than in the follicular phase of the cycle. This higher temperature is the result of the increased secretion of progesterone following ovulation. It takes a level of about 0.4 nanograms per milliliter of blood (ng/ml) to produce this temperature rise. In a non-drug-stimulated cycle, the average progesterone level on the day of the LH peak is about 2 ng/ml.

If a woman does not get pregnant, the progesterone rises to its highest point, about 15, during the middle of the luteal phase and then drops down to around 0 when menstruation begins. On the other hand, if a pregnancy occurs, the corpus luteum continues to secrete progesterone for about ten weeks. The level during those weeks averages around 25. After that, the placenta creates increasing progesterone levels, which can get as high as 125 ng/ml.

Beta hCG

A beta hCG test is used to determine whether a woman is pregnant. The test is extremely sensitive and can detect pregnancy as early as eight to ten days after ovulation. Usually, however, the test is done at least two weeks after ovulation or an artificial insemination. HCG levels rise rapidly during the beginning of a pregnancy. Typically, during the early part of the pregnancy, the level doubles every two days, although the doubling time can range between 1.5 and 3.5 days. Two standards are used to measure hCG: the second international standard (2nd IS) and the international reference preparation (IRP).

Sometimes women who have taken Profasi to trigger ovulation have small amounts of this hCG in their system, which can remain in the system for up to ten days. It is important not to test for a pregnancy until after this residual hCG has left your system so that you don't get your hopes up that you are pregnant when in fact you simply have residual Profasi in your system.

Women usually attain serum concentrations of 10 to 50 mIU in the week following conception. INCIID has created a chart showing how much hCG is in your system over the forty weeks of your pregnancy. You can find it at http://www.inciid.org/betas.html.

Prolactin Level

A doctor is unlikely to be interested in your prolactin level unless you have a milky discharge from your breasts, your periods are irregular, or you have a luteal insufficiency. Normally, prolactin, a hormone, is produced by the pituitary gland in large quantities only to stimulate the production of breast milk if you are pregnant or breast-feeding. High levels of prolactin also inhibit ovulation. So if you are not pregnant and your prolactin level is elevated, it could be causing your fertility problem.

Follicle Size

With the advent of vaginal ultrasound devices, it is possible to visualize not only the uterus and ovaries, but also the egg follicles that develop in the ovaries. The follicles appear as round, dark circles on the video screen.

Ideally, follicles should grow about 1 to 2 millimeters a day. The optimal size for mature follicles is between 18 and 23 millimeters in non-drug-stimulated cycles. When a patient is taking fertility drugs, she usually produces multiple follicles, which may differ in their rate of growth. But even a follicle under 18 millimeters can release a mature egg. According to Dr. Colin McArdle, a radiologist at Harvard Medical School, "mature ova [eggs] may be obtained from follicles between 12 and 34 mm."[16]

Doctors use the size of the largest follicle as their guide for follicle maturity. When the largest follicle reaches 16 millimeters, it is usually time for an hCG injection to prompt the follicles to release the eggs. Even after the hCG injection, follicles can continue to grow another 2 to 4 millimeters before releasing the egg. So a patient whose ultrasound revealed a largest follicle of 16 millimeters and then had an hCG injection may still release an egg from a 20 to 22 millimeter follicle.

GUIDE TO GIVING INTRAMUSCULAR INJECTIONS

Starting a program of treatment can be exciting as well as a bit scary. Most partners have never given injections before. Wives are often reluctant to be injected by their husband. That's understandable.

Despite these fears, we've found that most couples get through the injection phase just fine. After a few injections, in fact, the procedure becomes almost second nature, many of our clients report. One of the things that's helped them is getting clear instructions. Most infertility clinics offer injection-orientation classes led by a nurse. Couples about to begin Pergonal or other injection therapy watch a demonstration and receive a slew of information, usually quite rapidly. Participants may be reluctant to ask questions in front of a group. They fail to realize that a large portion of the audience probably has the same questions.

We have prepared step-by-step instructions designed to supplement any orientation class or one-on-one lesson you might participate in. If, after reading our instructions, you still have questions, call your doctor's office.

Throughout your infertility treatments, you will find yourself doing many things you never imagined doing. Giving or getting injections is but one.

MATERIALS NEEDED:

Alcohol   Box of alcohol pads

22-gauge syringes; 1½-inch for administering hMG, hCG, and progesterone injections

14- to 16-gauge syringes; for drawing progesterone more easily than with the 22-gauge syringe

hMG   a supply of ampules

Water   a supply of water solution ampules

hCG   one vial of water and one vial of hCG

Note: Insist that you are given a form of hCG that comes in two separate bottles. Do not attempt to work with the form of hCG that comes in an attached double-bottle unit.

Progesterone   a supply of vials

Note: Progesterone comes in two different oil bases: peanut oil or sesame oil. The typical base is peanut oil. If you experience discomfort when using the regular progesterone, ask your physician whether you should try the sesame oil variety.

hMG injection procedure:

1. Place the alcohol pad over the protrusion on the ampule. This will protect you if the glass splinters. Holding on to the pad, break the protrusion on the water ampule. Then repeat this procedure to break the protrusions on three Pergonal ampules.

2. Peel off the plastic wrapper from the 22-gauge syringe.

3. Holding the plastic cap that's over the needle, twist to make sure the needle is secured in the cylinder. Remove cap.

4. Pull out the plunger of the syringe and push it back in to make sure that it is drawing.

5. Carefully insert the needle into the water ampule. If the needle touches the outside glass of the ampule or any other object, it may become contaminated. Discard the needle and use another one!

6. Pull up the plunger of the syringe to draw entire contents out of the water ampule.

7. Insert the needle into the first hMG ampule. Inject one-third (or one-half if you're using two hMG ampules or the whole thing if you're using one). Repeat this procedure with the second and third ampules. This mixes the hMG with the water, creating a clear, sometimes foamy solution.

8. Insert the needle into the first hMG ampule. Hold the ampule horizontally. Tilt the syringe so that it is at a thirty-degree angle to the ampule. Place your thumb on the "wing-like" structure on the syringe and press the syringe against the ampule. With your index and middle fingers, pull up on the plunger to extract the contents of the ampule. Repeat this procedure with the second and third ampules.

9. Tap the cylinder of the syringe to get rid of any air bubbles.

10. Holding the syringe with the needle up, gently push on the plunger until a tiny bead of liquid appears on the tip of the needle.

11. Locate a spot on the buttocks for the injection. To find the location, spread your thumb and index finger against the hip bone. Locate a spot about six inches below this location. Use this spot for injections. You will be rotating spots each day. Find the comparable spot on the other cheek for the next day's injection. On the third day, you will return to the first cheek, but locate a spot slightly away from the site of the first day's injection, and so on.

12. Insert the needle all the way in, perpendicular to the plane of the buttock (not at an angle).

13. Hold the syringe with one hand and draw the plunger out slightly to see if any blood appears on the needle. If blood appears, it means you've hit a blood vessel and need to try again. If no blood appears, proceed.

14. Inject by pushing in the plunger fairly quickly. Pull out the needle fast.

15. Place an alcohol pad on the site for a few minutes.

HCG injection procedure:

1. Make sure you are working with two separate vials. Wipe the top of the liquid vial with an alcohol pad. Discard pad. Wipe the top of the powder vial with a different pad and discard the pad.

2. Hold the water vial upside down and insert the needle into the water vial. Pull back the plunger to extract 2 cc's of water.

3. Insert the needle into the hCG powder vial. Push in the plunger to inject water to mix with powder.

4. Hold the powder-vial mixture upside down. Make sure that the needle is below the level of liquid at all times to avoid getting air bubbles into the syringe's cylinder. Slowly pull back the plunger a little at a time to extract the entire contents of hCG mixture.

5. Follow the same procedure as above, beginning with No. 10.

CHAPTER 6

Using the Getting Pregnant Workout to Help You Through Treatment

ow that we've introduced you to the many treatment options to combat infertility, it's time to confront the emotional issues that are bound to crop up during treatment, if they haven't already. To help you through this phase, we have created a fictionalized couple, Amanda and Al Gambone, who are a composite sketch of dozens of couples we have met and counseled over the years. The Gambones' concerns are typical of infertile couples': finding a competent infertility specialist, educating and motivating themselves to begin injecting fertility medications, reducing sexual performance anxiety, remaining optimistic in the face of failure, and putting themselves first without feeling selfish.

DECISION-MAKING:
SELECTING A DOCTOR

For six months, Amanda and Al, both in their early thirties, have been following the advice of Amanda's gynecologist but have not yet conceived. They have kept careful temperature charts, used Clomid, monitored Amanda's LH surge, and made love every other day, just as the doctor instructed. Since their doctor can find no reason for their fertility problem, the Gambones are faced with a tough decision: Should they change doctors and, if so, to whom should they turn?

Like so many women, Amanda was initially reluctant to start from scratch with a new physician. She hated the idea of having to search one out, get used to him or her, repeat her medical history, and start treatment in unfamiliar surroundings.

But what began as a pleasurable part of their marriage has turned into a nightmare of scheduled, sometimes unemotional, intercourse for three weeks followed by devastation each time Amanda's period started. Their whole world seemed on the brink of collapse. Amanda and Al knew that her gynecologist, who does not specialize in infertility, had done all that he could do even though he would not admit it. Once they came to terms with that realization, the Gambones' next step seemed crystal clear: Find a doctor who could provide specialized fertility treatments.

They wanted a specialist who was not only knowledgeable about infertility and experienced in treating it, but one who was also compassionate and exhibited confidence in his ability to diagnose and treat their particular problem.

Training of the Infertility Doctor

Unfortunately, any doctor can hang out a shingle that says INFERTILITY SPECIALIST, and some with little or no infertility training do advertise themselves this way. The American Society for Reproductive Medicine (ASRM), the professional association devoted to the promotion of knowledge in fertility and allied fields, says that a variety of medical specialists—OB-GYNs and reproductive endocrinologists, among others—practice as infertility specialists. But medical schools don't train doctors to be "infertility specialists." These specialists are usually trained first as gynecologists or endocrinologists if they wish to specialize in female infertility. Doctors interested in male infertility first become urologists, andrologists, or endocrinologists. Once completing their primary training, doctors obtain additional training, usually in the form of a fellowship or a second residency, in the field of reproductive endocrinology, for example.

Also, many doctors who have been practicing their primary specialty—say, gynecology—for several years might take intensive infertility seminars, such as those sponsored by the ASRM. Not all "infertility specialists" do this, however.[1] Even though Amanda's gynecologist advertises himself in the Yellow Pages, in newspaper ads, and on his shingle as an infertility specialist, he keeps patients under his care long after their needs outdistance his experience and training.

The message here is: Buyer beware. Don't let a doctor learn infertility treatment by practicing on you. He or she may be experienced with just a few treatments, like prescribing Clomid, and that's it. As Amanda is about to do, you should consider leaving your current doctor and looking for a specialist. At the very least, this new doctor should be a member in good standing of the American Society for Reproductive Medicine. To help you search, we refer you to the Doctor Interview Guide that appears later in this chapter.

What You're Looking For: Collecting Information

Like most women, Amanda has an image of the perfect infertility specialist. He should have excellent training, be available 24 hours a day and 365 days a year, stay current on all new treatments, possess the sensitivity of Marcus Welby, have an office down the street, and accept whatever insurance pays him or charge next to nothing. The chance of finding a doctor with all of these traits is nil, but, just like Amanda, you need to try to find a doctor who meets as many of your criteria as possible.

After deciding on some basic requirements, Amanda begins compiling a list of available specialists. Being the meticulous and contemporary woman she is and leaving no stone unturned, Amanda scoured all available sources, from the most "low-tech" (the Yellow Pages) to the wealth of available information on the Internet. Her research included information from her local chapter of RESOLVE Inc. (or other infertility education and advocacy organization), recommendations from friends and co-workers who have used fertility specialists, the list of clinics listed in the INCIID (Internet-based International Council on Infertility Information Dissemination) Mini Fertility Site Directory (http://www.inciid.org/docs.html), the Fertile Thoughts Physician Listing Directory (http://www.fertilethoughts.net/infertility/), and the latest membership directory of the American Society for Reproductive Medicine (ASRM),[2] which is available in print or on the Web at http://www.asrm.org. At the Society of Reproductive Endocrinology (SREI) Web site (http://www.socrei.org/), Amanda located several physicians in her state.

Amanda decided to be a "new millennium woman" and try to interact with other infertile couples by using the Internet to help her find a doctor located near her home. She posted the following message on one of the popular Internet infertility discussion groups: "LOOKING FOR AN RE IN INDIANAPOLIS. CAN SOMEONE HELP? Hi: As we are new to this place and have decided to go ahead with injectable meds and possibly IUI, I would be grateful if someone can suggest a good doctor in Indianapolis ASAP." Not surprisingly, Amanda received four responses (one six hours later, one seven hours later, one the next day, and another the day after). The first response read: "My RE, Dr. A., is on the Northside of Indianapolis by St. Vincents. He is a very conservative doctor. The office is open M–F and also on weekends for treatment and ultrasounds only. The lab for blood work is right next door. The number is 317-xxx-xxxx. Best wishes. P.S. I am 15 weeks pregnant now." The other responses, describing different practices, were equally supportive and helpful. Despite her gratitude for their helpful responses, Amanda remembered that many of the opinions, although personal and powerful, might not have been informed opinions. Amanda weighed all her information in compiling her list.

From all of her sources of information, Amanda makes a shorter list of six doctors who are within a sixty-minute driving distance of her home. Pen and pad at hand, she calls each doctor's office and, after these brief phone calls, narrows the field down to three. Amanda found that one of the six clinics she called put her on hold and never got back to her. A second clinic was all "machine"—no interaction with a live human being. The third clinic she eliminated couldn't give her an appointment for six months. She decided that she would interview the three remaining doctors on her list using the interview guide in the next section. Amanda knew that by carefully shopping for the right doctor, she is sparing herself the grief of hopping aimlessly from doctor to doctor, hoping the next one will be better than the last.

Using the Interview Guide that follows, which includes the pronunciation for common infertility medical procedures, Amanda interviewed three doctors.

DOCTOR/CLINIC INTERVIEW GUIDE

Medical Training/Infertility Specialty:

1. How many physicians work with this practice? (Obtain this information for each physician in the practice.)
2. In what area was your primary training?
3. Are you an infertility specialist? Are you board certified or board eligible in reproductive endocrinology?
4. What is your training in infertility?
5. Did you do a residency or a fellowship in reproductive endocrinology?
    a. Where did you acquire your specialty?
    b. If yes, where did you do it?

Experience:

1. Have you ever done any of the following procedures:
    a. Diagnostic laparoscopies (la-pah-RAH-skoh-peez)
    b. Hysterosalpingograms (hih-stuh-roh-sal-PIHN-joh-gramz)
    c. Hysteroscopies (hih-stuh-RAH-skuh-peez)
    d. Intrauterine inseminations (ihn-trah-YEW-tuh-rihn ihn-seh-mih-NAY-shuhnz)
    e. Intracervical inseminations (ihn-trah-SUHR-vih-kuhl ihn-seh-mih-NAY-shuhnz)
    f. In vitro fertilization procedures (ihn VEE-troh)
    g. Egg-donation procedures

Logistics of Treatment:

1. What percent of your practice is devoted to infertility?
2. Will I see pregnant women in the waiting room?
3. Can I do most of my testing/treatment in the office or do I have to go elsewhere?
4. Do you do ultrasounds in your office?
5. What lab work is done in your office and what information do you have sent out?
    a. Estradiol
    b. Progesterone
    c. FSH
    d. Beta hCG (pregnancy tests)
    e. Semen analysis
6. Where do your patients get their medication?
7. Are there multiple doctors in the practice?
8. Can I select a primary-care doctor?
9. Do you arrange for doctor coverage when you are on vacation?
10. Which hospital are you affiliated with?

Hours:

1. What are your office hours?
2. Do you have early-morning, late-afternoon, Saturday, Sunday hours?

3. What are your callback hours? Do you have call-in hours? Do you call patients directly or establish a voice mailbox your patients call in to receive information?
4. Do you respond to electronic mail inquiries? How fast?
5. What kind of flexibility is there for scheduling specialized treatment?
6. I work from __ to __ and need to have my work done early/late, lunchtime. Can you accommodate me?
7. Do you see your patients promptly or should I expect to have a long wait?

Financial:

1. What are your fees for the following procedures:
   a. E2
   b. Ultrasound
   c. IUI
2. When does payment need to be made?
3. Do you arrange to bill the insurance company directly?

FACTORS TO TAKE INTO CONSIDERATION

Factors Al and I consider important:

Notes about each doctor:

1. Doctor's level of expertise

All three are competent doctors

2. Success statistics (how many people with problems like ours got pregnant)

Como has a "cult" reputation. Heard that Gold inflates his success statistics.

3. Cost of this doctor's services

All are very expensive.

4. Doctor's "bedside manner"

Como is a charmer. Murphy is sweet. Gold is cold.

5. Individualized treatment (e.g., will the doctor tailor treatment to my case or will he use a protocol similar to one used for all other patients?

Gold puts everyone through the same mill. Murphy will do anything you want. Como has some flexibility but not as much as Murphy.

Factors suggested by friends and acquaintances:

1. Is the practice limited to infertility?

Murphy has pregnant people in the waiting room. Como prohibits pregnant women or babies from coming to his office. Gold's practice is limited to infertility, but he allows kids in the office.

2. Does this doctor provide seven-day-a-week coverage?

Murphy and Gold do. Como doesn't but arranges for someone else to do inseminations when he's not available.

3. Is this doctor willing to work with us in terms of insurance coverage?

All seem wiling to work with patients.

4. Does this doctor have flexibility in the times when he schedules procedures?

Murphy only does inseminations in the morning. Other two seem more flexible.

5. Office appearance

Murphy keeps *Parenting* magazines and "duckies" in the waiting room. Has TV blaring all the time. Como's office looks like a classy French boudoir. Gold's office has that "industrial" look.

Factors suggested by articles and books I read and postings on the Internet:

1. What sorts of facilities does the office have for the husband to produce a semen sample?

Como has none; expects you to do it at home and bring it in. Gold has a special room with a VCR and "dirty magazines." Murphy has a bathroom with a lock.

2. How quickly can I get an appointment?

Como has a six-month waiting list. Murphy has a two-week wait. Gold seems able to take anyone at any time.

3. How quickly does this doctor give test results to patients?

Gold gets results to you immediately. Other two take longer.

4. How easy is it for the patient to speak with this doctor?

Gold filters all calls through his staff. Murphy and Como return calls fairly quickly.

5. How much time does it take to travel to and from this doctor's office?

Murphy is ten minutes away. Gold is forty-five minutes away but has a parking lot. Como is one hour away, but you must park in a parking garage.

Next, Amanda assigned a "grade" from 1 to 10, with 10 being the best, to each doctor for each factor.

Factor	Grade for COMO	Grade for GOLD	Grade for MURPHY
1. Doctor's level of expertise	9	8	7
2. Success statistics (how many people with problems like ours got pregnant)	10	7	7
3. Cost of this doctor's services	2	4	5
4. Doctor's "bedside manner"	8	5	8
5. Individualized treatment (e.g., will the doctor tailor treatment to my case or will he use a protocol similar to one used for all other patients?)	7	3	9
6. Is the practice limited to infertility?	10	9	5
7. Does this doctor provide seven-day-a-week coverage?	4	8	7
8. Is this doctor willing to work with us in terms of insurance coverage?	10	8	10
9. Does this doctor have a flexible schedule?	8	8	8
10. Office appearance	10	7	4
11. What sorts of facilities does the office have for the husband to produce a semen sample?	2	10	7
12. How quickly can I get an appointment?	1	9	8
13. How quickly does this doctor give test results to patients?	3	9	6
14. How easy is it for the patient to speak with this doctor?	7	2	8
15. How much time does it take to travel to and from this doctor's office?	2	5	9

Then Amanda assigned a weight, from 1 (not at all important to her) to 10 (crucial) to each factor. Each person decides what is important to him or her. How Amanda weighs a factor may be very different from how you weigh a factor. She multiplied the weight by the grade to get a *factor score* for each doctor. When she finished, she had scores on each of the fifteen factors for Como, Gold, and Murphy. Finally, she added up each factor score and got a total score for each doctor. Here is how she did it:

FACTOR	WEIGHT for this Factor	Grade for COMO	Factor Score for COMO	Grade for GOLD	Factor Score for GOLD	Grade for MURPHY	Factor Score for MURPHY
1. Doctor's level of expertise	10	x 9	= 90	8	80	7	70
2. Success statistics (how many people with problems like ours got pregnant)	10	x 10	= 100	7	70	7	70
3. Cost of this doctor's services	2	x 2	= 4	4	8	5	10
4. Doctor's "bedside manner"	4	x 8	= 32	5	20	8	32
5. Individualized treatment	9	x 7	= 63	3	27	9	81
6. Is the practice limited to infertility?	9	x 10	= 90	9	81	5	45
7. Does this doctor provide seven-day-a-week coverage?	9	x 4	= 36	8	72	7	63
8. Is this doctor willing to work with us in terms of insurance coverage?	9	x 10	= 90	8	72	10	90
9. Schedule flexibility	4	x 8	= 32	8	32	8	32
10. Office appearance	5	x 10	= 50	7	35	4	20
11. Facilities for husband to produce semen sample	2	x 2	= 4	10	20	7	14
12. How quickly can I get an appointment?	9	x 1	= 9	9	81	8	72
13. How quickly does this doctor give test results to patients?	3	x 3	= 9	9	27	6	18
14. How easy is it for the patient to speak with this doctor?	5	x 7	= 35	2	10	8	40
15. Travel time to office	7	x 2	= 14	5	35	9	63
Total Score			658		670		720

Based on the total scores, Amanda could plainly see that her best choice was Dr. Murphy. She called immediately and was able to make an appointment the following week.

Here's a blank chart to help you in your doctor selection. Photocopy it. Follow the steps. If you would like to download a copy of this template you can find it at http://www.gettingpregnantbook.com. Once you've made your choice, you can begin to Be a Partner in Treatment and Make a Plan. Remember, the steps are:

- List factors
- Gather information
- Assign grades
- Assign weights
- Multiply weights by grades to get Factor Scores
- Add up Factor Scores to get each Total Score
- Pick the choice with the highest Total Score

Factor	Weight for this Factor	Grade for Dr. 1	Factor Score for Dr. 1	Grade for Dr. 2	Factor Score for Dr. 2	Grade for Dr. 3	Factor Score for Dr. 3
Total Score							

ACTIVITY: PREGNANCY QUEST JOURNAL: INVESTIGATIVE REPORTER: CONCERNS ABOUT OVARIAN CANCER

One of the biggest concerns our clients voice as they embark on a course of medication is how this medication will affect their overall health. In the previous chapter we summarized some information about the relationship between taking fertility medications and developing ovarian cancer. We presented our take on the published studies. As we stated in the previous chapter, personally we concluded that the benefits to us far outweighed the risks we were taking. On the other hand, we took steps to minimize our risk by having Helane schedule annual ovarian scans and a battery of blood tests including CA-125 (a cancer screening test).

Despite the fact that many doctors think these steps are unnecessary, this annual "ritual" helps us feel more confident in our decision to use fertility medications.

You must make your own decision about whether to use injectable fertility medications. One of the best ways to help you make this decision is to participate in the *Investigative Reporter* activity.

- Gather medical information. Sources include: popular magazines, scientific/medical journals, Internet articles.
- Gather your family-history information. In particular, inquire about female reproductive history cancer-related instances.
- Participate in an Internet "ask the doctor" forum. One place to start is INCIID (http://www.inciid.org).
- Interact with peers who are making this decision or who have already made it. Sources include: Local RESOLVE chapter members and Internet discussion forums like INCIID's (http://www. inciid.org).
- Take a notebook divider and label it *Fertility Medication Information*. Insert it in your Pregnancy Quest Journal binder.
- Print out all the information you have gathered. Put it in your Pregnancy Quest Journal binder.

This activity follows from the "rational-emotive" approach we discussed in Chapter 2 in the Getting Pregnant Workout. What you've done at this point is to gather some of the necessary "rational" information. The next step is another "rational" activity: creating a cost-benefit analysis. Your next step will be to respond emotionally to the rational information you've collected. The final step will involve disputing some of the irrational fears you may have so that you can move forward. Use the information you now have in your journal for the next part of the activity.

Amanda used our approach to create her journal. We present her material below, which you can use as a guide in creating your own journal.

Concerns	Disputing My Concerns
The injections hurt.	They do hurt, but the hurt is brief.
The drugs are expensive.	My insurance may pay some of these costs. Unfortunately, for me to get pregnant will be costly.

There is a chance I will get cancer.	There is always a chance, but the odds are very much against it.
I could hyperstimulate.	There is a chance, but with good monitoring by my doctor the odds are very small.
I could end up with three or more babies.	My doctor understands this concern and will cancel a cycle if I've made too many follicles.
By taking these medications I am admitting to myself that we are having trouble conceiving.	I must face this fact if I want to up my odds of getting pregnant.
It seems so unnatural to get pregnant this way.	It is unnatural but it works. Also, more and more people are undergoing infertility treatment every year.
I can be trapped endlessly many doing inseminations.	I am going to make a plan to limit how many times I do this.
If I do this I am taking the first step on the road to IVF.	I have to admit this, but I hope this step will be sufficient to get me pregnant.

Now that you have this information, begin to create a journal entry. Find your special place and begin to write, allowing your emotions to flow freely and in an uncensored way. Remember: You are writing for yourself, not to impress anyone else. You may choose to share what you wrote with your partner or anyone else, but you certainly don't need to do so.

LISTENING/LEVELING: TALKING ABOUT INJECTABLE FERTILITY MEDICATIONS

Almost every couple engaged in infertility treatment uses some form of injectable fertility medication. Every night, countless husbands are opening glass ampules, mixing powder and liquid, filling syringes, and injecting FSH/LH into their wife's buttock. These men may not be gleeful about what they are doing, but they are certainly dutiful because they know that the drug will stimulate their wife's ovaries to produce multiple egg follicles, thus upping their odds of getting her pregnant.

Amanda and Al were open with one another about their hopes and trepidations. Al was afraid of killing Amanda by injecting an air bubble into her accidentally. As she had written in her Pregnancy Quest Journal, Amanda was worried that fertility medications might increase her chances of getting ovarian cancer. She also wasn't sure if she trusted her klutzy husband, who can barely turn on the dishwasher, to act as her combination chemist and nurse. But the Gambones couldn't afford the luxury of hiring a trained medical professional to give the injections, so they opted to Work as a Team and face their fears head on. To accomplish this, they mentally rehearsed the injection skills, and added some Getting Pregnant Listening and Leveling.

"I Trust You but I'm Scared." "So Am I."[3]

Using the following exercise, Amanda and Al were able to get in touch with their emotions and understand better what each was going through. Amanda read the italicized text to Al, who, using his mental imagery skills, would close his eyes and listen. After she finished the passage, Al would look at her and tell her what he thought about the passage. Amanda then would use the active listening skills she learned in the Getting Pregnant Workout until she truly understood how he felt.

"Close your eyes and picture the following scene: You are about to give me an injection of Humegon. You are preparing the medication. Using an alcohol pad, you break open three vials of Humegon and one of water. You stand the vials up carefully. You peel off the plastic wrapper from the syringe. You make sure the needle is secured in the cylinder. You pull out the plunger and push it back in to make sure that it is drawing. You carefully insert the needle into the water ampule. You pull up the plunger of the syringe to draw up the entire contents of the vial. You insert the needle into the first Humegon ampule and inject one-third of the water into this ampule. You insert the needle into the second ampule and inject another third of the water. Now you insert the needle into the last ampule and inject the remaining water.

"You insert the needle into the first Humegon mixture and draw it up. Now you do the same with the second ampule. You draw up the remaining solution. You tap the syringe to make sure there are no bubbles. You slowly push in on the plunger until a small bead of liquid appears on the tip of the needle.

"Now you approach me. You locate a spot on my buttock. You insert the entire needle perpendicular to the plane of my buttock. You hold the syringe with one hand and draw the plunger out to see if any blood appears on the needle. There is none. You then push the plunger in quickly to inject the Humegon. Now you pull out the needle quickly. You cover the site of the injection with an alcohol pad."

Amanda then asks Al to make a *true statement* about what he's feeling concerning Humegon. When he has made that statement, Amanda asks him yes-or-no questions, beginning with "Do you mean . . . ?" to clarify further what he's feeling. She continues to probe in this manner until Al responds "yes" a total of three times. You may have to ask as few as three questions or as many as twelve. Remember, your job is to listen to your partner, to ask good questions, to accept his responses, and to validate all his "yes"s.

Here is what Al and Amanda said. Remember, husbands' concerns and responses are as individual as they are, so if you try this exercise, don't feel you must mirror Amanda and Al exactly.

AL: "This whole thing is upsetting me."

AMANDA: "Do you mean that you want me to give up on the Humegon and IUI?"

AL: "No."

AMANDA: "Do you mean that you wish we could have a baby naturally?"

AL: "No."

AMANDA: "Do you mean that you're afraid that you don't have the coordination to do this?"

AL: "Yes."

AMANDA: "Do you mean that you're afraid that you'll cause me pain?"

AL: "Yes."

AMANDA: "Do you mean that you want to hire a nurse to give these injections?"

AL: "No."

AMANDA: "Do you mean that you're afraid that you'll inject me with air bubbles?"

AL: "Yes."

By the end of their dialogue, Amanda has a better understanding of what's bothering Al. Now they switch places, remembering that once Amanda has made her statement, she can answer only yes or no to Al's questions.

AMANDA: "I'm afraid of doing the Humegon shots."

AL: "Do you mean you want someone else to inject you?"

AMANDA: "No."

AL: "Do you mean you think I'm totally uncoordinated?"

AMANDA: "No."

AL: "Do you mean you think that I might break the needle in your buttock?"

AMANDA: "Yes."

AL: "Do you mean you think I'll inject you in the wrong place?"

AMANDA: "Yes."

AL: "Do you mean that you think this will ruin our marriage?"

AMANDA: "No."

AL: "Do you mean you are worried that I will resent you if I can't go out with the boys if you're scheduled to have an injection?"

AMANDA: "Yes."

DAYDREAMS WITH A PURPOSE: COPING WITH THE DEMANDS OF TREATMENT

Amanda and Al discovered that mental imagery could provide them with some very concrete assistance in meeting the demands of their treatment. Besides helping them mentally rehearse injections, relax their minds, and reduce stress, mental imagery also helped Al produce a semen sample on demand.

In most IUI cycles, the woman is the focus 95 percent of the time. The husband's big moment arrives when he produces a sample to be used for insemination. Although it takes only a few minutes, his contribution is pivotal. It is no wonder, then, that Al felt so pressured that he had difficulty producing a sample. The thought of failing to perform terrified him. He feared he wouldn't get aroused, that he'd lose his erection, or, worse yet, that he'd miss the cup. He suffered from performance anxiety, a feeling akin to stage fright.

One way to help alleviate performance anxiety is to produce a sample well before the insemination—one that can be frozen. Even though frozen sperm has a statistically lower success rate than does fresh sperm, it can be useful if all else fails. Another consideration that can reduce performance anxiety concerns where the sample is to be collected: at home or in the doctor's office. If you live more than an hour from the office, your husband should probably produce the sample there. If you live close by, let your husband make the decision. Some doctors provide rooms with erotic videotapes; other doctors just provide bathrooms or an examination room with a locking door. The very act of helping your husband Make a Plan to produce a sample will lower his anxiety.

Amanda found that Al felt less pressured when she encouraged him to create fantasies to help him become aroused on insemination day. In fact, Al and Amanda created fantasies and tried them out a week or so beforehand. Al would remember the most successful fantasy and re-create it to help him produce a sample.

Another way Amanda helped Al get aroused is by recording a fantasy audiotape, which he listened to on his Walkman. The Gambones Worked as a Team to concoct a particularly arousing fantasy. Some wives, if they feel brazen enough, make a surprise tape for their husbands. Many find this exercise fun, a welcome relief from the rigors of infertility treatment. It is important to tell your husband that his sexual fantasy life is an important part of his participation in your pregnancy quest.

HELPING YOURSELF STAY OPTIMISTIC: HANGING IN THROUGH REPEATED CYCLES

Treatment can work only if you faithfully follow the regimen prescribed by your doctor. But you are not a machine. You have worries, doubts, and other concerns that can interfere with your ability to follow protocol. Moreover, it's hard to sustain enthusiasm and motivation, particularly when you learn that you face yet another month of treatment.

What motivates you to get out of bed at the crack of dawn so you can make it to the doctor's office by 8:00 A.M. and be at work by 9:00? What prevents you from giving up? The obvious answer to these questions is: *You.* But sometimes you need help. Optimism and motivation can become increasingly elusive as failed attempts to conceive mount up. And at some point you may want to stop burdening your friends and relatives with your fertility problems. But you can still allow others to help you through the trials of fertility treatment by using your imagination.

Circle of Friends: A Series of Motivational Imagery Activities

From the beginning, Amanda felt that she had no one to turn to when Al could not be by her side; all her important friends and immediate family lived far away, and her beloved grandmother, who had always been her staunchest ally, had recently died.

Her fertility specialist had suggested she try six cycles of Humegon and intrauterine inseminations before moving to any more advanced assisted reproductive techniques. Amanda knew that course of action almost guaranteed at least one failed attempt, since the best Humegon/IUI statistics she read showed that only 14 percent of women get pregnant each month. After six months, Amanda had a 60 percent chance of becoming pregnant.[4]

To cope with the anxiety of this reality, Amanda conjured up visions of her grandmother by her side. Seeing her grandmother's smiling face in her mind's eye gave Amanda the confidence, strength, and motivation to endure almost anything.

Here is a series of three interrelated activities to help you adapt Amanda's experience to your personal situation. To derive the greatest benefit from these activities, read the descriptions of all three before engaging in any one of them. Record, or ask your partner to record, the italicized texts onto audiotape.

CIRCLE OF FRIENDS

Directions: The first part of this activity represents the beginning of your active search for people to assist you in remaining optimistic through repeated treatments. The following text can be recorded for you to listen to. If you have recorded the text, turn on the tape recorder now.

Together we are going to develop a circle of friends who are your supporters. This group can consist of your relatives, colleagues at work, childhood friends, neighbors, friends who belong to your church or temple, or any other friends who are meaningful to you. These people can be from your past or present life. They can be people who are living or dead, as long as their memory is strong and clear. You can select a religious figure, a person from history, or a contemporary individual whom you admire.

Allow yourself to think about people who you know can be your supporters in getting pregnant. Do not worry now about thinking of numbers of people; one or two or even three are fine. Picture each of those persons, one at a time. You may first find that person inside your head, or even in front of you, looking at you. That person can be whispering in your ear. Remember, that person can appear to you anywhere you want him or her to be. Get a clear picture of that person in your mind's eye.

Now imagine that the person is talking to you, coaching you in preparation for the treatment you are about to undertake. Try to hear and remember what the person is saying. Sometimes even words are not important, but rather the feeling you get when the person is with you. Allow yourself to see and hear all the people you've thought of. Take as much time as you want. [You may wish to pause the tape recorder here.] *When you are finished, open your eyes, read the following directions, and fill in the form that follows.*

Directions: For each group of lines, fill in names of the people who came to mind when you allowed yourself to find your supporters. If you did not find someone for a particular category, go on to the next category. If someone comes to mind while you are filling in the form, you may add that person, even though he or she did not surface during the time you were concentrating on developing your circle.

A. Relatives
    _____
    _____

    _____

B. Colleagues at Work
    _____
    _____

    _____

C. Childhood Friends
    _____
    _____

    _____

D. Neighbors
    _____
    _____

    _____

E. Friends from Church or Synagogue
    _____
    _____

    _____

F. Other Meaningful Friends
    _____
    _____

    _____

G. Someone You Admire, Respect, or Revere from Religion, History, or Contemporary Society
    _____
    _____

CREATE YOUR CIRCLE

Directions: Before you begin this part of the activity, look over your list of people. In the next part of the exercise you will be asked to recall the people on your list. Try to remember as many people as you can, but don't worry if you feel you won't be able to remember them all. Next time you do the exercise, you may remember more or different people, or even add a new one. If you have recorded the following text on a tape recorder, turn on the tape recorder now.

Get into a relaxed frame of mind. Allow yourself to recall the people who are part of your group of supporters. Don't worry if you can remember only one or two people. Start with those. If you remember more as you go through this activity, you can add those people to your circle.

Picture each of these persons seated in a circle. Now walk into the center of the circle and take a seat. Look around. Slowly focus on the face of each friend—one by one. Picture each person smiling at you and telling you how much he or she wants what you want for you. Really allow yourself to look at and hear each person. As each person smiles at you and speaks to you, you feel yourself becoming stronger and more optimistic. When you feel ready, stand up and leave the circle knowing that these friends and their various strengths are with you. When you have left the circle, turn off the tape recorder. But try to keep a part of each person with you in your heart for as much of your day as possible.

INVISIBLE FRIEND

Directions: For this part of the activity, you will select one or two specific people to take with you when you need support. You may find their support helpful when you need motivation to get up early in the morning to travel to a clinic. You may need their support when you are about to undergo a procedure. And you may especially need their support and encouragement when you have to bounce back after a failed procedure. If you have taped the activity, turn on the tape recorder now.

In this first activity you will use your friend to help you with an upcoming treatment. Allow yourself to be relaxed. Select one of your friends, who was sit-

ting in the circle, to prepare herself or himself to accompany you to your next treatment. In your mind's ear, have a conversation with your friend about the procedure you are about to experience. This friend is extraordinarily supportive, and everything he or she tells you makes you feel strong. Try to focus on several of the key sentences that your friend tells you. He or she may tell you, for example, "You can do anything you set your mind to." Or "Remember how you worked so hard to get what you wanted? You did it then and you can do it now." Or "Remember how you made it through that last treatment? You can do anything you set your mind to." After you have drawn strength from these phrases, allow yourself to believe that your friend can come with you and talk to you during the difficult time of your next procedure. Believe that he or she can come with you and believe that your friend can give you the strength you need to get through the treatment.

Practice imagining you and your friend conversing once or twice a day for a week or so before the treatment. Each day you picture you and your friend talking, your friend's words will have a more powerful influence on you. On the day of your procedure, your friend will exert a powerful influence over you and the success of your treatment.

In the next part of this activity, you will use your friend to help you be strong and hang in after a procedure that failed. Allow yourself to be relaxed. Select one of your friends, who was sitting in the circle, to support or console you after a failed treatment. In your mind's ear, have a conversation with your friend about the procedure that failed. Your friend is extraordinarily understanding and gives you an opportunity to feel sad. But he or she also tells you things that make you feel strong. Try to focus on several of the key sentences that your friend tells you. He or she may tell you, for example, "You had setbacks before and you bounced back. You did it then and you can do it again. Every time you keep trying, the odds of success get better." After you have drawn strength from these phrases, allow yourself to believe that your friend will be there to understand your pain and support you whenever you need her or him.

Practice imagining you and your friend conversing once or twice a day for a week or so while you recover. Each day you picture you and your friend talking, your friend's words will have a more powerful influence on you. Gradually, your friend's words will heal the hurt of the failed procedure.

TAKING CHARGE OF YOUR SOCIAL LIFE

Just when Amanda thought she was feeling strong, she received an invitation to a friend's baby shower. The invitation triggered a cascade of tears, which left Amanda shaken for hours. The mere thought of walking into an infantwear department to buy a gift made her quiver. But how could she disappoint her friend by being conspicuously absent from the shower?

Just as fertility patients must be assertive with their physicians at times, so must infertile people learn to be assertive in the social arena. Even the most well-meaning friends and relatives can pressure you without realizing it. This pressure may be real or imagined on your part, particularly when it comes to holidays and pregnancy-related events. We know of one infertile woman who became physically ill during her niece's christening and had to leave the ceremony.

To help you avoid such disasters, we've developed a series of activities to help you Manage Your Social Life and, in doing so, draw you and your partner closer to one another. These activities build on your GPST, mental imagery, and assertiveness skills.

No More Life on Hold: A Series of Socially Liberating Activities

Even though you may feel obsessed with your infertility treatments, you must still live in the real world. Pregnant women and people pushing baby carriages will cross your path almost daily. News of friends and relatives becoming pregnant and giving birth will also come your way. Infertile women have actually reported the urge to run over a baby carriage or shoot a pregnant friend. Stoic men with fertility problems have cried at the sight of a Little League game. Otherwise low-key couples report screaming matches over whether to visit a relative who just had a baby.

If the trials of daily life don't get to you, holidays and other special occasions can. To cope, you must first recognize and acknowledge the kinds of events that will cause stress for you or your partner. Only then can you plan your schedules to be as stress-free as possible. Careful planning is the key to taking charge of your social life.

IDENTIFYING TOUGH SITUATIONS

The following activity will help you identify situations you found difficult in the past, which helps you anticipate what might be stressful in the future. We've included three charts to get you started: one for you, one for your partner, and one for you as a couple. Take some time now to recall social and family situations you found awkward, unpleasant, or downright awful as a result of your infertility. To get you started, we begin each chart with situations that the Gambones found unpleasant. The exercise works best if you and your partner complete your own lists separately before completing the couple list together.

SOCIAL SITUATIONS: WIFE	
Easy Situations	**Difficult Situations**
1. Taking my sister's kids to the movies	1. Going to a baby shower of my friend, Connie, who conceived easily

SOCIAL SITUATIONS: HUSBAND	
Easy Situations	**Difficult Situations**
1. Attending a christening	1. Watching a Little League game

SOCIAL SITUATIONS: COUPLE	
Easy Situations	**Difficult Situations**
1. Going to a RESOLVE social function	1. Going to the family Thanksgiving dinner

PROS AND CONS

Next, list the pros and cons of participating in each of the situations you listed. Here is what Amanda wrote regarding her discomfort in going to Connie's baby shower.

SITUATION: GOING TO CONNIE'S BABY SHOWER	
Why I Should (go to the shower)	**Why I Shouldn't (go to the shower)**
1. Because I'm polite. My mother taught me that it's the right thing to do.	1. I'll want to cry when I think that she's having a baby and I can't have one.
2. She's my good friend. She came all the way from Cleveland to be one of my bridesmaids.	2. I'll resent her for her good fortune.
3. My friends will think that I'm rude and selfish if I don't show up for Connie's shower.	3. After I come home, I'll be in such a bad mood that I'll get into a fight with my husband.

Here's a chart for you to write pros and cons for your own situations. Before filling in the chart, photocopy it to use with your husband's list and your couple's list.

SITUATION: _____	
Why I Should _____	Why I Shouldn't _____

EMPTY CHAIR

Completing these charts should help you understand the kinds of demands you put on yourself. Sometimes people feel as though they have *no choice* about what they do, that they *must* do certain things, regardless of any emotional upheaval a situation might trigger. But you have more freedom than you might realize.

We are not trying to teach you to be selfish or irresponsible. We are saying: Be kind to yourself, and give your friends and relatives credit for their ability to empathize with your plight. You have very sound reasons for avoiding painful social situations. By "arguing" with the part of yourself that shackles you to social conventions, those reasons will become clearer. The inner-dialogue activity we present next is taken from Gestalt psychotherapy.[5]

Gestalt psychotherapists emphasize human *polarities*. That is, each person's psyche is made up of many parts, which have different and often opposing desires. According to Gestalt psychotherapists Erving and Miriam Polster, people should allow their various parts to make contact with one another. "This reduces the chance that one part will stay mired in its own impotence, hanging on to the status quo. Instead, [each part] is energized into making a vital statement of its own needs and wishes, asserting itself as a force, which must be considered in a new union of forces."[6]

Through the following exercise, you can give voice to your conflicting feelings through a form of debate. We use the baby shower as an example, but you can adapt the exercise to any situation you wish.

Directions: You are going to participate in a debate between two parts of yourself: One part says you *should* go to the baby shower, and the other part says you *should not* go.

Sit opposite an empty chair, which is facing you. Become the part of you that says, "I should go to the shower." Imagine that you are putting the part of you that says, "I should not go" in the empty chair. Tell yourself why you should attend. After this opening statement, go sit in the other chair. Refute your "should go" argument, telling your first part why she is wrong. Do this for a few minutes, then switch back to the other chair. In this way, you are creating a dialogue, of sorts, with yourself.

Here is a sample of what we mean:

Should Go:

You really should go to the baby shower. Your mother brought you up to be polite and do the right thing. She would be appalled if she knew that you didn't go to the shower. She would say: "What kind of daughter did I raise?" [Switch seats.]

Should Not Go:

You're so bogged down in always "doing the right thing." What about your needs? Must you torture yourself? Don't you deserve to be kind to yourself? You know how upsetting it will be for you to go to that shower. You know how nasty you'll be to your husband after you get back. [Switch seats.]

Should Go:

Don't keep making excuses for yourself. You can always find some justification to avoid your obligations. But you know deep down that you're being selfish. If everyone acted this way, nobody would ever do anything nice for anyone else. [Switch seats.]

Should Not Go:

But you know that you're not a selfish person. You've always gone out of your way to do nice things for other people. You do grocery shopping for your mother. You give money to charity. If you weren't dealing with your infertility, there's no question that you'd go. But this just isn't the right time for you. [Switch seats.]

Remember, these are not lines to memorize; they're merely an example to follow. You can use the Empty Chair activity anytime you want to argue with yourself about what you "should" or "should not" do. You might be surprised by the intensity of your feelings.

A FINAL WORD

We don't expect you to follow each and every element of the Workout throughout your pregnancy quest. Pick and choose the exercises that suit you at any given moment. The daily demands of infertility treatment can be quite time-consuming, and we realize that it's not always easy to stay with the Workout program. But even if you try to do just one or two of the exercises described in this chapter, you may find that it is possible to reduce the stress that accompanies most situations.

CHAPTER 7

The "ART" of Getting Pregnant: Assisted Reproductive Technologies

n 1978, the world's first "test-tube baby," Louise Brown, was born thanks to the pioneering efforts of Drs. Patrick Steptoe and Robert Edwards. Not surprisingly, Louise's birth revolutionized reproductive medicine and offered new hope to countless infertile couples.[1] Since her birth, tens of thousands of infants have been delivered as a result of *in vitro fertilization*, more commonly known as IVF. Since our last edition was published in 1993, IVF techniques are more sophisticated, more available, and are now considered standard fertility treatment.

IVF is one of several "alphabet soup" terms that will be discussed in this chapter. Medically, ART does not represent a quantum leap from the treatment you already may be trying. But psychologically, ART does represent a major step for infertile couples: the last hope of producing a child who is theirs genetically.

For some couples, ART is explored only after low-tech procedures have failed. Others, wanting to maximize their odds of success despite the increased cost, may go directly to ART without trying any of the low-tech procedures. Nevertheless, ART may still be a couple's last shot at parenthood because of its drain on their pocketbook as well as on their emotional life.

Medically, ART embraces many of the low-tech procedures and regimens covered in earlier chapters: Humegon injections, blood monitoring, ultrasound scans, semen samples, and maybe even a laparoscopy. What's different is that eggs are physically removed from the woman's body. Once removed, the eggs are mixed with sperm in a petri dish and allowed to fertilize, either on their own or with some specialized assistance, before being transferred into the womb.

Psychologically, people who attempt these procedures must come to grips with the fact that ART is a further cry from lovemaking than is artificial insemination. At least during an insemination sperm is introduced through your vagina, albeit via a tube and syringe. With ART, eggs and sperm disappear behind closed doors, hopefully returning as embryos several days later.

WHAT IS ART?

Assisted reproductive technologies make use of laboratory procedures to examine eggs and sperm and enhance their likelihood of being fertilized. Although there are several variations on ART, they tend to be referred to as in vitro fertilization (IVF). *In vitro* means "in glass"—to refer to glass laboratory dishes in which fertilization takes place. Like tissues that are called "Kleenex" and photocopying procedures referred to as "Xeroxing," assisted reproductive techniques are often referred to as IVF.

At this writing, there are approximately 350 IVF clinics operating nationwide, some freestanding, some hospital-based. (For a complete list of these facilities, see the Centers for Disease Control Web site, http://www.cdc.gov/nccdphp/drh/art97/index.htm.) Almost all of these clinics use the same techniques. Here is how ART works.

THE ELEMENTS OF ART

Downregulation

The use of the drug Lupron for "downregulation" of the pituitary gland's functioning was one of the most dramatic developments of IVF technology in the early 1990s. Downregulation means that Lupron temporarily inhibits the production of the pituitary hormones FSH and LH so that the doctor can artificially regulate your menstrual cycle. It also allows the doctors to control egg development and minimize the chance that you will ovulate your eggs before they can be retrieved. In addition, Lupron helps to increase the number of eggs you produce, as well as improving the quality of those eggs. Downregulation with Lupron takes eight to fourteen days. At this time, you will get your menstrual period and be ready to begin your superovulation medication. You will continue taking Lupron while you are also taking the superovulation medication. Lupron is injected once a day into your thigh or stomach with a tiny needle.

Ovarian Stimulation

Ovarian stimulation is probably one of the most publicized and most anxiety-provoking aspect of ART. Perhaps the anxiety stems from fears that the use of drugs will somehow cause birth defects in future offspring. Studies show this is not the case. A second concern is that taking these medications will increase your risk of breast and ovarian cancer. As we noted in Chapter 5, the research so far has failed to find support for the link between use of fertility medication and developing cancer. The third concern is that you will give birth to three or more babies. It is certainly true that cases such as the Iowa septuplets are rare events. These higher-order multiple births resulted from superovulation used with an insemination procedure, not from an ART procedure. Nonetheless, the American Society for Reproductive Medicine has placed the issue of multiple births high on its agenda.

Depending on the individual and how much medication she is given, superovulation drugs help ovaries grow up to a dozen or more mature eggs rather than the single egg that normally develops each month. Since most women ovulate naturally, you don't need these drugs to induce ovulation. Rather, you take these drugs to enhance the doctor's ability to obtain multiple eggs for potential fertilization. Infertility specialists agree that your chances of becoming pregnant improve if you produce many eggs. Multiple eggs potentially can result in multiple embryos. And by transferring several embryos to your uterus at once, the odds of at least one of them implanting and growing into a baby increase.

The list of medications used to induce superovulation includes Pergonal, Repronex, Humegon, Fertinex, Follistim, and Gonal-F. Pergonal, Repronex, and Humegon all contain a combination of two hormones: FSH and LH. Fertinex, Follistim, and Gonal-F contain almost pure FSH. Some of these drugs are injected intramuscularly into your buttocks; others are injected into your thigh or stomach. Although the intramuscular needle may look intimidating, the injections are virtually painless because the needle pierces fatty tissue and does not hit any nerve endings. Dosage varies depending on the IVF program and the patient, but you will probably be taking more medication each day than you did for a medicated insemination cycle. Expect to inject the fertility drug or drugs for seven to twelve days per cycle.

Taking larger doses increases the risk of "hyperstimulation syndrome." This severe hyperstimulation of the ovaries can cause nausea, vomiting, abdominal swelling, and rapid weight gain. Severe hyperstimulation can occur if you take large amounts of medication, have extremely high estradiol levels, and then use hCG to ovulate your eggs in preparation for an insemination. When the hCG shot is given, some of the many eggs may not ovulate. Instead, they may produce hormones called cytokines that lead to fluid accumulation responsible for hyperstimulation.

Ovarian hyperstimulation syndrome is not very common with ART. The reason is that doctors physically remove some of the estrogen-producing cells that will become part of the corpus luteum (the "yellow body" formed in the ovary following ovulation that produces the progesterone needed to sustain a pregnancy) and prevent the production of cytokines that might trigger hyperstimulation. Also, if scans and blood tests indicate that the patient is at high risk for hyperstimulation, the doctor refrains from administering hCG and cancels the cycle. Through careful monitoring, then, you can safely take high doses of fertility drugs and reduce, though not completely eliminate, the risk of ovarian hyperstimulation syndrome.

Monitoring: Blood and Ultrasound

Your response to the medication will be monitored via blood tests to determine your estradiol (the major ovarian estrogen) level and ultrasound scans of your ovaries. Undergoing this monitoring is a mixed blessing. It's a relief to know that your doctor is checking how fast your eggs are growing every day or every other day. Monitoring ensures that eggs grow as large as possible, but not so large that they are overripe or so mature that they ovulate before they are ready to be retrieved. But you pay a price for your doctor's vigilance. And we don't mean only money.

Most clinics want you to arrive early in the morning to have your blood drawn. Early often means between 6:30 and 8:30 A.M. Arriving at a distant clinic may mean leaving your home before dawn. And surprisingly, getting there early doesn't necessarily mean avoiding the crowd. Chances are you will be one of many women waiting to be monitored. While comparing notes with others can be a source of support, being amid so many infertile women also can make you feel depressed or overwhelmed. Also, starting your day at an IVF clinic and then going to work can make you feel nervous and preoccupied.

While you are still half awake, a nurse or a technician will stick a needle into a vein in your arm and then a doctor or an ultrasound technician will insert a probe into your vagina. The probe is used to obtain an ultrasound scan of your ovaries. Using high-frequency sound waves, the probe produces a picture of your ovaries and follicles on a video screen. To help you stay involved in your treatment, many clinics will give you a notepad and have you write down a series of numbers the technician calls out as she scans. "Twelve on the right." "Fifteen on the left." These are not football plays. They are the diameter—the millimeters—of the egg follicles that are being measured on the screen. The lead follicles must be at least sixteen to eighteen millimeters in diameter before they are ready to be aspirated.

Doctors need to obtain your blood early in the morning to allow sufficient time for a laboratory to analyze your hormone levels. Doctors get their lab reports early in the afternoon and use this information, together with your ultrasound results, to adjust your dosage for that evening's fertility drug injection. You will be notified of the doctor's decision later in the day. Some doctors phone you with the results; others ask that you call your assigned mailbox.

Figuring out the logistics of receiving a call from your physician with this vital information can be quite stressful, especially if you don't want to be called at work where colleagues or customers might overhear your conversation. You may worry that a message left on your answering machine could be unclear. You may want to speak personally to the doctor if you have questions or concerns. Or you might elect to sit by the phone to make sure that you don't miss the call.

In addition to telling you how many ampules of medication to inject that evening, some doctors also will tell you your estradiol level. Getting information about estradiol levels can be troubling. It's easy to obsess over the numbers, plaguing yourself with questions such as "Is it going up enough?" and "Am I doing okay?" If your doctor routinely shares estradiol levels, we recommend Getting Organized by keeping track of them in your Cycle Log. If your levels fail to match last cycle's levels, don't worry. It is not unusual for women to respond differently to the same doses of medication from month to month.

Sometimes, however, your doctor may decide to cancel your cycle because you have not responded optimally to the medication. The latest available statistics of the Society for Assisted Reproductive Technology (SART) indicate that approximately 14 percent of all ART cycles were canceled, mostly because of a poor response to medication. Don't give up hope. With so many medications to choose from, your doctor can either change medication or change dosage during a subsequent cycle. A canceled cycle, though very disappointing, avoids making you pay for an expensive egg harvest that would not result in a pregnancy.

Triggering Ovulation

When your doctor decides that your follicles have reached optimal development, he or she will prescribe an hCG injection. Like Pergonal, hCG is injected into your buttock and is not particularly painful. Egg retrieval will be scheduled thirty-four to thirty-six hours after this injection.

Egg Harvest (Follicle Aspiration)

Eggs are harvested primarily through a technique called *ultrasound guided transvaginal aspiration*. This procedure requires no incisions and uses sedation, which is usually intravenous. The doctor inserts an ultrasound probe into the vagina. When a mature follicle is identified, he or she guides a needle through the vaginal wall and into a follicle to be aspirated. All follicles of reasonable size are aspirated. This procedure usually takes between ten minutes and one hour. The follicular fluid containing the retrieved eggs is passed to an embryologist, who isolates the eggs under a microscope and assigns them a grade indicating their quality and maturity. For a detailed description of how embryologists grade eggs, see the embryology question-and-answer section of Chapter 15.

Doctors take care to ensure that you are physically comfortable during the retrieval procedure. For most women, anticipating the outcome—whether enough healthy eggs will be harvested—is more stressful than the procedure itself. Although a pregnancy can occur even when only a single egg is harvested, more eggs means that your chances of success are greater. Likewise, a harvest of eggs that are of inferior quality has a poor prognosis.

Fertilization

When you try to get pregnant on your own, you have to wait at least two weeks to learn whether your egg got fertilized. With IVF, you get important information within twenty-four hours after egg retrieval. This is because the site of fertilization is changed from inside the body, where it is invisible and unknown, to outside the body: a dish in the laboratory.

Each harvested egg is placed in its own plastic dish filled with a special IVF culture medium. Your husband's or a donor's sperm cells that have been washed and specially prepared are also placed into the dish. Each dish then goes into an incubator. After about eighteen hours in the incubator, an embryologist will check the eggs to determine whether they are fertilized. In about twelve hours, an egg that was fertilized will divide and become a two-celled embryo. A little while later, the embryo may divide again into four cells. Two to three days after retrieval, multi-celled embryos are transferred into your uterus through the vagina. The transfer is similar to an IUI procedure. Embryos of good quality are stored in frozen form for possible transfer in a subsequent cycle.

Rarely Used Techniques: GIFT and ZIFT

The GIFT Alternative

Some doctors believe that the fallopian tube is a better, more natural site for fertilization to occur because there may be certain fluids in the tube that help stimulate fertilization. To help infertile couples achieve this goal, medical science has come up with GIFT—gamete intrafallopian transfer. During a GIFT procedure, gametes (sperm and egg cells) are injected into one or both fallopian tubes. If all goes well, fertilization takes place in the tube and the embryo enters the uterus and implants, just as it would in natural, unassisted reproduction. Today, very few GIFT procedures are done. GIFT has the same success rate as IVF but requires laparascopic surgery and general anesthesia. For details, see our Web site (http://www.gettingpregnant-book.com).

The ZIFT Alternative

ZIFT—zygote intrafallopian transfer—involves the transfer of a zygote, the medical term for a fertilized egg before it begins to divide. Like GIFT, ZIFT is not used very often nowadays.

New Advances: Intracytoplasmic Sperm Injection (ICSI)

One of the most important recent advances in infertility treatment is intracytoplasmic sperm injection, also called ICSI. ICSI was pioneered in Belgium in the early 1990s. Prior to the availability of ICSI, a man with poor motility, low sperm count, poor-quality sperm, or sperm that had trouble penetrating eggs had to face the prospect of using donated sperm, adopting, or living without children. Now, with ICSI, even if your partner has sperm problems you can get pregnant through IVF with the addition of ICSI.

Eggs are harvested in an IVF procedure. Fresh or frozen sperm samples are used in the ICSI procedure to fertilize these eggs. The eggs are viewed under a high-contrast microscope. The embryologist uses a device called a micromanipulator that allows her to execute extremely precise movements. The embryologist sometimes uses an extremely thin glass tube called a pipette to hold a single sperm. How can an embryologist catch just one sperm? First she slows it down with a drop of a special chemical solution. Then she pinches its tail to immobilize it so it won't move around after it is injected into the egg. The immobile sperm is sucked up into an injection pipette. Meanwhile the egg is held in place using gentle suction to its outer covering applied through a holding pipette. Then, while the egg is held in place, the sperm is injected through the zona pellucida (outer covering) and into the cytoplasm (the living matter within a cell excluding the nucleus) of the egg. After it is injected, the injection pipette is withdrawn and within one minute the hole seals naturally and the egg resumes its original shape. Obviously, to do this procedure the embryologist needs to be highly skilled. The same ICSI procedure is repeated on all the eggs that are good candidates for ICSI. After the sperm have been injected into the eggs, the petri dishes containing the injected eggs are placed in an incubator for about fourteen hours. Then the embryologist checks to see whether the sperm have succeeded in fertilizing the eggs.

SPECIAL WAYS TO RETRIEVE SPERM

Sometimes a semen analysis fails to find any sperm in the ejaculate. Although this used to be the end of the line, now there are methods for extracting sperm from the epididymis (an organ in the male lying above and behind the testicles) using a procedure called MESA, microepididymal sperm aspiration, or PESA, percutaneous sperm aspiration of the testes, in a procedure known as TESA, testicular sperm aspiration, or TESE, testicular sperm extraction. Sperm obtained from these procedures can be frozen and then thawed and used in ICSI, or they can be extracted just before the retrieval and used as fresh sperm.

A urologist or a skilled fertility specialist performs the sperm-aspiration procedure. If the plan is to use freshly aspirated sperm, you will need to plan carefully to coordinate the timing of the aspiration and the retrieval. Since it is often difficult to know in advance exactly when the retrieval will take place, you may find such coordination particularly stressful. The aspiration may be done twenty-four to forty-eight hours prior to egg retrieval. This time frame provides an opportunity for the sperm to gain motility. Fortunately, research studies have demonstrated that thawed sperm obtained from MESA were usually just as effective as fresh sperm in producing pregnancies when used in an ICSI procedure.[2] Knowing this, you can avoid the logistical nightmare of waiting to have your eggs retrieved while your husband is also undergoing surgery. You can have him present to hold your hand after you recover and, in some cases, spare him the ordeal of having another aspiration procedure should you wish to do a subsequent IVF cycle with ICSI.

Typically, the urologist will first try to extract the sperm from the epididymis. He will use local or general anesthesia to perform the operation. If he cannot obtain sperm from the epididymis, he can perform a testicular biopsy to obtain the sperm. The disadvantage of testicular extraction is that sperm obtained from the testes do not freeze as well as sperm obtained from the epididymis. If both the epididymal and the biopsy procedures are done one after the other, the procedure can take up to three hours. If only the testicular-aspiration procedure is done, it can be performed with local anesthesia and takes a relatively short time. PESA can be performed on an outpatient basis using IV sedation and local anesthesia. In one type of modified PESA, a one-centimeter incision is made in the scrotum and sperm are aspirated through a twenty-four-gauge needle.[3] Men undergoing this procedure report that there is relatively little post-operative pain.

ARE THERE RISKS WITH ICSI?

There is concern that ICSI may allow abnormal sperm to fertilize an egg. It is believed that nature eliminates many sperm with genetic defects by rendering them incapable of penetrating the egg to fertilize it. But if an embryologist pokes a hole in an egg and sticks a sperm inside, he or she may inadvertently enable a genetically defective sperm to fertilize the egg.

Embryologists do not know whether the sperm they are injecting are genetically defective. So patients are left wondering whether the laboratory silver lining that enabled them to get pregnant may be hiding a cloud of genetic defects that will appear after the birth of their baby.

Several studies have been conducted to assess whether children born as a result of an ICSI procedure are normal. The Belgian group that developed the ICSI procedure did the first study.[4] This study evaluated 877 children born from ICSI procedures at two months, one year, and two years after birth. They found twelve cases of abnormal karyotypes (the chromosomal characteristics of a cell), all transmitted from the father. They speculated that these chromosomal aberrations were probably "linked directly to the characteristics of the infertile men treated rather than to the ICSI procedure itself."[5] They concluded that the 2.6 percent of major malformations in the children who were born is within the expected range in the general population. Nevertheless, they urged that patients contemplating the use of ICSI be counseled about potential risks.[6]

There have been several assessments of this first study. In one study involving ICSI follow-up,[7] researchers at Cornell studied 578 babies born after ICSI from procedures performed between 1993 and 1995. They found that 1.6 percent had major congenital abnormalities at birth and 1 percent had minor abnormalities affecting the urinary tract. They concluded that this proportion of abnormalities is "lower than the congenital abnormality rate seen in births in the general New York population."[8] Finally, in 1999 Great Britain established a National Registry of all babies born as a result of ICSI. As of 1999, there were 3,000 British babies born by means of this procedure. Hopefully, follow-up studies of these children will provide information about the risks of ICSI.[9]

The Belgian group continues to conduct follow-up research on ICSI. In a 1998 paper, they studied the mental development of 201 children at age two and found that their mental development was comparable to that of children born from standard IVF procedures.[10] And more recently, a British study of 123 singletons between one and two years old focused on mental and physical development in ICSI babies versus children conceived naturally.[11] These babies were comparable to those conceived naturally with the single exception that they had poorer eye-hand coordination. These researchers plan to follow up on this population again when the children are five years old.

ASSISTED HATCHING

To become pregnant, a sperm must fertilize an egg and the embryo created from this union must be able to implant in the endometrium.

ICSI solves the first part of this problem, but help is needed to get past the second hurdle. Until the time of implantation, eggs and embryos are surrounded by a protective protein "halo" called the zona pellucida (ZP). The ZP protects the embryo from attack by white blood cells, from bacterial infection, from physical damage by the environment, and from premature implantation in the fallopian tube. Some have speculated that embryos created in vitro can have harder ZPs than those created in the fallopian tube,[12] and the longer they remain in vitro, the harder their ZPs get. Also, women older than thirty-eight or women with elevated Day 3 FSH levels seem to have embryos with harder ZPs. If the embryo is to implant, it must first "hatch": ooze out of a hole in the ZP.

Scientists are not exactly sure how embryos hatch on their own, but they speculate about several mechanisms that may help. First, they think that some chemical created either by the embryo itself or by the female reproductive tract may eat away a part of the ZP and help the embryo to hatch. A second possibility is that, as the cells of the embryo grow inside the ZP, they exert pressure on the ZP like a balloon being blown up. This expanding pressure may cause a rupture in the ZP that enables implantation.

In the embryology laboratory the embryologist can use several techniques to help the embryos hatch. Assisted hatching can be done mechanically by dissecting the ZP using a technique called partial zona dissection (PZD). It can also be done using a laser, or chemically using acid in a technique called zona drilling (ZD). The chemical procedure is done by holding a six-to-eight-celled embryo in a dish using a holding pipette and making a small hole in the ZP using a second pipette containing an acidic solution. Then the excess acid is rinsed off, the embryo is put in an incubator, and several hours later it is transferred into the uterus. An even newer method uses a piezo-micro-manipulator together with a needle that responds to piezoelectric pulses to create a tiny hole in the thinned ZP. The embryos treated this way are not rinsed and are replaced in the uterus soon after this treatment.[13]

Does hatching increase the chances of a pregnancy? Research results suggest that sometimes it can increase the likelihood of a pregnancy and sometimes it can decrease it. Assisted hatching is most useful for women over age thirty-eight, for women with a high Day 3 FSH, and for embryos with thick zonas. If you do not fit into one of these categories and you use assisted hatching, it may lead to premature hatching and disintegration of the embryo. On the other hand, if you fall into one of the three categories above, hatching can increase the chance of your success. Be a Partner in Your Treatment. Talk with your physician and determine whether assisted hatching is right for you.

Blastocyst Transfer

When embryos grow in petri dishes in the laboratory, most stop dividing before they reach the size they would be when they implanted in the uterus if conception occurred naturally. Embryologists need to transfer these embryos before they die in the petri dish, so they transfer them one or two days after fertilization. These embryos are small, usually at the eight-cell stage, and the endometrium may not be ready for them to implant. What is needed is a way to grow these embryos in the laboratory for five days until they reach the blastocyst stage (30–150-celled stage of embryonic development). At the blastocyst stage, the embryo has outer surface cells called the trophectoderm, inner cells called the inner cell mass, and a central fluid-filled cavity. If this blastocyst implants and continues to develop, the trophectoderm will become the placenta and the inner cells will become the fetus.

Since only about 25 percent of embryos will survive to blastocyst stage, if all embryos were allowed to develop for five days, few patients would have embryos available to transfer. In contrast, about 85 percent of patients have larger than two-celled embryos that can be transferred on Day 2. Not all blastocysts are equally viable. Embryologists are currently studying ways to identify the most viable ones. Perhaps embryos created from the eggs of young fertile donors have the greatest likelihood of benefiting from blastocyst transfer. The high-quality oocytes retrieved from these donors increase the likelihood that the resulting embryos will survive to the blastocyst stage.

Efforts are under way to develop an approach that will enable embryos to develop to the blastocyst stage in vitro. At the time of this writing, researchers have had mixed success using transferred blastocysts. Some studies report increases in ongoing pregnancy rates for all their patients. Other studies find no difference in ongoing pregnancy rates using blastocysts as compared with standard embryos transferred several days earlier. It is also possible that the reason blastocyst transfer has higher success is that only the most viable embryos survive to blastocyst stage. Had those same embryos been transferred on the second day, they might also have resulted in a pregnancy.

RISKS AND BENEFITS OF BLASTOCYST TRANSFER

The risk of blastocyst transfer is that, by allowing embryos to remain in the laboratory until Day 5, many or perhaps all of them will not survive until the blastocyst stage. Had these embryos been transferred on Day 3, perhaps some would have implanted.

On the other hand, because blastocysts are more likely than two-to-eight-celled embryos to implant, doctors are able to transfer only one or two blastocysts as compared to the three to six less-developed embryos that are typically transferred. By transferring one or two blastocysts, it is possible to avoid the risks of getting pregnant with three or more embryos and thus avoid the Hobson's choice of a multifetal pregnancy reduction.

Preimplantation Genetic Diagnosis

Anyone thinking of getting pregnant hopes that she will give birth to a healthy baby. But because pregnancy has been harder to achieve, infertile women probably worry more about this than others. And there is reason to be worried. It is estimated that one in twenty members of our population are affected by a genetic disorder.[14] Additionally, as a woman gets older, her eggs are more likely to suffer from chromosomal abnormalities. Although eggs containing abnormalities can often be fertilized, they are likely to produce embryos that are genetically defective. Often a pregnancy created from these embryos will result in a pregnancy loss. Indeed, more than half of all pregnancy losses are the result of chromosomal abnormalities. Usually the problem is the result of having either one too many or one too few chromosomes, a condition known as aneuploidy.

Most cells in our bodies carry *two* sets of twenty-three chromosomes, one set obtained from our mother and the other from our father. Sperm cells and egg cells are different: They each contain only *one* set of twenty-three chromosomes, half the usual number, and are therefore called *haploid*. Two special chromosomes determine the gender of the child: X and Y chromosomes. Women (and mothers) always have *two* X chromosomes. Men (and fathers) always have *one* X *and one* Y chromosome. Because the sperm has only *one set of chromosomes* (it is haploid), a sperm cell may have either the X chromosome or the Y chromosome. On the other hand, despite the fact that the egg also only has one set of chromosomes, that one set will always contain an X chromosome. So the gender of a child will be determined by whether the sperm that fertilized the egg carried an X chromosome or a Y chromosome. As you can see, it is the male partner who determines the gender of the offspring resulting from fertilization.

Testing Embryos Before They Are Transferred

Embryologists can use one of two different techniques to do preimplantation diagnostic testing. One approach looks for *chromosomal* problems. The other technique looks for *genetic* defects. Currently there are only a few facilities in the United States that perform these techniques. Costs are about $5,000 and are typically not covered by insurance.

As the embryo develops, the number of its cells increases. The embryologist can make a gap in the outer covering of the embryo and gently remove one or two of the cells of the developing embryo and test them. She then returns the embryo to the incubator so it can continue to develop. While it is developing, she can look to see if there are too few or too many chromosomes. The process rarely damages the embryo.

The embryologist analyzes the cells using a technique called *fluorescence in-situ hybridization*, which has the acronym FISH. Different fluorescent colors attach to each chromosome. Embryologists are particularly interested in examining chromosomes 13, 18, 21, X, and Y. Because of FISH, it is possible to distinguish each of these chromosomes by its color. The process of testing the cells involves repeatedly heating and cooling them as they are glued to a slide. The process actually destroys these cells.

Be aware that sometimes (though it is rare) the cells extracted from the embryo to detect translocations (transfer of a chromosomal segment to a new position) may die during the procedure, making it impossible to obtain any useful information. Also keep in mind that once in a while (in less than 10 percent of cases), the test may provide no information or may provide ambiguous information.

The FISH technique is useful in detecting which chromosomes are present and which are absent in the nuclei of the cells being tested. The technique can also detect translocations (the fusion of part of one chromosome onto another) as well as aneuploidy. This technique can be used to screen for defects related to chromosomes. For example, trisomy 21 (trisomy means having three copies of a given chromosome in each somatic cell rather than the normal number of two), or Down's syndrome, is a condition that can be detected through FISH. If FISH can detect this condition, it can prevent the need to grapple with a decision about whether to abort a baby diagnosed with this condition through amniocentesis or raise a child with a handicap. Other related trisomy conditions that can be detected are trisomy 18 (a condition that can involve severe mental retardation and features such as cleft palate) and trisomy 13. In both of these conditions, children usually die before they reach their first birthday.

FISH is useful for ruling out other potential problems. These are genetic problems that are sex linked. Some genetic defects are found only on the Y chromosome. Since females do not inherit a Y chromosome, they cannot be affected by this disorder. In addition, some defects occur only on the X chromosome. Since females have two X chromosomes and males have only one, a man having a single recessive disease allele (any of the alternate forms of a gene) will develop this condition. On the other hand, a female must have two copies of the recessive allele in order for this disease to be expressed. Consequently, the ability to detect whether an embryo is male or female can provide useful information when there is concern about transmitting a particular sex-linked genetic disorder.

But FISH is not an appropriate technique for detecting genetic disorders. For that, the embryologist needs to use a PCR (polymerase chain reaction) technique. Currently, only about ten genetically based disorders can be detected—some through PCR and others that are sex linked—through FISH. This represents a minute fraction of the diseases attributed to genetic defects. Currently PCR performed on cells prior to implantation can detect the following genetic disorders: cystic fibrosis, Duchenne's and Becker's muscular dystrophy, Huntington's disease, beta-thalassemia, Marfan's syndrome, and sickle-cell disease. The Human Genome Project will undoubtedly increase this number manyfold. We hope that the next few years will see many break-throughs in techniques that will enable embryologists to detect prob-lems and avoid the heartbreak of a problem that occurs when you finally get pregnant when you thought you couldn't.

Embryo Transfer

Embryo transfer requires no anesthesia, although some patients prefer to have a mild sedative. The transfer procedure is very similar to what happens during an intrauterine insemination.

You will be asked to lie on a table or bed with your feet in stirrups. The doctor will use a catheter loaded with one or more embryos that have been suspended in a drop of culture medium. The doctor inserts the catheter into the cervix and deposits the embryos into the uterine cavity. The procedure takes ten to twenty minutes. Some clinics recom-mend that you remain on your back for two to four hours following the transfer.

Medically, an embryo transfer is fairly simple. Emotionally, it is rather complex. As these embryos enter your body, you may begin to think you are pregnant. After all, your body now contains fertilized eggs. Many women grow convinced that they have finally succeeded, that they are now "with embryo." Unfortunately, implantation is the aspect of ART that is least understood. Despite their ability to fertilize and transfer embryos, doctors are frustrated by their inability to exer-cise comparable control over the implantation process. Everyone involved must wait apprehensively for the next twelve days to see whether a pregnancy has occurred.

Post-Transfer Hormonal Support

Even though doctors cannot ensure that your embryos will implant successfully, they can help increase the odds. They know that an ample supply of progesterone increases the likelihood of a successful pregnancy. When a woman becomes pregnant on her own, the corpus luteum produces progesterone, which helps keep the uterine lining conducive to pregnancy. Sometimes, however, ART procedures can affect the ovary's progesterone production. Because of a diminished internal supply of progesterone, you must get it externally. You can take injections, use vaginal suppositories, use Crinone gel, or even take pills to get the needed supply of progesterone. You will use progesterone supplements up until you have your pregnancy test. If the test result is positive, you will continue to take progesterone for eight to ten weeks, or as long as your doctor deems necessary.

Cryopreservation

One option that most clinics make available is cryopreservation: freezing the excess embryos. In order to freeze embryos successfully, steps must be taken to protect them from damage during the freezing process. The embryologist needs to prevent a buildup of ice crystals inside the embryo that could expand and damage the cells. She does this by using propanediol or glycerol, which acts as antifreeze. She also uses a sugar solution to extract excess water through osmosis. Once the embryos have been protected using these methods, they are placed inside a plastic "freezing vial or straw." Then the embryologist labels each straw with the recipient's name.

The straw is placed in a special machine that gradually lowers the temperature to about −40 degrees Celsius. Then the straws are placed in a liquid nitrogen tank. At IVF New Jersey, where we consult, the lab has special backup power generators so that in the event of a power outage power will be available to maintain the proper temperature needed to preserve the embryos. Everyone at that practice was relieved that this backup was in place several summers ago when the local power utility instituted planned power brownouts to preserve scarce energy during a particularly brutal heat spell.

If you have cryopreserved some of your embryos, you can thaw them out for use in a future cycle. You may choose that option if, unfortunately, your fresh embryo transfer did not result in the birth of a baby. You may also choose this option if you did give birth to a baby and several years later want to have another pregnancy.

Many of the excess embryos created during an IVF cycle are not suitable for freezing. The experience of the embryologists at IVF New Jersey has taught them that poor-quality embryos (those with greater than 25 percent fragmentation or with an inappropriate number of cells) will not survive the freeze and subsequent thawing-out process.

Patients wishing to use thawed frozen embryos can use one of two procedures: In a natural cycle the physician monitors the cycle to detect the LH surge and then transfers the embryos three or four days later. The other alternative is to use estrogen and progesterone to prepare the uterine lining and then transfer the embryos. With either of these methods you need to make fewer visits to the clinic to be monitored than you would if you were taking fertility medications in preparation for a fresh cycle.

New developments in cryopreservation techniques are enabling about 80 percent of frozen embryos to survive the freeze-thaw process.* However, the latest available statistics from the CDC indicate that 18.6 percent of all frozen embryo transfers result in a live birth. For comparison purposes, the figure for live births resulting from fresh transfers is 29.7 percent.[†]

*For a discussion of these techniques, see Schmidt, C. 1991 "Cycle of Replacement for Frozen Embryos: Natural or Artificial," in *In Vitro Fertilization and Embryo Transfer: A Comprehensive Update*. Santa Barbara, CA: UCLA School of Medicine, 174–206.
[†]Centers for Disease Control. February 2000. *Assisted Reproduction in the United States: 1997 Results*.

Frozen embryo transfers can create some unusual questions. Consider this case, reported in the November 1991 issue of *Fertility and Sterility*:[15] In March 1985, a doctor in Australia collected eggs from a woman, fertilized them, and obtained six embryos. Three were transferred immediately, and the remaining three were frozen. One of the freshly transferred embryos developed into a baby girl who was born in December 1985. In January 1987, the same woman received one of her frozen embryos, which developed into another baby girl, born in October 1987. Finally, in November 1989, the woman had the last two frozen embryos thawed and transferred to her womb. In September 1990, the woman gave birth to a baby boy.

So what are these babies? Are they triplets or three single children? From the point of view of a biologist, they are triplets, since they were conceived simultaneously. But from the parents' point of view, these children are singletons, born years apart. For the infertile couple, they are a blessing regardless of when or how they were conceived.

How healthy are babies conceived from frozen embryos? A study in the British medical journal *The Lancet* reported on the experience of one Scandinavian clinic that followed children born from cryopreserved embryos.[16] They matched 255 children conceived from frozen embryos with 255 children conceived from fresh embryos and 252 children made "the old-fashioned way." There were no significant differences in the number of problems in any of these groups. Six children in the cryopreserved group had major malformations compared with eight children in the fresh embryo group and nine children who were conceived spontaneously.

Pregnancy Testing

The most taxing phase of ART procedures is waiting for the results of a pregnancy test. Twelve days after embryo transfer, your doctor will take a blood sample and analyze your hCG level. If hCG is detected in your blood, you are pregnant. In the next chapter we offer an activity to help you stay hopeful but realistic during this difficult waiting period.

Multifetal Pregnancy Reduction

IVF programs have been perilously walking a line between transferring too few or too many embryos. Transfer too few and the patient has low odds of getting pregnant. Transfer too many and she risks a multiple pregnancy with the possibility of having to undergo a multifetal pregnancy reduction, a procedure where one or more fetuses is aborted so as to increase the chance that at least one healthy baby will be born.

Doctors and patients want to avoid a pregnancy with three or more fetuses. Such a pregnancy can put the mother at risk for problems such as pregnancy-induced high blood pressure, anemia, blood clots, or severe postpartum bleeding. The babies may also be at risk. When a woman carries three or more babies, they are at higher risk for premature birth, low birth weight, chromosomal anomalies, or other birth defects.

Multifetal pregnancy reduction, sometimes referred to as selective reduction, is a relatively recent technique. Although it was pioneered in 1986, it did not come into widespread use until the early 1990s. The decision to use this technique is a difficult one, and many couples facing this choice wrestle with guilt and a great moral, ethical, or religious dilemma. In many ways they face a more upsetting decision than one faced by a couple experiencing an unwanted or unplanned pregnancy. A multifetal pregnancy is the result of a planned intervention—the transfer of a large number of embryos. Had the doctors not tried so hard to ensure that the couple would get pregnant and replaced three or fewer embryos, it is likely that the couple would not face this choice. The practice of transferring many embryos and then using selective reduction has come to the attention of people opposing abortion, and protests at fertility clinics have taken place. Those people who oppose abortion may begin not merely protesting but also lobbying against ART because, in their minds, it increases the likelihood of abortions. If your ethical or religious convictions would not permit you to have a fetal reduction and you would not want to carry and raise triplets, you should share this information with your doctor when planning your procedure.

HOW REDUCTION IS DONE

Multifetal pregnancy reduction is performed in the first trimester. The reduction can be carried out in one of three ways: transabdominally, transcervically, or transvaginally. The abdominal approach is most commonly used. Typically, a specialist other than the physician who does the IVF procedure performs the procedure.

The details of the procedure are somewhat gruesome. In the transabdominal approach the physician uses an ultrasound machine to guide a needle into the chest of the fetus. He injects potassium chloride into the baby's heart to get it to stop beating. Sometimes the heart starts beating again after it has stopped and a second injection is required. After the baby dies, it is usually reabsorbed into the mother's body. Sometimes, when a reduction is done late, a small amount of tissue from the dead baby is present at the same time when the mother delivers her liveborn. If a transcervical approach is used, the lowest embryos are reduced by suction. With any of these procedures there is a risk that you may lose the entire pregnancy. In fact, one study assessing this risk found that 8 percent of women using this procedure lost the entire pregnancy.[17]

SUCCESS STATISTICS OF ART PROCEDURES

Many patients seeking ART overestimate their odds of success. Part of our job at IVF New Jersey is to help these couples become more realistic. (One couple we counseled thought they had an 80 percent chance of getting pregnant on their first ART attempt.) By understanding that the odds are always against you for any given cycle, you can avoid becoming overly distressed if the procedure fails.

It's important not to blind yourself with unrealistic hope. But we also urge you not to despair over the statistics. In the next chapter we will give you some activities to help you balance hope and despair and to assess realistically your odds of success with repeated ART attempts.

SOME FINAL THOUGHTS

Some people are reluctant to try ART because they view it as unnatural or as meddling with nature. Others are reluctant to give up on ART despite repeated failures. For them, abandoning treatment means giving up on their dream. Regardless of where you are on this spectrum, expect to encounter a certain degree of emotional turmoil as you venture into the world of high-tech infertility treatment. The next chapter can help you cope.

CHAPTER 8

Helping Yourself Through ART— Financially and Emotionally

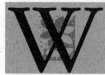hen Kristen's doctor suggested she take Clomid after failing to conceive after twelve months of trying, Kristen was shocked. How could I manipulate my menstrual cycle like this? she thought. As time went on with no pregnancy, Kristen slowly accepted the logic of her doctor's advice and began taking Clomid. When Clomid didn't work, Kristen's doctor recommended that she advance to Pergonal.[1] But again, Kristen was reluctant.

"I can't believe I'm doing some of the things I'm doing now," Kristen told us during a counseling session. "I said I'd never take Pergonal, and then I did. Six months later, the doctor told me I needed to have inseminations. I said, 'No way, I'll never do it' . . . and I did it."

Kristen also had recoiled at the thought of advanced reproductive treatment (ART). But eventually she did that, too.

What allowed Kristen to change her attitude, to move her "line in the sand" in order to do something she previously considered repugnant? According to psychologist Kurt Lewin,[2] the key was Kristen's ability to remove roadblocks that initially prevented her from trying something new.

Generally speaking, people feel most comfortable maintaining the status quo. For example, it's easier to stay in a job that is not boosting your career than it is to quit and look for something more fulfilling.

Likewise, it is far easier to repeat cycles involving Pergonal injections and intrauterine insemination (IUIs) month after month than it is to abandon the familiar routine and take the emotional and financial risks involved with ART. If you have been engaging in low-tech treatments for six months to a year and still haven't had a baby, you have reached a set of crossroads—and a daunting one at that. Your choices: Continue your current treatment, move to more advanced treatment, or give up trying to become pregnant altogether. If everything else has failed and you still want to give birth, ART may be your only viable alternative.

MOVING FROM LOW-TECH TO HIGH-TECH TREATMENT

As much as you want to be pregnant, the idea of taking massive doses of fertility drugs and then having your eggs plucked out of your ovaries might paralyze you with fear.

In addition to fear, there are three other major roadblocks encountered by most people considering ART: insufficient finances, job stress, and lack of support from family and friends. In this chapter we will show you how to break through those roadblocks. We also will teach you how to remain optimistic but realistic while engaging in these exciting new treatments.

Identifying Roadblocks

Let's look at two diagrams that we helped Kristen prepare. The act of making the diagrams helped Kristen conquer her fears and move from Clomid to Pergonal, and then to add inseminations to her treatment regimen.

Kristen was stuck in the Clomid-treatment status quo. She was telling herself: "Pills are one thing, but injections are something else. I am drawing the line at Clomid." Kristen needed to Change Her Thinking. She used Getting Pregnant Self-Talk (GPST) to help move her line in the sand. She told herself: "Injections are a small price to pay for having a baby. I will take Pergonal."

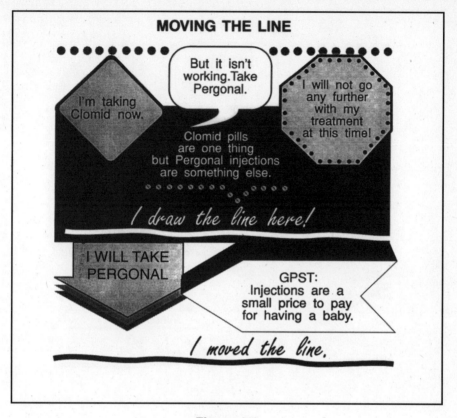

Figure 8.1

Unfortunately, Kristen did not get pregnant with Pergonal alone. Her doctor said she needed to combine Pergonal and artificial inseminations with her husband's sperm. Kristen balked. Here's a diagram of her thoughts and how she Changed Her Thinking to "move the line" once again.

Kristen used the same approach to help her move the line to try ART. You can use Kristen's method to help you change your mindset—to help you try the more advanced treatment your doctor may be suggesting. On page 205 is a blank form for you to fill out that can help you move on.

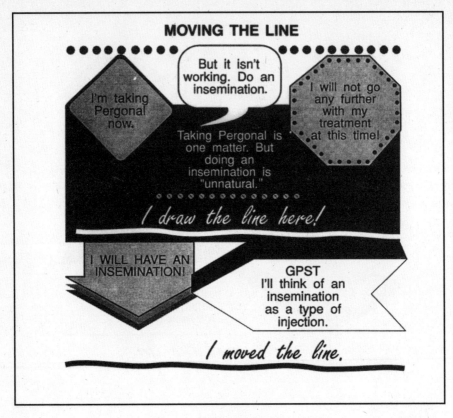

Figure 8.2

Having changed her attitude, Kristen now needed to remove the roadblocks to ART and get psyched up for the rigors of high-tech treatment. Like Kristen you need to:

- Educate Yourself about medical insurance for infertility;
- Manage Your Social Life by garnering the support of your family and friends;
- Make Effective Decisions; and
- Motivate Yourself to hang in despite setbacks: Don't Give Up.

To accomplish these goals, we ask you to draw upon the skills you mastered in the Getting Pregnant Workout.

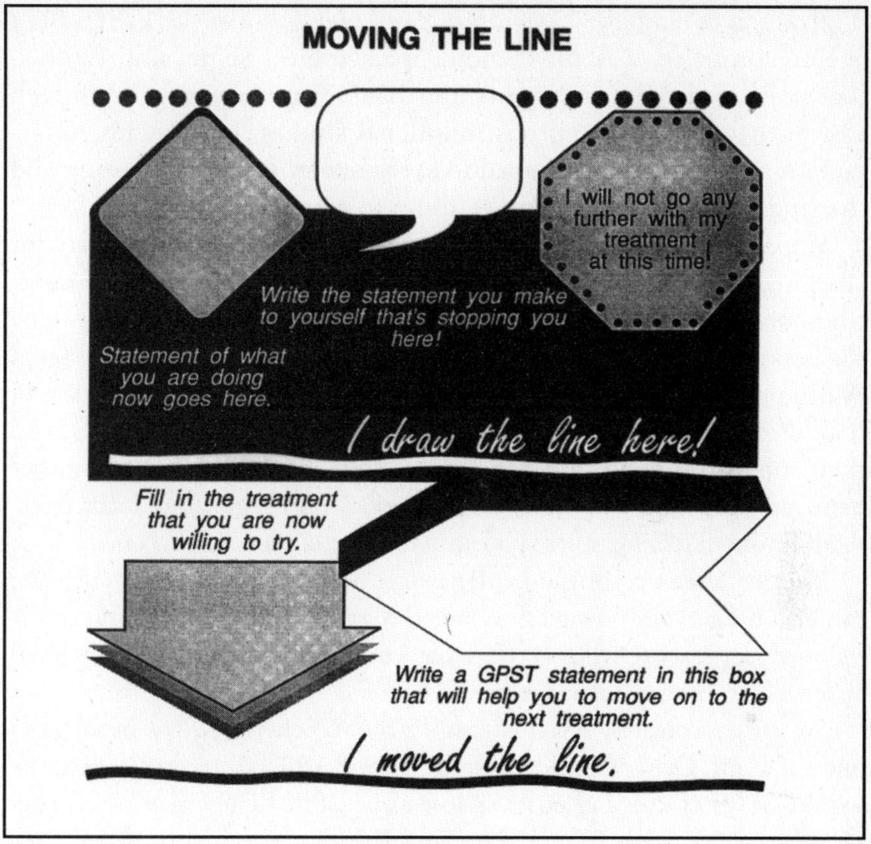

Figure 8.3

BLOOD AND MONEY: PAYING FOR INFERTILITY TREATMENT

By the time you've begun thinking about ART, you've probably gotten used to having blood taken out of your arm for various tests. While parting with a vial of your blood has become second nature, parting with your money gets more and more difficult as infertility treatment goes on. Even if you are insured, many polices have limited benefits for infertility treatment. For most people, the high cost of ART becomes the major roadblock to getting pregnant when they thought they couldn't.

Scores of patients we have interviewed ranked money as the number one or number two factor (behind psychological or physical trauma) that prevented them from pursuing ART. Every aspect of high-tech treatment costs money: drugs, hormonal studies, ultrasounds, interpretation of results, professional fees, the operating room, freezing and thawing embryos, and sperm washing, to name a few.

You can't completely begrudge infertility doctors and technicians for charging so much. Thanks to their knowledge and training, many infertile couples are getting pregnant. Certainly you want your doctor to be the best that money can buy. But you also wish his fees weren't so steep. When presented with the bill, it is easy to succumb to the unfairness of it all: People lucky enough to get pregnant the "regular" way can spend their money on baby furniture and college funds. You, on the other hand, are spending your hard-earned money on Pergonal and surgeries. And, unlike fertile couples, you aren't even guaranteed success.

We can offer no simple explanations for the inequities of life. We can encourage you, however, to face the issue of money in a pragmatic manner, separating your grief over your infertility from a rational approach to money management.

For many couples, ART is simply too expensive to try more than once, if at all. Other couples who can afford ART fail to investigate the various ways of keeping costs as low as possible. They may be embarrassed to work with their doctor and insurance company to enhance their reimbursements. Instead of fighting for what rights or services are theirs, they withdraw, give up, and mourn their predicament. They are engaging in what psychologist Martin Seligman, author of the national best-seller *Learned Optimism*, calls learned helplessness.[3]

In contrast, we urge you to Be Assertive and leave no avenue unexplored that might help you loosen ART's financial pinch. While the following section emphasizes ART insurance coverage, it also pertains to coverage for low-tech infertility treatments.

Insurance and Infertility Coverage

Insurers and infertile couples always seem to be battling over costs. Until infertile couples took on the roles of advocates, few, if any, insurers automatically paid for infertility treatment. In the last several years, however, infertile couples have been successfully lobbying state legislatures to pass laws requiring insurers to cover their medical bills.

As of April 2000, twelve states have enacted infertility-insurance legislation: Arkansas, California, Connecticut, Hawaii, Illinois, Maryland, Massachusetts, Montana, New York, Ohio, Rhode Island, and Texas. Specific information about legislation for each of these twelve states can be found at the Web site of the American Society for Reproductive Medicine (http://www.asrm.org).

What Can You Expect?

In a RESOLVE of Central Jersey newsletter, attorney Raymond Godwin summarized differences among various state laws dealing with infertility insurance. According to Godwin, "Other differences include, for example, the length of time a couple has experienced infertility (Arkansas: two years; Maryland: five years) before coverage is allowed; the exemption of employers with a certain number of employees (California: fewer than 20; Illinois: fewer than 25); and whether only the husband's sperm can be used with IVF and GIFT."

If you live in any of these twelve states, you probably have a better chance of having some of the costs reimbursed than if you live elsewhere. But if you do not meet all the conditions set forth under the law (i.e., length of time you've been trying to have a baby, medical condition, or use of your own gametes), the law may work against you. On the other hand, insurance may in fact cover your diagnosis and treatment, even if you live in one of the other thirty-eight states.

At the time of this writing, the majority of insurance carriers cover between 50 percent and 80 percent of "conventional" infertility treatments.[4] In terms of in vitro fertilization, 41 percent of commercial health-insurance carriers provide coverage. One in four do so as a standard practice, and the remainder do so on a case-by-case basis.[5]

For lesser, low-tech procedures, most BlueCross and BlueShield plans cover much of the diagnostic testing. As long as the insurance company can justify a treatment as leading up to the diagnosis of an illness or condition, the company will reimburse you for surgeries, blood tests, diagnostic tests (like the HSG or endometrial biopsy), and ultrasound scans.

Insurance companies do not consider infertility to be the illness itself; their argument is that most procedures bypass rather than cure the problem and are "experimental" in nature.

But don't lose hope or make assumptions. There are various ways to find out definitely what, if any, infertility tests and treatments your policy covers. One couple we know assumed that their insurance would not reimburse them for $700 of out-of-pocket expenses for Lupron during an IVF cycle. The insurer had initially turned down their claim, but the couple resubmitted it, pointing out that the FDA had recently approved Lupron for the treatment of endometriosis, a recognized contributor to infertility. The argument was convincing enough that the insurer reimbursed their $700.

Finding Out What Your Insurance Company Covers

Determining which infertility treatments your policy covers can be tricky. On one hand, you want accurate information. On the other hand, you risk alerting your insurer to the fact that you are about to undergo infertility treatment. If you are covered by a group plan, you cannot be disenrolled for medical reasons. But if you have individual coverage, there is always the possibility that the insurer will try to cancel your policy if it anticipates costly claims on the horizon. There are ways, however, to make inquiries about coverage without jeopardizing your policy.

The first step is to read your claims booklet carefully. This booklet may contain statements like "the treatment of infertility is not provided through the general policy, but may be part of a rider clause negotiated by a specific group." Your personnel manager should be able to give you a copy of the rider. Even though infertility treatment (particularly in vitro procedures or even inseminations) may not be covered, try to find out if diagnostic blood tests and ultrasound procedures are, and, if so, how many are covered. From the booklet you may be able to deduce which diagnoses are more likely than others to be reimbursable.

You also will want to know what percentage of treatment costs are typically covered by the policy. Sometimes, instead of paying a percentage of a medical bill, some companies offer a flat fee. They may, for example, pay up to $45 for any blood analysis, even if your analysis costs $100. Try to find out what the general fee schedule is, particularly if you have ever seen the following explanation (or one like it) from the insurer when it only partially reimbursed you: "This charge has been declared over and above the customary fees charged by medical professionals in your area." Finally, try to find out about deductibles and at what ceiling your coverage changes. Many companies begin to offer a higher percentage of coverage when your co-payment ceiling is reached. For example, our carrier pays 80 percent of specific charges until the total bill reaches $2,000, at which point they cover 100 percent of certain charges. Also try to find out which drugs may be covered. Injectable fertility medications are all costly. Some insurers cover them, others do not. Some policies have an annual dollar limit for prescriptions. If you are lucky, your policy includes a liberal prescription plan that covers almost all prescription medications (except birth-control pills), with a small co-payment by you. If your claims booklet fails to answer all your questions about covered medications, your pharmacist, who deals with numerous insurance carriers every day, may be able to answer some of your questions.

If you are still baffled after reading the claims booklet (some of them are notoriously vague and confusing), schedule an interview with the benefits representatives or personnel managers at your and your husband's workplaces. Begin at the workplace that provides your primary coverage, and then move to the workplace that provides your secondary coverage. Even if you've chosen to keep your fertility problem a secret from your boss and co-workers, we encourage you to level with your benefits representative, urging him or her to maintain your confidentiality. By giving the representative specifics about your condition, you are apt to walk out of the meeting knowing exactly how much—if any—money you will personally have to fork over for your treatment. Also, knowing exactly how many of those treatments are covered can help you Make a Plan.

Another good source of information is a co-worker or friend who has the same policy you do and has undergone infertility diagnosis and treatment. This individual should be able to give you the "lowdown" on the insurer's payment record and can alert you to any land mines. Even if this person is only an acquaintance, remember that there is an allegiance of sorts among infertile people. Having suffered and survived the experience, most of us are eager to help and comfort others in any way we can.

You may have no choice but to call your insurance company, which probably provides a toll-free number for its beneficiaries. If the insurance representative tells you something is covered either by the general policy or under a rider to that policy, write down the representative's name, exactly what he or she told you, and the date and time of your call. If possible, have the representative confirm your conversation in writing. This letter can become invaluable should you need to appeal a claim denial in the future. Some insurers require a letter from your doctor estimating the cost of an ART treatment prior to considering any claims related to that treatment. The request for such a letter doesn't necessarily mean your claim will be turned down. It's a tool insurance carriers use to budget for their future outlays. We also encourage you to read the detailed question-and-answer section that focuses on insurance in Chapter 15.

Reducing the Stress of Financial Strain

"Going in the hole" to finance infertility treatment is stressful and can provoke marital strife. If you and your partner have agreed to set aside money for important life goals, your suggestion that you allocate that money for ART can spur an argument about priorities, for example. Even if your heart is set on ART, your husband might argue that the money you spend on treatment will render you unable to afford an adoption should the procedure fail.

To minimize or even prevent these conflicts, we urge you to employ the skills described in the Getting Pregnant Workout. You and your spouse must Listen and Level with one another about how to handle this financial crisis. We further recommend using the decision-making exercises described earlier in this book to decide whether to pursue ART or to spend that money on adoption.

At this point you may decide that "enough is enough." The money crisis may be the straw that breaks the camel's back. You may have been able to bounce back from failed cycles, cope with injections and medication, and deal with the disruption in your social life. But spending your last penny or borrowing money you may never be able to repay may just be more than you can handle. If you are unable to continue treatment because the costs are beyond your means, you are not giving up—you are merely being realistic. But if, somehow, you are able to hang in financially, you need to consider ways to finance your ART treatment.

How Deep Are Your Pockets?

Before you begin an IVF cycle, make sure you have enough money to pay for it should the insurance company fall through or fail to cover fully all your medical bills. You may want to sell some stock, dip into your savings account, borrow money from a bank or relative, skip a vacation (or two), or otherwise modify your lifestyle to shore up the necessary funds.

In examining your current financial wherewithal, first look at your savings accounts, CDs, and money market funds and decide if you can liquidate any of these assets. Are you expecting any lump sums this year, such as an inheritance or a lawsuit settlement? One couple told us they waited until they got their tax refund every year and used that money for several Pergonal/IUI cycles.

Next, explore loan programs at your workplace or through the bank where you do business. Family or friends may be able to lend you money at very low interest. Some lucky couples have well-to-do family members who are happy to make a monetary contribution toward their pregnancy quest. As a very last resort, you can charge ART to your Visa or MasterCard. While this option gives you quick money, don't forget that consumer-credit interest rates are extremely high.

Before you borrow money, even at low interest, try to think ahead about how you will pay back the loan. And brace yourself for the possibility that you may wind up making loan payments for a procedure that failed to get you pregnant.

An alternative to dipping into your savings or borrowing money is to take an extra job or become involved in a project that generates money, such as selling Tupperware or baking something special for a local gourmet shop. If you choose this route, discipline yourself to put your entire extra paycheck into a "getting pregnant account" each week. Also, begin and finish your additional job prior to undergoing high-tech treatment. Maintaining an additional job at the same time you are involved in ART can raise your level of stress to the point where it may diminish your chances of becoming pregnant.

Reducing the Cost of ART

A different approach to making ART more affordable is getting your doctor or IVF clinic to reduce fees. Recently, some of the larger clinics have developed "scholarship" programs and sliding-scale fees based on the couple's need and ability (or inability) to pay. Such programs are designed to assist infertile people who desperately want treatment but who have exhausted their insurance coverage and personal resources. Clinics tend to favor couples who have already completed several cycles there and who are believed to have a good potential for success if they try one or two more times.

One plan to reduce costs is to find a clinic that offers a "money-back guarantee." This procedure is called "risk sharing." In this case, the clinic usually allows only women who are "good candidates" (i.e., under age forty with a normal Day 3 FSH level, etc.) to undergo IVF paying a higher-than-normal rate. If they do not become pregnant, they receive either part of their money back or another IVF cycle for free. If they become pregnant on the first cycle, they have paid more than the usual cost and the clinic keeps the extra. In effect, couples who *do* become pregnant on the first try are subsidizing the cost for couples who do not. The clinic is also sharing in the risk and, for this reason, this practice is limited to "good prognosis" candidates. (Pacific Fertility Center in San Francisco is one clinic that has such a program.)

Another approach is to ask your practice to accept, as full payment, what your insurance picks up. If your insurance will pick up part of the cost and you anticipate that you'll have trouble making up the difference, you might be able to persuade your doctor or clinic to accept as payment in full whatever your insurance company is willing to reimburse. Always talk to the doctor before you begin a cycle about any arrangement of this sort.

Finally, some women who have produced many eggs in a previous IVF cycle may be able to work out an agreement to finance their next cycle by donating any extra eggs made in that cycle in exchange for free medication or a lowering of fees.

Preparing Your Bills to Submit to Insurance

Many infertility doctors and programs are willing to "work" with insurance companies and couples to help obtain the maximum coverage to which their patients are entitled. Toward this end, many doctor's offices and clinics employ a benefits counselor to help patients navigate the insurance maze. Be sure to discuss your ideas and concerns with this individual before your bills are prepared.

Here are some tips:

- Don't list "infertility" as a diagnosis. Instead use the cause of your infertility, such as endometriosis, endocrine dysfunction, ovarian failure, tubal occlusion, fibroids, polycystic ovaries, or low sperm count. The reason is that insurers are more apt to cover treatment for precise diagnoses than they are treatment for infertility.
- Break down a particular procedure into its smallest components. Instead of insemination, for example, which may or may not be covered by your policy, the bill should reflect a series of less costly items such as cervical dilation, mucus check, sperm washing, office visit, etc. Always use as many treatment codes (called CPT codes) as possible.
- Specify dates. If you are having a series of ultrasound scans, blood tests, or office visits, make sure each bill states the date and the individual costs for each instead of lumping all the scans and tests into a single day's billing.
- Don't overlook the potential of being reimbursed for office visits. If you are seeing your doctor frequently, ask the billing manager to vary the CPT code number of the office visits. Office visits are listed with numbers such as 90020 (initial visit), 90060 (office visit), 90080 (comprehensive visit), and other numbers in between 90020 and 90080. Insurance companies are more likely to cover CPT codes that are in the middle range (not initial consultation or comprehensive office visit), code numbers such as 90030, 90050, or 90060.

- If you are undergoing various procedures over a two- or three-week period, submit insurance claims on different forms in separate envelopes.

Try not to view insurance companies as the "bad guys." It's more beneficial if you play their "word game," using their parlance in all your verbal and written contact. Remember, your claim is handled by a person who is administering a rigorously designed policy. By following insurance-industry rhetoric, you won't call undue attention to your claim. Also remember: Never lie. Outright cheating is insurance fraud. Your goal is to enable your claims to be considered easily and quickly.

Keeping Track of Insurance Payments

Almost all doctors demand payment at the time of treatment and let you play the waiting game with the insurance company. If you submit claims in the manner we recommend, within a few weeks your reimbursement checks will begin to trickle in. In some cases, you may have to resubmit claims to major medical or your secondary insurer. It is at this point where the "shoe box" organization system—the one where you stick everything into a box—grows into a hurricane of paperwork. The number of claims at different stages of processing can become overwhelming and extremely stressful, especially if you lose or misplace a bill or correspondence.

Lori, a participant in one of our support groups, shared with us her relatively simple system of keeping track of insurance claims. She set up three file folders.

- Folder 1 contains bills that have not been submitted to insurance yet. It is labeled BILLS TO BE SUBMITTED.
- Folder 2 contains bills that have been submitted but no word has been received concerning their payment. It is labeled BILLS PENDING.
- Folder 3 is for bills that have been reimbursed. It is labeled BILLS REIMBURSED.

As soon as Lori gets a receipt from her IVF clinic, she fills out an insurance form and immediately photocopies both the form and the receipt. The photocopies are for her records—to be used should any question arise or should anything get lost in the mail. If she can't mail in the claim that day, she places the originals and the photocopies in Folder 1.

After she mails in the claim, the copy of the receipt goes into Folder 2. When the reimbursement check arrives or the doctor receives payment from the insurer, Lori staples the check stub or record of payment to the copies of the receipt and the insurance form and transfers all documents to Folder 3. Lori told us that Getting Organized in this manner helped her keep track of a very complicated process and gave her a welcome sense of control.

Contesting a Claim

If you are undergoing long-term infertility treatment, chances are you eventually will exceed your coverage limit. When this happens, you can contest or appeal the denial of your claim. There are two basic ways of accomplishing this: by telephone or by letter.

Appealing by Phone: Before you make your call, have handy all the relevant information: your policy number, copies of the bills, and notification of denial. Ask the insurance representative to explain why your claim was denied. If the representative is unsure, ask to speak to his or her superior. If the superior cannot make a determination, ask what information you and your doctor must submit to ensure that the claim is covered.

Appealing by Letter: Your letter should state clearly that you want your claim reevaluated because your doctor maintains that the treatment was medically necessary. If you received reimbursement for the same treatment previously, mention that unless the contract stipulates a cash ceiling or a number limit on treatments, insurance cannot stop paying for that procedure if the medical necessity continues. Even if there is a number limit, say, three IVFs, explain that the prior procedures were diagnostic in nature and that the information gleaned from those procedures suggested modifications in the current treatment. In addition to your letter, most insurers also require a letter written by your doctor explaining why he or she believes continued treatment is necessary.

PSYCHING YOURSELF UP BEFORE, DURING, AND AFTER TREATMENT

Many psychologists tell their infertile clients to be pessimistic. "Don't get your hopes up because if the procedure fails, you will be too disappointed," they warn. Perhaps these psychologists fear that they will somehow be blamed if the procedure fails to result in a pregnancy.

We encourage our clients to be hopeful. We find it hard to imagine how anyone would endure the ordeal of infertility treatments if they believed from the outset that all the pain and sacrifice was to be in vain.

While we tout optimism, we also ask our clients to adopt the realistic view that the procedure might, indeed, fail. We believe that having a good balance of hope and realism has helped our clients cope better with the despair brought on by a failed ART attempt or insemination. Staying hopeful is time-consuming and takes work, but the "work of hoping" can have a positive impact on your emotional and physical health.

A key ingredient to our philosophy is one of the strategies that permeates this book: Don't Give Up. Infertility specialists agree that both low- and high-tech treatments take time to work, and while your chances of pregnancy are fairly low for each individual cycle, the chances increase dramatically when these attempts are repeated. The vast majority of our clients firmly believe that optimism and hope enabled them to withstand the rigors of treatment.

This is not to say you should continue battling infertility until you are emotionally and financially bankrupt. But neither should you engage in treatment if you aren't able to temper your pessimism with hope. Hope is a powerful motivator. But hope needs to be realistic—not blind.

Models of Hope

People vary in how much weight they give to hope and its counterpart, despair. We present three cases, each of which balances the prospect of success and possibilities of failure in different ways. Consider these three characters, each of whom is about to have a second ART procedure. Try to decide which of these models best describes you.

Rosie Sunshine Rosie sees everything through rose-colored glasses. Her hopeful outlook filters out all information that pertains to potential failure. When Rosie undergoes an ART procedure that has a 30 percent pregnancy rate, she tells herself: "I know it will work." She never considers the 70 percent chance that it will fail. She never prepares herself for despair in the event of failure. While she is pleasant company, Rosie is deluding herself. Surely she cannot continue ignoring negative information indefinitely. If her ART procedure fails, her strategy of unabridged optimism could collapse, crushing her will to give it another try. *Rosie hopes for success and denies the possibility of failure.*

Gladys Gloomsbury Gladys's outlook is steeped in pessimism. Facing the same ART procedure that Rosie tried (with its 30 percent chance of success), Gladys focuses solely on the 70 percent chance of failure. She says, "I'm sure this procedure won't work for me. Other procedures have failed in the past; why should this one work?" In her mind, she changes the failure rate from 70 percent to 100 percent. Psychologically, Gladys has given up. She avoids any information that might remind her that there is a three-in-ten chance of success. Her point of view bodes ill for the future. *Gladys excludes hope from her life and focuses on impending failure.*

Olga Optimistic Olga pays attention to both success and failure rates. When Olga participates in the ART procedure discussed above, she tells herself: "I'm real hopeful that this procedure will work. Sure, there's a 70 percent possibility that it won't work this time. But there's also a 30 percent chance that it will work. And if it fails, I can always try again." She permits herself to entertain negative information, but invests energy in the positive elements. Hers is a mature hope. *Olga hopes for success but accepts the possibility of failure.*

Obviously, the healthiest strategy is Olga's. Like Olga, you need to have hope, but not at the expense of distorting reality. Olga is savvy without being so negative that she can't get out of bed or so positive that she has already furnished the nursery. If you are feeling more like Gladys or Rosie, here are some ways you can begin to see your world through Olga's eyes.

Using the Odds to Help, Not Hinder You

As you begin to incorporate hope into your life, you must first learn your personal odds for success. Consider the following scenario: You are about to undergo an IVF procedure. Your doctor estimates that your odds of becoming pregnant through IVF are 30 percent for each attempt. Now, 30 percent is not a high probability. In fact, it means that you have a 70 percent chance of failure.

But your doctor also tells you that you must be patient and give IVF a chance. "If it doesn't work the first time," he tells you, "try it again. I know that your insurance will pay for at least three attempts. I think you should consider trying IVF three times before giving up." He also points out that, although the odds are only 30 percent on any given try, in three tries the odds increase to about 66 percent.[6] So if you play the odds, after three attempts you will have almost a 66 percent chance of success and only a 34 percent chance of failure. Clearly there is a chance of failure, but the odds of ultimate success are certainly worth shooting for.

Next you must change the way you look at the odds to have them work for you, not against you. We have developed a simple exercise called Counting Backward to help couples accomplish this goal. Counting Backward helps you Change Your Thinking. Beginning with your first IVF procedure, say to yourself, "By the end of the year, I have a good chance of being pregnant." Then, if your first IVF does not lead to a pregnancy, say "One down, only two more to go until my odds of being pregnant are very high." With each failed procedure, focus on how your pregnancy is now more likely to happen rather than focusing on how many times you have failed. The odds, as well as how you look at them, are an important piece of information that can help keep you reality-based yet hopeful through repeated attempts at getting pregnant through ART. This tactic works equally well with inseminations and other low-tech treatments.

Hoping Through a Procedure: Working at Being Realistically Optimistic

The work of hoping is an ongoing process. One important facet of the work of hoping is sequencing the focus of attention from the possibility of failure to the likelihood of success—throughout the progression of treatment. Through sequencing, you can balance hope and realism and avoid being overwhelmed by the enormity of what you are doing. Because so many infertile couples feel they are on an emotional roller coaster, we use that metaphor to divide that roller-coaster "ride" into four phases:

- Before the procedure: standing on line to board the roller coaster
- During the procedure: riding the roller coaster
- Waiting for results: getting off the ride and waiting to feel either invigorated and elated or sick to your stomach
- Reassessing before the next treatment: psyching yourself up to get back in line for another roller-coaster ride

Here's how sequencing might go for the IVF procedure, with its 30 percent chance of success:

- *Before the procedure,* think about the potential for success (30 percent) and failure (70 percent). By doing so, you can start on level ground. Say, "Realistically, the odds are more in favor of failure than of success. I'm prepared for that. But I do know that I have a chance for success. Maybe this will be my month."
- *During the procedure,* work at being as hopeful as possible. Since you've already allowed yourself to entertain the possibility of failure, you have protected yourself emotionally. Now is the time to let yourself rise to the peak of hopefulness. During the procedure, be as hopeful as possible. Concentrate only on the possibility of success. Repeat to yourself, "I know this will work."
- *While waiting for the results,* you must be hopeful but also begin to prepare yourself again for the possibility of failure. You feel yourself slowly descending from the summit of hope you attained during the procedure. The potential for failure begins to loom large again. Work at focusing predominantly on the positive side, but also entertain a few negative thoughts. Try to say, "I've got a good chance. I know it might fail, but I hope this will be my month."
- *If the procedure fails,* let your negative thoughts flow freely, even if they pull you to the depths of despair. This is your legitimate

time to grieve. Give yourself permission to feel sad. At the same time, try to muster some positive thoughts. After a while, those positive thoughts will help you accept the failure and become strong enough to try again. Tell yourself, "I'm so disappointed that it didn't work last month. I need time to deal with this. I'm not giving up, but I'm not ready to make any plans."

Couples who can equip themselves to handle the roller-coaster emotions of infertility treatment are the least likely to suffer the devastation that ill-equipped couples can experience when a procedure fails. By learning to balance hope and reality, you are developing a psychological arsenal to protect you from serious emotional wounds.

An Activity to Help You Sequence Hope and Despair

Directions: This activity will help you do "the work of hoping." It requires a significant investment of psychological energy, but the payoff is grand. It can release you from constant worry and brighten your morale. It may even help you get pregnant when you thought you couldn't.

STAGE I: PRIOR TO THE PROCEDURE

1. Collect information that leads you to believe that the procedure may fail. Record this data in a column labeled "Failure Ideas."
2. Collect information that leads you to believe the procedure will succeed. Record this data in a column labeled "Success Ideas."
3. Look over the list and make sure that you've included more information about failure than about success.
4. Now write a Getting Pregnant Self-Talk (GPST) statement that is hopeful but realistically reflects a balance between failure and success.

Here is a sample of how to do this. Look it over and use it as a model to fill in your own statements.

Stage of Procedure	Failure Ideas	Success Ideas	GPST Statement
Prior to procedure	Louise had 3 IVFs and she still isn't pregnant.	Bonnie kept saying she could never get pregnant, and she just gave birth.	I know it's a long shot, but maybe this is the month I'll get pregnant.
	I know the chances of failure this first time are quite high.	There are new procedures on the horizon.	If it doesn't work with a regular transfer this time, we hope to do a blastocyst transfer next time.
	Even if it works, there's still a chance of a miscarriage.		

STAGE II: DURING THE PROCEDURE

Prepare the statements you will use for this stage just as you did for Stage I. The only difference is that you reverse the balance between failure and success ideas. The table below illustrates how you do it.

Stage of Procedure	Failure Ideas	Success Ideas	GPST Statement
During the procedure	(No failure ideas. This is the point where you allow yourself to believe completely in success.)	My doctor has a high success rate with this procedure.	"I just know this is my month."
		My response to Humegon has never been better.	"I believe I'm going to get pregnant."
		Everything about this cycle is perfect.	"I deserve to have this work, finally."

STAGE III: WAITING FOR THE RESULTS

You now must become more realistic. Try developing an equal number of success and failure ideas.

Stage of Procedure	Failure Ideas	Success Ideas	GPST Statement
Prior to getting results	This wasn't my husband's best sperm sample. Maybe that's why it won't work.	My estradiol level was good this time.	"I need to keep hoping that it will work."
	Maybe my endometrium wasn't perfect. I have had difficulty before.	My nipples feel really tender.	"By doing this procedure, I'm upping my odds."
	Sometimes the first test is positive and then you get a negative result the second time.	I had some spotting. Maybe that means the embryo was trying to hook up.	"If it doesn't work this time, it can always work next time."

STAGE IV: IF THE PROCEDURE FAILS

At this point, you can give yourself permission to feel disappointed and very sad. Write down statements indicating how badly you feel. You might say, "It will never work" or "I must be kidding myself. Why do I go on with these treatments?" No statement at this stage is too negative. Allow yourself to grieve. But at the same time keep in mind that after you've given yourself sufficient time to mourn, you can psych yourself back up and board that roller coaster again. Remind yourself that the next ride can end differently.

Incorporating Hope into Your Treatment

We've helped you move the line in the sand to consider ART. We provided information to help you optimize your insurance coverage. We showed you ways to strike a healthy balance between being hopeful and being realistic.

The final push must be yours. As you embark on ART, it's your job to find the best way to meet the demands of treatment and to stay optimistic even in the face of failure. Photocopy the following chart. Fill in your charts at the various phases of your treatment. Throughout all the stages of your treatment, never forget that your goal—to conceive and bear a child—deserves every bit of effort you are putting into it.

Stage of Procedure	Failure Ideas	Success Ideas	GPST Statement

Calling It Quits

Even though you have managed your social life, coped with Humegon injections and repeated doctor's visits, and bounced back from a half-dozen or more failed IUIs, you may simply be unable to afford ART either financially or emotionally, under any circumstances. There is no shame in deciding that you've reached the end of the line. If you arrive at this conclusion, you must accept the fact that you may never give birth. It will take a great deal of time and emotional energy to get past this crisis. You and your partner should give yourselves time to heal. Work as a Team to support one another.

GETTING THE SUPPORT
YOU NEED

If you decide to pursue ART, it is vital that you elicit support from others, especially your parents, siblings, and in-laws. Sometimes families can be wonderfully supportive. Two days after one of our clients received an embryo transfer, her mother-in-law asked her to hold the telephone to her belly so she could offer the embryos verbal encouragement to implant. On the other hand, another client told us that her own mother refused to lend her money for ART even though she had set up trust funds for the client's two nieces.

To help sensitize your family to what you are going through, we have prepared a guide that you can fill in, photocopy, and give your family members. You may also download it from our Web site (www.gettingpregnantbook.com) and personalize it with your own information. Titled "About [fill in your name here]'s Infertility," the guide is designed to help open the topic for discussion. Write your name in the appropriate blank spaces to make the guide more personal. You may also rewrite the guide to express yourself in your own way. Following is a template of our guide.

About _____'s Infertility

Guide for Family and Friends

To: _____

Because you care about _____ and her happiness.

_____ knows that you love her and want her to be happy, to be her "old self" again. But lately she seems isolated, depressed, and obsessed with the idea of having a baby.

You probably have difficulty understanding why getting pregnant has colored virtually every aspect of her daily life. _____ hopes that by reading this booklet, written by psychologists with both personal and professional experience with infertility, you will better understand the pain she is feeling. The booklet also will tell you how you can help her.

Some Facts About Infertility

It may surprise you to know that one out of six women who wants to have a baby cannot conceive. There are many possible reasons for this dismal statistic: blocked fallopian tubes, ovarian failure, hormonal imbalances, toxic exposure, husband's low sperm count, to name just a few. Moreover, after a woman turns thirty-five it becomes difficult to have a baby primarily because many of the eggs she has left are defective.

All these barriers to pregnancy are physical or physiological, not psychological. Tubes don't become blocked because a woman is "trying too hard" to get pregnant. Antibodies that kill sperm will not disappear if a woman simply relaxes. And a man cannot make his sperm swim faster by developing a more optimistic outlook.

Well-Meaning Advice

When someone we care about has a problem, it is natural to try to help. If there's nothing specific we can do, we try to give helpful advice. Often we draw on our personal experiences or on anecdotes involving other people we know. Perhaps you recall a friend who had trouble getting pregnant until she and her husband went to a tropical island. So you suggest that _____ and her husband take a vacation too.

_____ appreciates your advice, but she cannot use it because of the physical nature of her problem. Not only can't she use your advice, it also upsets her greatly. Indeed, she's probably inundated with this sort of advice at every turn. Imagine how frustrating it must be for her to hear about other couples who "magically" become pregnant during a vacation simply by making love. To _____, who is undergoing infertility treatment, making love and conceiving a child have very little to do with one another. You can't imagine how hard she's been trying to have this baby and how crushed she feels every month when she learns that she's failed again. Your well-meaning advice is an attempt to transform an extremely complicated predicament into a simplistic little problem. By simplifying her problem in this manner, you've diminished the validity of her emotions, making her feel psychologically undervalued. Naturally, she will feel angry and upset with you under these circumstances.

The truth is: There's practically nothing concrete you can do to help _____. The best help you can provide is to be understanding and supportive. It's easier to be supportive if you can appreciate how being unable to have a baby can be such a devastating blow.

Why Not Having a Baby Is So Upsetting

Women are reared with the expectation that they will have a baby someday. They've thought about themselves in a motherhood role ever since they played with dolls. A woman may not even consider herself part of the adult world unless she is a parent. When _____ thinks she cannot have a baby, she feels like "defective merchandise." Not having a baby is literally a matter of life and death. In the Bible, Rachel was barren. She said to Jacob, "Give me children or I die" (Genesis 30:1). Commenting on this, some sages said, "One who is childless is considered dead." So powerful are the feelings connected with barrenness that the person feels dead or wants to die.

Worse, _____ is not even certain that she will ever have a baby. One of the cruelest things you can do to a person is give them hope and then not come through. Modern medicine has created this double-edged sword. It offers hope where there previously was none— but at the price of slim odds.

What Modern Medicine Has to Offer the Infertile Woman

In the past decade, reproductive medicine has made major break-throughs that enable women who in the past were unable to have children now to conceive. The use of drugs such as Humegon can increase the number and size of the eggs a woman produces, thereby increasing her chances of fertilization. In vitro fertilization (IVF) techniques extract a woman's eggs and mix them with sperm in a "test tube" and allow them to fertilize in a laboratory. The embryo can then be transferred back to the woman's uterus. There are many other options as well.

Despite the hope these technologies offer, they are a hard row to hoe. Some high-tech procedures are offered only at a few places, which may force _____ to travel great distances. Even if the treatment is available locally, the patient must endure repeated doctor's visits, take daily injections, shuffle work and social schedules to accommodate various procedures, and lay out considerable sums of money—money that may or may not be reimbursed by insurance. All of this is preceded by a battery of diagnostic tests that can be both embarrassing and extremely painful.

Infertility is a highly personal medical condition, one that _____ may feel uncomfortable discussing with her employer. So she is faced with coming up with excuses whenever her treatment interferes with her job. Meanwhile, she is devoting considerable time and energy to managing a mountain of claims forms and other paperwork required by insurers.

After every medical attempt at making her pregnant, _____ must play a waiting game that is peppered with spurts of optimism and pessimism. It is an emotional roller coaster. She doesn't know if her swollen breasts are a sign of pregnancy or a side effect of the fertility drugs. If she sees a spot of blood on her underwear, she doesn't know if an embryo is trying to implant or her period is about to begin. If she is not pregnant after an IVF procedure, she may feel as though her baby died. How can a person grieve for a life that existed only in her mind?

While trying to cope with this emotional turmoil, she gets invited to a baby shower or a christening, learns that a friend or colleague is pregnant, or she reads about a one-day-old infant found abandoned in a Dumpster. Can you try to imagine her envy, her rage over the inequities in life? Given that infertility permeates practically every facet of her existence, is it any wonder why she is obsessed with her quest?

Every month, _____ wonders whether this will finally be her month. If it isn't, she wonders if she can muster the energy to try again. Will she be able to afford another procedure? How much longer will her husband continue to be supportive? Will she be forced to give up her dream?

So when you speak with _____, try to empathize with the burdens on her mind and on her heart. She knows you care about her, and she may need to talk with you about her ordeal. But she knows that there is nothing you can say or do to make her pregnant. And she fears that you will offer a suggestion that will trigger even more despair.

What Can You Do for _____?

You can give her support and not criticize her for any steps she may be taking—such as not attending a nephew's bris—to protect herself from emotional trauma. You can say something like this: "I care about you. After reading this booklet, I have a better idea about how hard this must be for you. I wish I could help. I'm here to listen to you and cry with you, if you feel like crying. I'm here to cheer you on when you feel as though there is no hope. You can talk to me. I care."

The most important thing to remember is that _____ is distraught and very worried. Listen to what she has to say, but do not judge. Do not belittle her feelings. Don't try to pretend that everything will be okay. Don't sell her on fatalism with statements like "What will be will be." If that were truly the case, what's the point of using medical technology to try to accomplish what nature cannot?

Your willingness to listen can be of great help. Infertile women feel cut off from other people. Your ability to listen and support her will help her handle the stress she's experiencing. Her infertility is one of the most difficult situations she will ever have to deal with.

Problem Situations

Just as an ordinary room can be an obstacle course to a blind person, so can the everyday world be full of hazards for an infertile woman—hazards that do not exist for women with children.

She goes to her sister-in-law's house for Thanksgiving. Her cousin is breast-feeding. The men are watching the football game while the women talk about the problems with their kids. She feels left out, to say the least.

Thanksgiving is an example of the many holidays that are particularly difficult for her. They mark the passage of time. She remembers what came to mind last Thanksgiving—that the next year, she would have a new son or daughter to show off to her family.

Each holiday presents its own unique burden to the infertile woman. Valentine's Day reminds her of her romance, love, marriage—and the family she may never be able to create. Mother's Day and Father's Day? Their difficulties are obvious.

Mundane activities like a walk down the street or going to the shopping mall are packed with land mines. Seeing women pushing baby carriages and strollers strikes a raw nerve. While watching TV, _____ is bombarded by commercials for diapers, baby food, and early pregnancy tests.

At a party, someone asks how long she's been married and whether she has any kids. She feels like running out of the room, but she can't. If she talks about being infertile, she's likely to get well-intentioned advice—just the thing she doesn't need: "Just relax. Don't worry. It will happen soon," or "You're lucky. I've had it with my kids. I wish I had your freedom." These are the kinds of comments that make her want to crawl under the nearest sofa and die.

Escape into work and career can be impossible. Watching her dream shatter on a monthly basis, she can have difficulty investing energy in advancing her career. All around, her co-workers are getting pregnant. Going to a baby shower is painful—but so is distancing herself from social occasions celebrated by her colleagues.

The Bottom Line

Because she is infertile, life is extremely stressful for _____. She's doing her best to cope. Please be understanding. Sometimes she will be depressed. Sometimes she will be angry. Sometimes she will be physically and emotionally exhausted. She's not going to be "the same old _____" she used to be. She won't want to do many of the things she used to do.

She has no idea when, or if, her problem will be solved. She's engaged in an emotionally and financially taxing venture with a low probability of success. Overall, only about one-third of people using special fertility treatments succeed in having a baby. The odds are even lower for women over forty. The longer she perseveres, however, the greater her chances of pregnancy become.

Maybe someday she will be successful. Maybe someday she will give up and turn to adoption, or come to terms with living a childless life. At present, though, she has no idea what will happen. It's all she can do to keep going from one day to the next. She does not know why this is her lot. Nobody does. All she knows is the horrible anguish that she lives with every day.

Please care about her. Please be sensitive to her situation. Give her your support—she needs it and wants it.

CHAPTER 9

All About Third-Party Pregnancy

he paths to parenthood are varied and expanding year by year. In our past, questions used to be "Who's the father?" and "Who's the mother?" Now we hear, "Whose eggs?" "Whose sperm?" and "Who carried the baby?" Soon, with new experimental procedures, the questions will become more complicated than ever. In a cytoplasm transfer, for example, two women provide parts of an egg. So if a donor and a recipient each provide parts of an egg and the baby is carried by a surrogate, how many "mothers" are there? Infertile couples will have to grapple with some very complex answers to some simple questions.

Even today's questions are pretty perplexing. Although all the procedures described in this chapter and the two following chapters are very different solutions for very different medical problems, they share one essential characteristic: They involve at least one other person in addition to you and your partner—a third party. Instead of two people making a baby, at least three or more people (or their sperm, eggs, or uterus) make the baby. And once this third party becomes involved, our clients describe new thoughts and feelings that emerge about the limits of medical intervention, their relationship to each other, and parenting.

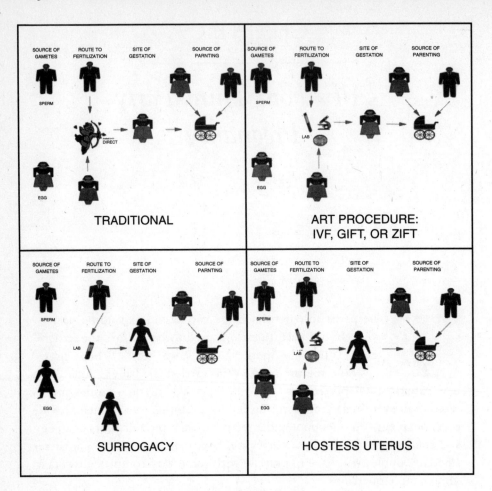

Figure 9.1

PATHS TO PARENTHOOD

This figure depicts the various paths to parenthood.
Each path involves four variables:

- The source of the gametes
- The route to fertilization
- The site of gestation
- The source of parenting

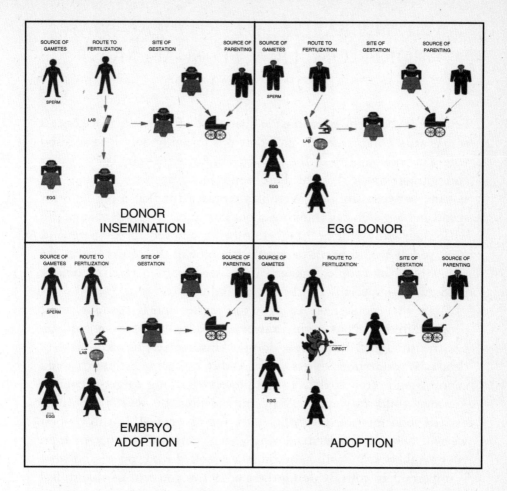

The figures allow you to compare each of the options and show you the differences among the different paths to parenthood. For example, compare egg donation and adoption. In egg donation, Tim and Nora provide the gametes. Nora is *not* Tim's wife. The gametes are fertilized in the lab and the resulting embryo is placed in Lily's uterus. Lily gestates and gives birth to the baby. Lily and Tim (the husband and wife) are the parents of the baby. In comparison, in adoption, Nick and Nora provide the gametes. Fertilization takes place naturally in Nora's body. Nora gestates and gives birth to the baby. She then gives the baby to Lily and Tim (husband and wife), who become the baby's parents. PLEASE NOTE: These figures depict "traditional" family units. However, other arrangements are also possible, such as the adoption of a baby by partners who are not married, by partners of the same sex, or by a single parent.

MAKING BABIES THE "REGULAR" WAY: MORE COMPLICATED THAN MOST PEOPLE REALIZE

Few think about the monumental changes that will take place once a third entity enters into the unit that was formerly only husband and wife. For the majority of the population, having a baby comes easily and without much thought. Sure, some lucky people can "plan" the spacing between siblings. Were it a requirement that a couple must spend an hour each day thinking about how their lives will change and what their baby will be like before being allowed to get pregnant, most people would begin to experience some of the concerns that are encountered by couples engaged in assisted reproductive technology procedures—especially third-party procedures.

Since they don't have to give the matter much thought, most people thinking about having a baby are excited and focus mainly on positive thoughts. But people doing a third-party procedure have to think about questions others don't. And it is these questions that add concerns and often anxiety to the process of trying to get pregnant. You may think to yourself, Why am I feeling this way? I should be excited about getting pregnant, not upset or worried. In this chapter we will help you understand why your experience is different from your neighbor's. We will help you take a look at who you are and what is important to you. By doing these activities you will be able to feel in control of your situation and enjoy as fully as possible the experience of getting pregnant when you thought you couldn't.

FACING YOUR OWN THIRD-PARTY ISSUES

Certainly if you decide to have a baby on your own, no one asks you how you feel about parenting. Possibly, in what now must seem the distant past, you did take a pop quiz or two from a women's magazine that on a very simple level helped you and your partner get ready to make a baby. We're certainly not going to ask you to complete a pop quiz on the topic of third-party pregnancies. Unlike some "classic therapists" who may have told you that the reason you are not conceiving is that your subconscious is telling you you're not ready to have a baby, we aren't questioning your motives or your readiness. Instead, we ask you to search your soul as a way to prepare yourself to grapple with the many decisions you may have to make.

You're probably thinking to yourself, or maybe even saying aloud, My situation is not nearly so complicated as the ones you just wrote about! What's the big deal? I'll just use an egg donor/sperm donor/surrogate and have a baby. And, in fact, there are many medical doctors who view these third-party procedures merely as that: procedures. They see donor insemination, egg donation, and even surrogacy as the next step in getting pregnant when you thought you couldn't. These procedures are the next medical step. But the implications of the medical procedures are enormous. Unfortunately, people often jump right into these procedures without ever allowing themselves to get in touch with what they are really thinking or to experience their gut feelings about them.

You may have bought this book believing that you would not involve the services of a third party, but, for reasons that are becoming increasingly clear, you gradually have come to the realization that you must. That's why you are reading this chapter. Or you may have bought this book because you heard that it had an excellent discussion of third-party issues. No matter which, we always recommend that you come to embrace these procedures, not view them as second best. The series of activities that follow will help you uncover feelings and thoughts you didn't know were there.

Identity Dimension

When you start to use a third party, a part of you is taken out of the equation. What part has been lost and how great is that loss? Can a third party replace any of what will be lost and does it matter if she or he cannot replace it? To answer this question you must think about who you are and what is important to you.

In addition, doing a third-party procedure is uncommon behavior. Over and above the fact that a part of you will not be transmitted to your baby, you have to cope with the fact that you are engaging in an unconventional conception. Our discussion of the dimensions that follow will help make sense of what is happening.

How you feel about yourself and your role in the procedure really provides us with clues of potential trouble before the fact. Is your identity tied up with being pregnant or having your wife pregnant? Do you want to be a parent more than you want to be pregnant? Are you able to engage in a procedure that is viewed by some people as weird?

Each person doing a third-party procedure is a unique individual. You may meet people, in person at your clinic, or on-line through a bulletin board, chat room, mailing list, or newsgroup, who are doing a third-party procedure. These individuals may have strong opinions about how they feel, felt, or might feel about doing a third-party procedure. Remember, you are a unique individual with your own personality, needs, and reactions. Don't believe that because someone else had a particular emotional response you will have a similar response. The best way to predict how you will respond is to know yourself. In this section we will give you a series of probes to help you get to know yourself better and then project how you will handle these situations.

Control and Trust

Some of the third-party situations require giving up some degree of control. For example, some clinics that do anonymous egg-donor procedures do not allow you to meet the donor or see a picture of her. Recipients working with such a clinic must trust the egg-donor coordinator to know what you want and to find someone who satisfies those needs. Some recipients can live comfortably with giving over this control to the donor coordinator. Others feel uncomfortable not being in control of this situation. These people might prefer to use a known donor.

If you are thinking about doing a gestational-carrier procedure, remember that the carrier will have your baby in her womb for nine months. She will need to have proper nourishment, live a healthy lifestyle, go in for regular medical checkups, and so on. Unless you move in to her house and be with her twenty-four hours every day, you will not have control over what she does for those nine months. Can you cede this control to her and trust her to behave the way you expect her to?

Think about yourself. Can you identify any situations in your life when you were required to give up control of a situation that was very important to you? Were you able to do that? Discuss this question with your significant other. What insights can he or she provide to help you have a realistic assessment of yourself?

Conformity and Conventionality

Third-party procedures are instances of unconventional conception. You will be party to unconventional behavior. Do you view yourself as unconventional? Are there other areas in your life where you behave unconventionally? Are you in a profession where you are surrounded by conventionality (you meet few outwardly unconventional bankers, for example). The implications of your answers are either that you may feel comfortable informing others that you are doing a third-party procedure or that if you choose not to tell others but they somehow learn what you did, you will not feel ashamed. If you feel uncomfortable with the notion that others would be aware of your unconventional choice, then you will need to hide this information. How comfortable would you feel having to conceal the information and perhaps be constantly vigilant that others not find out?

Spirituality Dimension

In his book *Not Yet Pregnant*, Arthur Greil refers to infertility as "an experience of biographical disruption."[1] People experiencing such disruption engage in a search for meaning. For many people, the search for an answer to the question, Why me? leads to an immersion in spirituality, faith, religion. But religion is a hard row to hoe for infertile people. Seeking solace in religion often results in being hit with a "triple whammy." First, if you are religious you may believe that the world is governed by a Higher Power who rewards goodness and punishes wrongdoing. If this is the case, then you may wonder, What did I do wrong? You may feel guilty and seek atonement. But that search may be fruitless. Many religious leaders will counsel that God's ways are mysterious and we cannot know why He has meted out the portions we have been given. If you can accept this perspective, you can maintain your religious involvement.

But now you face a second obstacle. So much of the activities of religious institutions revolve around family activities. It is difficult to attend a religious service and hear about church family picnics or pancake breakfasts or communions or bar mitzvahs and be able to participate in this aspect of organized religion. But if you somehow manage to steel yourself against the anguish of feeling that you do not belong when you attend these events, you still have to deal with the third obstacle: violation of religious prescriptions.

Each religion has rules and regulations related to activities involved in assisted reproductive technology. We will *briefly* digress into a discussion of some of these rules and regulations. It is intended to help you understand how this aspect of your identity may influence how you deal with a third-party procedure. Since we cannot possibly cover all of the questions you may have, we will refer you to sources that may provide you with additional answers.

Religious View of Infertility

The first and most fundamental question that you will have to deal with is, Does my religion permit me to do a third-party procedure? The answer to this question requires an answer to an even more fundamental question: Does my religion permit me to utilize assisted reproductive endocrinology procedures? Our search for answers to these questions has taught us that there are no simple cut-and-dried answers.

The official Catholic position is expressed in a document entitled *Instruction on the Respect for Human Life in Its Origins and on the Dignity of Procreation*.[2] That document sets out the Vatican position on assisted reproductive technology. The doctrine expressed sympathy for couples who are unable to have children, but it rejected many aspects of assisted reproductive technology, including third-party procedures. According to this document, a child must be conceived through an act of love, which is expressed as sexual intercourse only. This position ruled out artificial insemination, even with the husband's sperm. The document also suggests that the use of third-party gametes can damage family relationships. Surrogacy, therefore, flies in the face of the Vatican. Nevertheless, individual priests have offered spiritual counseling that has enabled practicing Catholics to utilize the services of reproductive endocrinologists to do procedures, even those involving third parties.

For Protestants there are no doctrinal prohibitions against procedures designed to produce a pregnancy, but there may be difficulties associated with procedures such as selective reduction that involve potential destruction of a life. We suggest that you take advantage of the numerous Internet resources that can help you find answers to and support for your religious questions and concerns. A good place to start finding Christian support and answers is at Hannah's Prayer (http://www.hannah.org).

The Jewish religion is comprised of a number of different branches that differ in their views of what is permissible. Traditional Judaism, often referred to as Orthodox Judaism, adheres to Halachah, a religious code of laws defining what is and is not permissible. This code is enormously complex and includes majority and minority positions. Because of this complexity, each case has to be considered according to its unique aspects. The recommendation of many Jewish religious authorities is for each patient to consult her rabbi for guidance in her particular case. The most pressing question Jewish patients have asked is: Should I use a Jewish or a non-Jewish [sperm or egg] donor? There are conflicting religious opinions in this matter, and the best course of action is to consult a rabbi whose opinion you accept. Additionally, a good place to find useful information and support is at a Web site called ATIME (*A Torah Infertility Medium of Exchange*) (http://www.atime.org/home/home_frames.html).

Self-Confidence

Do you consider yourself a self-confident individual, or do you question your self-worth? Every parent has moments of friction with his or her child. Every child has a moment when he or she tells a parent, "I hate you" (often because they cannot stay up late to watch a show, borrow the car, eat unlimited ice cream, put a ring in their nose, etc.). When your child says "I hate you," will you chalk it up to her being a kid, or will you think, If this child had been biologically connected to me and my spouse, he (or she) wouldn't feel this way? Your response to this situation will be influenced by whether you feel confident in yourself or doubt your self-worth.

A SERIES OF JOURNAL-WRITING ACTIVITIES

Musing About Your Baby: A Theatrical Model

A pregnancy is a scientific/medical occurrence. A baby is more than that. He or she is also a social phenomenon replete with symbolism. Each child occupies a unique niche in its parents' psyches. It is important for you to determine what your pregnancy and your child means for you. We will discuss a variety of dimensions on which you can locate the image of the child in your mind. Where in this psychological space you locate your child will determine how you handle the possibility of a third-party pregnancy.

Do you remember the soliloquy Billy Bigelow sang in the musical *Carousel*? Billy has just found out that he is going to be a father, and the fantasies he has had and the realities of his life come together in a powerful theatrical moment. Here is how the song begins:[3]

> *I wonder what he'll think of me!*
> *I guess he'll call me "the old man."*
> *I guess he'll think I can lick*
> *Ev'ry other feller's father—*
> *Well, I can! I bet that he'll turn out to be*
> *The spit an' image of his dad;*
> *But he'll have more common sense*
> *Than his puddin'-headed father ever had.*
> *I'll teach him to wrassle,*
> *And dive through a wave,*
> *When we go in the mornin's for our swim.*
> *His mother can teach him*
> *The way to behave,*

But she won't make a sissy out o' him
Not him!
Not my boy! Not Bill! Bill . . .
My boy, Bill—
(I will see that he is named after me, I will.)
My boy, Bill!
He'll be tall
And as tough as a tree, will Bill!
Like a tree he'll grow,
With his head held high
And his feet planted firm on the ground. . . .

In this soliloquy Billy sums up his image of his child, his image of himself, and his motives for having a child. His first image focuses on a son. Billy entertains the image of a boy "tall as a tree." His boy Bill is strong and can fight and defend himself. He can picture Bill as a champion prizefighter or as president of the United States. As for most prospective parents, much of his initial image of Bill is based on his image of himself. Bill is "the spit an' image of his dad." But Bill is also the new and improved version, not "puddin'-headed" like his dad. He wants a son to go fishing with. He wants to live out his fantasies through Bill's accomplishments.

But suddenly he wakes himself from his reverie, thinking, "Say, why am I takin' on like this? My kid ain't even been born yet!" But that doesn't stop him. He goes back to his fantasy until a substitute fantasy overtakes him: the 50 percent chance of having a girl. "Wait a minute! Could it be? What the hell! What if he is a girl?" Bowing to this possibility, he alters his image to accommodate a pink and white girl who adores her daddy. Quickly and earnestly he creates a girl fantasy and happily becomes the father of a perfect little girl.

In the past you have probably allowed yourself to soliloquize like Billy Bigelow when you contemplated having a baby. Right now you're finding it hard to let go, to some extent, of that particular image. Most people create an image of themselves, their ideal child, their partner, and what they believe is the meaning of children in their lives. When the pregnancy is a "traditional" one—one that does not involve a third party—most people can find satisfaction in whatever child they have, even if that child is not exactly the one they imagined.

For example, Billy's child can be a she and Billy can still be happy. When you began your pregnancy quest you were probably happy in your ruminations about your baby: your ideal image of what you and your partner could produce and raise. But as you begin to contemplate using a third party, *something* changes. In our work at IVF New Jersey, we hear about that something daily and have ourselves experienced it. In order to try to understand what that something is, we will give you an opportunity to participate in an activity we call Our Son Will. To prepare you for this activity, we will share what our client Sylvia wrote. As you read what she considered important, you too may reflect upon some aspects of identity that play an important role in influencing how you think about the baby you will be adding to your family.

OUR SON WILL

Directions: Sit down in a quiet space. Bring a paper and pencil. You may even decide to include this list in your Pregnancy Quest Journal, which you began in Chapter 2.

Close your eyes and try to form a mental image of the child you are longing to have. Start with a visual image. Your image can be of a child at any age. It could be an infant, a toddler, or even a teenager or a grown individual. Perhaps the image is blurry at first or you have no image at all. Stay with the process. Try to bring that image into closer focus. What do you see? Is the face coming into focus? Are you seeing any special parts of this child's body? Hands? Feet? Fingers? Ankles? Eyes?

Your image need not be only visual. It can also be kinesthetic. Can you feel the sensation of this child? Is it soft, muscular, squeezable? Can you smell this child? Do you smell a baby smell? What about an auditory image? Can you hear this child? Do you hear cooing, or speech, or singing?

Once you form this image, hold on to it and use it to help with the remainder of this activity. Keeping this image in mind, write ten adjectives or phrases to answer the question, Who is my child? Your answer may be a trait; it may be a feeling. Each person will answer this question differently. In fact, you and your spouse may even have very different answers to this question.

SYLVIA'S EXAMPLE AS A MODEL

To get you started, we will share what our client Sylvia Franklin-Stone wrote about her child.

My child:

- *is thin*
- *has a beautiful singing voice*
- *looks just like his daddy*
- *loves me very much*
- *is stubborn just like me*
- *is athletic*
- *is not good at math*
- *has a wonderful sense of humor*
- *is popular with his classmates*
- *is a poor eater*

Sylvia surprised herself when she considered what she had written. Even though the image in her mind was of a baby, the phrases she wrote were of a child at different stages of development. The thin lad in her first response was a teenager. She heard his beautiful singing voice (#2) as it rang out during hymns in her church. She also saw him arguing with her and her husband, Dave, about the curfew they imposed on him (#5) and recalled how she had argued the same way with her own parents. Imagining him surrounded by a flock of admiring classmates (#9) brought back memories of her years in school as a girl who was never popular with classmates and her powerful wish for things to be different. In short, Sylvia realized that this as yet unformed child had an extremely complex relationship with her experiences, memories, wishes, and fantasies.

Identity Review: Musing About You

The next step for you in figuring out the something that drives you—and almost everyone else contemplating a third-party pregnancy—crazy is an identity review. Probably you've not had much chance to think about yourself, but it's important for you to understand what you think are both your good qualities and your bad ones. Interestingly, as many women or men embark on this exercise they begin to feel overwhelming sadness. Particularly if you are the one whose genes or body may not be part of this pregnancy, you may wonder if your partner will reject you. Didn't he marry you because you were so pretty/smart/athletic, so his kids will be too? Before you allow yourself to "go there," try to complete the following activity, called Who Am I?

WHO AM I?

Directions: Just as you did in the previous activity, make a list of the ten most important characteristics that describe you. Use as many sense modalities as you can. Focus on yourself. Get an image of all those characteristics—both good and bad—that make you you. Think about what your partner, your parents, your friends, your colleagues know about you. When you have a clear composite picture, write down your list.

WHAT SYLVIA WAS THINKING

We'll return to Sylvia again. As Sylvia tried this activity, she was having trouble figuring out what really was at her essence. So many Sylvias came to mind. As she began her internal search, Sylvia was confused and wanted to understand this complex mix of images and emotions. We helped her sort these out. Here is what we asked her to think about.

We asked Sylvia to think about how she saw her child linked to herself and her ancestors in time. Did she herself feel strongly linked to her ancestors? Did she see herself passing on important traits that her ancestors bestowed upon her? Golden voices had always been a hallmark of the Franklin family. Grandpa Stephen was a soloist in the community chorus, and her dad was featured in his UPenn barbershop quartet. Sylvia herself was almost always chosen to sing lead roles in her school plays. So imagining this child with a golden voice seemed so natural and reflected an important link in her ancestral chain. But could a donor provide that link? Could anyone assure her of this? What if this child was tone deaf? Could he really be a Franklin? Sylvia realized that an excellent singing voice was an important characteristic of her hoped-for child because it would enable him to take his place in the familial lineage. His voice was a link to the past and also to the future. Here is what Sylvia wrote:

Sylvia:

- *is a devoted daughter*
- *is funny*
- *is a successful and well-respected lawyer*
- *has a beautiful singing voice*
- *has thin ankles*
- *is very energetic*
- *is committed to women's rights*
- *loves to read*
- *is self-sufficient and doesn't look to others for help*
- *is optimistic*

We asked Sylvia mentally to superimpose the description of herself on the description of her child. She did this and was surprised at what she saw. She immediately recognized several qualities that formed her core identity, which she had projected onto her child. Her sense of humor, she realized, was such an integral part of her identity. She noted that her image of her child was that he was funny. She wondered, Is a sense of humor transmitted genetically? Dad was funny. Was I born funny or did I model myself after Dad? She had no answers. Indeed, we told her we had no knowledge of whether there was a genetic component to humor. But she did realize that she hoped her child would be similar to her in this core identity feature.

We asked her whether she considered her husband, Dave, particularly funny. She realized that although he appreciated a good joke, Dave himself did not have much of a sense of humor. "What," we asked Sylvia, "if your child is like Dave?" Upon reflection, Sylvia realized that because of her optimism, history of career success, and self-sufficiency, she always believed that she would *make* her child funny. So did this mean that she could influence her child by the way she parented him or did she have to depend on genetics as well?

Sylvia thought about how she considered herself a devoted daughter and wondered whether she would be unable to sustain this view if she failed to create a child who continued the Franklin chain of excellent singers. Sylvia realized how much her image of her child was intertwined with her image of herself. She also realized that many of her core identity aspects she expected her child to possess might be beyond her ability to control or influence.

Your Motives for Having a Child

We sometimes hear of a therapist who tells infertile clients that the reason they are not becoming pregnant is because they have all the wrong reasons for wanting to have a baby. Of course this theory is ridiculous—as if wanting a child because you hope the child will carry on your talents instead of wanting a child because you hope to create a unified whole family will make any difference to your eggs or your sperm or your uterus.

So as we ask you to analyze your own reasons for wanting a child, it is for the purpose of helping you come to grips with how a third party might affect these motives.

WHY DO I WANT A CHILD?

Directions: Find a quiet space. Sit down with a paper and pencil. You can write this list in your Pregnancy Quest Journal. Relax and allow your thoughts and feelings to have full range. Now write down all the reasons you want to have a child.

HOW SYLVIA ANSWERED

We asked Sylvia to write answers to the following question: Why Do I Want to Have a Child? She wrote:

I want to have a child because:

- *I want to create something wonderful, a person whom I can mold to be a good human being who will make a difference in this world*
- *I want to continue the lineage of the Franklin family*
- *I want to experience a part of myself, the nurturing, caring person I have never yet experienced*
- *I love children—their innocence, playfulness, and spontaneity, and want to experience the novelty and joy I can have interacting with a child*
- *someday I will die, but I can live on through my child and my child's children*
- *my relationship with my husband, Dave, is that of spouses. It is a wonderful relationship but I want to expand it into a parental relationship where we are a family and relate to each other in our parental role*
- *as much as Dave loves me, his love is different from the kind of love and affection I can get from a child*
- *as much as I've achieved as a successful lawyer, I still don't feel that I have achieved full status as an adult until I have a child*
- *I am very involved with my church and my religion. Somehow I feel that not having a child is a curse—that I must have done something wrong and I'm being punished for it. Moreover, I feel that without a child I cannot participate in so many of our church's activities—so many of them center around the family.*

What Are You Ready to Give Up?

The next step in your personal assessment is to look at all three lists side by side and see how they fit together. Clients often tell us that they are surprised at how the lists seem to mesh or not to mesh. Although regular people beginning regular pregnancies aren't asked to think about these inconsistencies, we believe that you really should clarify how you see your potential baby, yourself, and your parenting goals as you begin to think about using a third party to extend your family.

We asked Sylvia to place her three lists side by side and see how they fit with one another. How did her view of herself, her image of her child, and her motives for having a child fit with one another? Could she satisfy her motives for having a child even if the child she had differed from the one in her mind's eye? Where was there room for give? She needed to answer these questions before she could go the third-party route to having a child. But before she embarked on this phase of the activity, there was one more issue we needed to address with Sylvia.

Entitlement: The Next Biggest Stumbling Block

The last stumbling block that most couples must grapple with is their debilitating feelings of entitlement. Because of what has happened to them medically and because they must face the fact that they must use a third party and not their own genes, many couples believe that they have been dealt a lousy hand. And because of this bad luck, couples believe that they are entitled to some sort of compensation. Couples feel that they now have permission to make any request they want and those who work with them must help them fulfill their wish.

Initially as we worked with couples trying to select a donor, we were struck by how driven these couples were. Since we ourselves had been at that juncture, we knew the desperation and sense of urgency that plagued us. But when we were undergoing egg donation in the early nineties, the variety of programs and options available were nothing like what is available now. In response to the expanding need, donors, sperm banks, donor brokers, and medical practices capitalize on couples' ever-increasing sense of entitlement. "Quality donors: brilliant, handsome/beautiful, everything you want and more, ready immediately." (All this for a fee, of course!) As couples, many of whom are older and successful in their careers, read these ads, they are placed in business or shopper mode and act accordingly.

Unfortunately, couples take one of our Pointers, Educate Yourself About Infertility, one step too far. They feel that their situation is even worse than anyone else's, that they have both money and information and they want service now! And, of course, they want the best donor money can buy. We have worked with many who have said to us, "We are bright and successful, we've had a series of terrible experiences. We want a donor who will make a baby who is as good as or better than we are. Here's the money. Make it happen immediately."

You too may believe that you are entitled to compensation for your bad luck. You may feel that for the big-time bucks of this procedure you are entitled to the ear of the egg-donor coordinator or the manager of the sperm bank. You may feel that here is your chance to produce a child who has all the good traits of your spouse and ones that surpass even your own. The sense that you are entitled to get a donor who can make a baby who is so perfect is what we see as the primary stumbling block in moving ahead. It's what makes those looking for a sperm donor get longer and longer profiles as well as baby pictures and videos.

Women we counsel often request a donor who is like them in every way but without a weight problem. They think choosing a donor is like visiting a Web site and requesting that car but in a different color. Poof! It happens on the screen. But not with people and not in real life. You cannot "commoditize" a human being! Donor B may have a better health history but not be as tall as Donor A. Donor C has a master's degree but is slightly chunky. And offering more money will probably not get you all those things anyway, because rarely does one person have everything. This is a major flaw when thinking about a third-party procedure, and the quest for perfection can make it impossible for women to get a donor or do the procedure because no donor or surrogate is perfect.

Last year a couple hired an attorney who headed up a national search for a tall, beautiful blond woman with an elite college education and extremely high SAT scores. They offered this ideal candidate $50,000 to be their egg donor. We think that the whole $50,000 (and, more recently, $100,000) donor search was the epitome of entitlement. The thinking goes, Since we are tall and brilliant and we have so much money, and because it happened that our eggs are no longer viable and that is a terrible thing, we are *entitled* to offer as much money as we want to get the tallest, smartest donor—even taller and smarter than we are. Even though the donor procedure began because altruistic donors gave their eggs for a small fee, now that's not good enough for us. We could get a fat, stupid, short donor and then the baby wouldn't be one we wanted. Because of our situation, we're *entitled* to ask for what we want in a donor and advertise and pay and reject.

HOW SYLVIA WORKED THROUGH HER ISSUE
OF ENTITLEMENT

During the course of hours of discussion and reflection, Sylvia became aware that she felt she was "entitled to" have certain things because of what she was "deprived of." She felt she had been penalized by not being able to use her genes to create her child. Had she been given the same rights as other women to create a child using her own genes, she would be willing to accept whatever child she gave birth to. But now that she had been deprived of this opportunity, she was entitled to a "perfect child" as compensation. Rather than thinking just of being pregnant and having a baby, she now was obsessed with what sort of baby she would have. She could trust herself to create a baby who would satisfy her. But this stranger—could she be trusted to give Sylvia the baby she was entitled to? What did letting go and giving up control to a third party imply?

Our work with Sylvia helped her understand what she hoped for and what she feared as she contemplated using a third party. It also helped her let go of these feelings of entitlement to the perfect child. It wasn't easy to let go of this sentiment, but she did it. This is the sort of counseling that many couples find helpful as they move to a third-party pregnancy. Having moved past this phase, we turned to our exercise of reshaping the image of Sylvia's child to one that could likely be created using a donor and still satisfy her motives for having a child.

WHAT YOU CAN DO TO MOVE AHEAD

We know how hard it is to give up your dream of your child—the one you held deep in your heart. For us, it was the one with Helane's dimples and brains and wonderful sense of humor. Now that we have been lucky enough to be blessed with two healthy, beautiful, and bright children, we love who they are as people, not because they are Helane's reflection. They are much like Helane because she is their mother, but they are ultimately like themselves. What the donor gave them was possibilities and a variety of wonderful potentials. What we gave them was life and a great chance of becoming all they can be.

As we work with couples, we help them get back to what motivated them to think about becoming pregnant in the first place. We tell them our story and share with them how our kids are turning out. We help them know that a donor can never replace them but can at best be a stand-in for the procedure. We encourage them to work together with the sperm bank or the donor broker or the practice to find them the best available donor, but always to keep in mind that the best donor is the donor who will ultimately allow them to become pregnant. So the tallest, smartest, blondest, $50,000 donor is not a good donor if the procedure is not a success. And there is no guarantee that any characteristic, even the recessive one nobody knew about, won't turn up in the child of even the most selective recipient couple. A surprise red-haired child or a six-footer or someone with perfect pitch or smiling blue eyes—ultimately these traits or skills are merely aspects of a beloved child who is the result of amazing medical feats. What could be more wonderful?

CHAPTER 10

Egg Donation: Braving the New Frontier

f you are reading this chapter you are probably beginning to think about what it might be like to become a recipient. You may already be sure this is for you. Or you may just be beginning to consider what this procedure entails and are grappling with the many complex issues of a third-party pregnancy.

Most clients come to see us after they have already decided that their next step is egg donation. Many of them, like you, have been trying to get pregnant for many years. Most have tried follicle-stimulating medication and IUIs or IVFs unsuccessfully. Many may have had one or more miscarriages. For most of you, egg donation, even though it's the next step, is a major procedure with an expensive price tag and a high success rate (an almost 70 percent chance of becoming pregnant and a 60 percent chance of carrying the baby to term)[1] that provokes numerous questions.

You may be asking yourself a variety of questions. Will I love this baby? How can we be 100 percent sure the donor isn't lying about her medical history? What if the donor wants to see the baby? Or even try to get custody of the baby? What if I tell my child that she's a donor baby and she rejects me—and then wants to meet the donor? We explore these and similar questions in this chapter.

THE HISTORY OF EGG DONATION

Egg donation is a relatively new procedure. The first documented egg-donor pregnancy was in 1984. In its early stages, egg donation was done in two ways. The first attempts involved a procedure called a lavage, which means washing. During a lavage procedure, a woman, who provided the eggs, was inseminated with the recipient husband's sperm. Several days later the embryos were washed out of her uterus and placed into the uterus of the recipient. Needless to say, this procedure was fraught with difficulties. Often, instead of washing out the embryos the donor stayed pregnant. Or, because the lavage needed to occur so early in the pregnancy, the procedure took place needlessly because fertilization had not occurred. Neither outcome was the desired one, since the recipient rarely became pregnant.

The next stage in the development of the modern egg-donation procedure occurred just as IVF centers expanded but before freezing techniques had become widespread. IVF patients who had cycled previously and were known to produce many eggs donated their "excess" eggs to another couple, usually for a reduced cost for their own cycle. Because synchronization was fairly chancy (before Lupron became available), often several couples were "on standby" in the hope that one woman might be mid-cycle at the same time as the woman who was donating her eggs. Success rates for egg donation remained low. And once clinics could provide couples with the chance to freeze their embryos, this source all but dried up.

Two new developments in IVF technology changed the procedure of egg donation and allowed it to develop into such a major procedure. One was the use of Lupron to help prevent LH surges in IVF patients. This same medication allowed doctors to synchronize cycles between recipients and donors. Also, once eggs were retrieved vaginally with IV sedation, as opposed to through a laparoscopy, donors could volunteer to undergo this procedure without the risks of general anesthesia. As a result of these two new developments, the number of egg-donation procedures increases each year. RESOLVE Inc. estimated that in 1996 approximately 1,700 babies were born from egg-donor procedures.

EGG DONATION: THE MEDICAL DETAILS

The medical aspect of egg donation is very similar to what happens in an IVF procedure. The difference is that the action is split between two players: you and the donor. The donor does what any IVF patient would do up until her eggs are retrieved. The recipient utilizes a special medical protocol designed to ready her endometrium to accept an embryo.

Cycle Synchronization

The key factor here is to ensure that both the donor and the recipient be at mid-cycle at about the same time. The protocol to achieve synchronization is fairly standard. The table below gives an example of a standard protocol if the recipient still has ovarian function. If the recipient has no ovarian function, synchronization can occur more easily.

Day of Recipient Cycle	Day of Donor Cycle	Recipient Protocol	Donor Protocol
	Day 21	Begin taking Lupron, continuing until donor gets hCG injection	Begin Lupron
	Next 6 days	Still taking Lupron	Continue taking Lupron
	Next day	Continue Lupron, begin estrogen	Continue taking Lupron
	Day 1 of period (within next 6 days)	Continue Lupron and estrogen	Continue taking Lupron
	Day 3 of new cycle	Continue Lupron and gradually increase estrogen dosage	Continue Lupron, begin taking Pergonal
	Day 12 of new cycle	Continue Lupron and estrogen	Stop Pergonal, stop Lupron, take hCG injection
	Day 13 of new cycle	Stop Lupron, continue estrogen, begin progesterone	

Day of Recipient Cycle	Day of Donor Cycle	Recipient Protocol	Donor Protocol
	Day 14 of new cycle	Continue estrogen and progesterone	Eggs retrieved. End of involvement.
2 days later		Day 3 embryo transfer; continue estrogen and progesterone.	
2 days later		If doing blastocyst transfer, continue estrogen and progesterone.	
Day 12 after IVF		Pregnancy test; if positive, continue estrogen and progesterone for next ten weeks.	

In essence, Lupron shuts down both the donor's and the recipient's natural FSH/LH function so that their cycles can be artificially stimulated. Everybody's cycle is slightly different, but these factors remain fairly constant:

- Both donor and recipient continue taking Lupron throughout the entire protocol, until the donor gets her hCG injection.
- The donor should not begin taking Pergonal until the recipient is taking estrogen for at least four days.
- The length of the artificial follicular phase (taking estrogen) of the recipient is not important; what is important is when the recipient adds progesterone.
- No transfer can take place unless the endometrium is adequately prepared with estrogen and progesterone.
- Estrogen can be taken in the form of injections (Delestrogen), patches (Estraderm), or by mouth (Estrace), as long as the estrogen is natural, not synthetic. Usually the program prescribes one or the other.

- Progesterone can be taken by injection, in vaginal suppository form, or as vaginal gel; any form is acceptable as long as the progesterone is natural, not synthetic.

Sometimes prior to going through the actual cycle, the recipient must participate in a test cycle to ensure that her estrogen and progesterone levels can be manipulated with drugs. Although a successful test cycle does not guarantee a successful procedure, it rules out certain donor candidates. At various points during this experimental cycle, you will have your blood tested and your endometrium scanned with ultrasound. You will complete this cycle with an endometrial biopsy.

COMMON THEMES: WHAT YOU MAY BE THINKING AND FEELING

Common themes emerge from the stories couples tell us about their lives. As you decide about whether you want to do egg donation, it's important to know that other people have experienced feelings similar to yours and have had similar thoughts.

The Need to Give Yourself One Last Chance

We always tell women thinking about egg donation that they will know when they are ready to move on. A reputable clinic will advise you about what procedure they think you should select and what your potential chances are of becoming successful with your own eggs or with the eggs of a donor. They should never, however, force you to choose egg donation.

Some couples are ready the day they find out that the woman has an elevated Day 3 FSH. Others need time to integrate fully the meaning of this information. Still others need to try their eggs one more time. The knowledge in your head that you're better off statistically using donor eggs doesn't always make it to your heart. The best decision for you is what you feel is right.

We really like what Cathleen and Bill decided to do. Cathleen is older than Bill. She's forty-one; he's thirty-seven. After several attempts at using the fertility medication Follistim and having insem- inations, Cathleen was ready to undergo a donor-egg procedure. Not Bill. "I love Cathleen. Everyone loves Cathleen. I married Cathleen because of how wonderful and loving she is. I want her to try to have her baby, not somebody else's. There's nobody like her."

What Bill says is true. There is nobody like Cathleen. Certainly no donor could replicate Cathleen, but she could certainly enable Cath- leen and Bill to be parents. Cathleen is ready; Bill is not. What this couple did was compromise. Cathleen agreed to try one more stimula- tion cycle. If she did not stimulate on the medication, Bill agreed to move on to a donor egg. Cathleen did try one more cycle. As in pre- vious cycles, Cathleen did not respond to even "industrial strength" medication. The cycle was almost canceled, but Bill insisted that, even though there was only one egg, they have an insemination. Bill's hopes were high, but unfortunately Cathleen did not become pregnant. They are now waiting for a donor to help them fulfill their dream.

What's interesting about this story is that the one-last-time request was made by the husband, not the wife. In our experience, it's more often the woman who needs this cycle to close the chapter on her own eggs. In either case, though, it's important for the partner who needs this to be heard. It may be impossible to proceed with this last-ditch cycle—for money reasons, for timing reasons, or even for medical rea- sons. Our point is that when you try donor eggs, you must embrace this procedure as the best one in your current circumstances. Because you must muster all your emotional strength as well as shoulder so much financial burden, you must be ready to move forward full steam ahead!

Grieving for the Lost Biological Connection

Perhaps the most common theme is the one of loss. One couple told us a classic story that was filled with loss. Karen and Joe, both in their early forties, had been married for about two years when they came to talk to us. Karen told us how excited and hopeful she had been when she mar- ried Joe: "I never thought I'd find the right man. He likes me to be a strong woman and knows how important my job is to my sense of myself. I told him all about my dreams to have a baby that would be like me—and like my whole family. We all have curly red hair and play a stringed instrument. I thought someday I would have a curly redheaded kid who plays the violin. I love my family so much I couldn't wait to have a baby for me—and for them. Now the whole thing is lost—the baby, the picture. I'm so sad. I don't think I can bear that loss."

Perhaps you feel like Karen. Your dream of a family was one that was carefully nurtured since you were a girl. When they discover that their eggs will not be part of the process, many women feel a tragic loss, not just of eggs, but of possibilities and dreams. You may also be experiencing a perceived loss of your youth. Even though you may still have your periods, the doctors tell you that you are slowly moving toward menopause. You are being told that you have "old eggs," even though people still tell you how young you look. Until you found out about your eggs, you even felt young.

Before you can openly accept and nurture a third-party pregnancy, it's important to grieve for the genetic line you will be unable to pass on to the next generation. If you are the one whose line will not be passed down, you must say good-bye, in a sense, to that baby—the one who would have had your dimples or your curly red hair. Only by working through your grief can you recognize the many nongenetic characteristics you can give your baby.

You probably have asked yourself, Why me? Why can't I have the same opportunity other parents have to pass down their traits? There are no answers to these questions. Sometimes life is not fair; we urge you to make peace with this injustice. Also, realize that deprivation sometimes fosters a greater appreciation for the other opportunities you have. Perhaps because you cannot pass down some of your traits you will work harder than other parents to set examples for your baby that will teach him or her to be a warm, loving person.

One way we help couples cope with their mixed feelings about what is lost and what is gained is to engage in a fairly ritualized type of activity. A form of GPST, this activity can help you bid farewell to the baby who could have been and embrace the baby who could be. The following activity was developed by one of our clients to help her Change Her Thinking and gain a new, healthy perspective on having children using an ovum donor. You can also use the activity if you are doing a traditional surrogate procedure. With slight modifications, your husband can also use it before you undergo a sperm-donor procedure.

GIFTS FOR MY BABY

Preparing the List of What You Cannot Pass Down Genetically

The first part of the activity helps you to determine what you cannot give your baby and then to "put these traits away." In the next part, you determine what gifts you can give by the way you raise your baby and concentrate on these qualities.

List the names of each relative who had a feature you hoped to pass down to your baby. These features can be physical traits, mental abilities, or characteristics of temperament. Next to each person's name, list the feature you wanted to pass down. We will give an example.

What I Cannot Pass Down Genetically

NAME OF RELATIVE	FEATURE I HOPED TO PASS DOWN
Aunt Joan	Her wavy brown hair (a physical characteristic)
Dad	His mathematical mind (a mental ability)
Mom	Her boundless energy (a temperament characteristic)

Now do the same for your own features that you hoped to pass down to your baby.

Me	My manual dexterity
Me	My creativity

Now fill out the form titled "What I Cannot Give My Baby."

What I Cannot Give My Baby

I believe I have wonderful traits and abilities that I could have passed on genetically to my baby. Many of these traits and abilities came from _____, (an) important person(s) in my life. In preparation for what I am about to do, I am giving myself time to think about all that is good and wonderful and special about _____. I like to think that I am like _____ and can carry _____ with me in my heart. Not just through _____'s genes, but also through what _____ taught me, which helped me to become who I am.

I also believe that I have much that I could have passed on genetically to my baby. I am a _____ person. I have great _____ and a good _____. I hoped that my baby would be all of this—and more—but I will not be able to give my baby my genes. I feel sad that I cannot genetically contribute to my baby. But I will provide for this baby the best uterine environment and transfer what I can in utero. And by the way I raise him or her, I will ensure that this baby can have the best of me. Together with my husband, _____, we will raise a baby with a love of life.

Signed _____

Date _____

Now take the signed and dated document "What I Cannot Give My Baby" to a quiet place where you can be alone. Read the document out loud. When you have finished reading, take a few minutes to look at what you have read. Form a picture of this document. Take a special envelope, place the document inside it, and seal it. Then, gently and lovingly, put it away in a special place.

Preparing the List of What You Can Give Your Baby by Example

Now, list the things you can give to your baby by the way you raise her or him and by the example you set for your baby. We will provide some examples.

What I Can Give My Baby:

my honorable character

my love of art

Now, on the form below, "Setting Examples: My Gifts to My Baby," fill in the information you just listed in the appropriate place. Then sign and date the form.

Setting Examples: My Gifts to My Baby

I believe that I have many gifts I can give to my baby. By setting an example, I can teach him or her to be _____, to love _____, to value _____, and to know how to _____. I can raise my baby with love and build up our baby's sense of self and love of humanity.

Signed _____

Date _____

Find a special place where you can read aloud "Setting Examples: My Gifts to My Baby." Take a long look at the document and form a picture of it in your mind. Then place it in an envelope in a special place you reserve for important and valued documents.

Dealing with the Lingering Feelings of Loss

Even after completing these exercises, you will have moments of grief. You will remember the items you listed in "What I Cannot Pass Down Genetically." Don't fight these feelings. Allow yourself to "go with them." Then relax yourself with your deep breathing and picture the "setting examples" document and the second ritual. Let the positive statements override the negative thoughts by concentrating on or even rereading the list of gifts you can give your baby.

Anger at the Unequal Contribution

Many women tell us that their gut response to hearing that they need to use an egg donor is anger that their partner will be passing down his genes and they won't. They feel so furious that they will not only have to undergo all the medical treatment and carry the baby, but they will also have to give up all genetic connections to this baby.

We like to share the way Rita and George thought about this inequality before the procedure. "I'm worried," explained Rita at our first session. "I'm afraid the baby will look just like George, talk just like George, think just like George, and love George more than it loves me. I'm like a human incubator and a for-hire wet nurse. I might as well get somebody else to grow the baby. I feel out of the loop here. I want to be pregnant, but maybe not this way."

We urged Rita to explore her feelings about being left out and her thoughts about not wanting to be pregnant with an egg-donor baby. Interestingly, through our discussions, Rita found that she often felt in competition with George and that this theme of competition appeared in many of the stories she told about her relationship to her siblings and herself in her job. Rita also discovered that she always saw her parents as being constantly at war with each other and with the children. Rita seemed to think that all families were like her own.

We helped Rita think about a family as a cooperative unit. We urged Rita to think about what would be her unique role in this pregnancy and how she could raise this baby together with George. We also asked Rita to think about what she loved about George and why she married him in the first place. Once Rita began to reframe how she thought of parenthood—not as a battle but as a collaborative project—Rita and George felt ready to proceed.

Lack of Control of the Situation

So many couples tell us that the most difficult aspect of the egg-donation procedure is their inherent lack of control. Once you involve a third party in the procedure, so many questions arise: Who is the donor? Why is she a good match for me? Did she lie about her medical history? Is she taking her medication? How is she responding to it? How many eggs will she make? Will the sperm fertilize these eggs? Will she come for the baby? Who is this person anyway? As couples consider egg donation, they tell us that they fear the lack of control and all the unknowns it entails.

In fact, recipients tell us that they often feel neglected and uninformed because everyone—the doctors, the nurses, the egg-donor coordinator—is worrying about the donor and not about them. You too will be worrying about her and can really do nothing about the situation. You, who have masterminded the whole infertility quest, will now be in the background wondering about who is giving her injections and whether she really hasn't taken a drink. You'll be listening for weather reports and worrying that there will be snow or rain and she won't be able to make it to the clinic. Nobody will worry about you, because we all know you will take your medication and show up for the procedure.

If you really think about the whole nature of "regular" baby making, you may realize that much of that situation, particularly what the baby will be like, is out of parents' control, too. Even in the most planned, fertile life, the sex and appearance and characteristics of the baby, as well as precisely when the baby will be born (except in a scheduled C-section), are never under our control. But we have come to relish these unknowns and not think about them.

Egg donation has few real-life models, however. Rarely would someone enlist the services of someone they have never met. Many recipients, who are often older and in high-powered careers, can't believe that they have to trust other people so much. Although recipients tell us that they are used to allocating responsibility, they are often doers, not people who wait. Recipients tell us that they fantasize about hiding outside the clinic to catch a peek at their donor.

WHO ARE RECIPIENTS?

As couples begin to consider using an egg donor, they tell us that they feel like outsiders—"completely different" from the rest of the world who gets pregnant easily. To help them understand where they fit in, we wrote an article that appears on the Surrogacy Web site (http://www.surrogacy.com) classifying the kinds of people who are recipients, which we excerpted below. As you read through the categories below, try to find one that most characterizes you. These categories emerged from factors that consistently appeared and reappeared in the stories of egg-donor couples who came to see us.

Recipients in each of the categories face different pitfalls, describe different sorts of difficulties, and voice different concerns. Knowing what may be hard for you and what could be easier can help you up the odds for yourself. Try to place yourself in the category that best describes you.

Group 1. The Modern Classic: A Fortyish Woman, Never Married, with a Previously Married Husband with Children from the First Marriage

Typically, the woman is in her late thirties to mid-forties, has an active career, and has spent much of her young adulthood building her career instead of finding a partner. She has found and married the man of her dreams, who has been married before and has children from the first marriage. Usually the woman expresses an intense desire to be a parent and to be pregnant, not to adopt. Often the husband is less passionate about the pregnancy quest, although he goes along with this procedure to satisfy his new wife. In fact, having a child is often a condition of the marriage, either implicitly or explicitly.

Often the woman feels angry because "nobody told me that I would have trouble getting pregnant." Because she feels young and her gynecologist told her that she is in good health, the woman feels that since she beat one set of odds in getting married, she will also beat the odds in getting pregnant when she's over forty. Her girlfriends, who are her support network, see her as "career woman extraordinaire," not "Mom." Her family is usually ambivalent or, at best, resigned to the idea.

Members of this group typically hide the fact that they are using an egg donor and therefore get little social support. When they get pregnant, both they and their husband are thrilled. Since they typically conceal their use of a donor, they tend to stay in contact with their donor coordinator as their source of support.

Group 2. The Trendsetters: A Fortyish Woman Married to a Thirtyish Man, Both of Whom Have Never Had Children

Women in this group are usually in their forties and married to a man who is five to fifteen years younger. Neither has children, and the man usually has not been married previously. Usually the woman feels enormous pressure to have a baby because she wants to fit in with friends who are often the peers of her younger husband. Though she looks young, she fears that her young husband will lose interest in her and find another woman, particularly because she cannot produce a baby "for my husband." She feels pressured to get started as soon as possible.

On the other hand, her husband often feels less pressure because he is young and has typically been married only recently. He says he married his wife because of all her wonderful characteristics, which he really would like to pass down genetically. Consequently, the couple reports much discord in trying to come to a decision about the donor in particular and the procedure in general. Typically, this couple decides to do the procedure, gets pregnant, and makes believe the donor part never happened.

Group 3. To Mother Again: A Fortyish Woman with Children from a First Marriage Married to a Younger Man Who Has Never Had Children.

Group 3 is similar to Group 2 except that the woman in this group has had a child or children from a previous marriage. The husband typically tells us that his new wife is a "wonderful mother" and that he was attracted to her, in part, because he admired these skills and hoped that he could participate, together with her, in making a "blended" family. The woman reports that she loved being a mother and would like to have a similar experience, this time, however, with a husband who would also participate in the parenting.

Typically these couples get very little social support from their family and friends, who lived through the difficult first marriage and the single parenting. They tell her to enjoy this relationship and be happy parenting her existing children. The husband has an instant family and all the emotional and financial obligations of that situation. Although some friends caution him about creating a new life, particularly if they know that the new baby will involve an egg donor, most get enthusiastic support from friends and family because they want what the couple wants.

Interestingly, the couple themselves are often split over their expectations for a donor. The woman, already a mother and having experience with the unique characteristics of each child, as well as loving a child while not loving its father, usually is very open to any donor possibility. The husband, usually still mourning the loss of the characteristics of the woman he loves, usually brings in a list as long as his arm. The battle that ensues between the couple is usually extensive.

Group 4. The Parents of an Incomplete Family: A Woman and Man Who Have One or More Children Together but Want More Children

The couple in Group 4 are experiencing secondary infertility. They have one or two children together and usually became parents at an age comparable to their friends. The wife mentions how much she enjoyed being pregnant and taking care of an infant or toddler. The husband mentions how much he likes being involved in the school and/or activities of their children. What makes these couples turn to egg donation is that they (almost always the woman and sometimes even the two of them) have a clear image of a larger family, usually made up of three, four, or even five children.

Though frantic to conceive, they usually don't tell extended family because they fear the family would tell them to "leave well enough alone"; they don't tell friends with several children because they fear these friends will tell them how hard it is to raise so many children; they don't tell infertile friends because these friends might view them as greedy. If their children are old enough to understand the donor process, they don't even tell them because they fear that this biological family might view the new baby as a "second-class citizen." They want a donor who presents as everything the wife is (which is usually quite an extensive list of requirements). And, at the same time, they want this donor now!

Group 5. The Two-Career Couple: Coming of Age a Decade Behind

This couple, both usually in their late thirties or early forties, has only recently married. Typically, neither partner has been married previously, or, if they were, neither has any children. Typically, they have very successful careers and have no expectations that they will have any difficulty having children. They married in order to produce wonderful children who will inherit all their parents' wonderful characteristics.

Usually they do not tell their friends and family what they are doing. Typically, they say that their family and friends support them in their pregnancy quest but think they are using the wife's eggs. We find that these couples are very difficult to satisfy in their choice of a donor. For them the donor is their "stand-in" and only a donor "as good as I am" will satisfy them.

Group 6. The Young Infertiles: Peer-Group Pressure Big Time

These couples got married when their friends got married, usually in their mid- to late twenties. Like their friends, they began early to try to have a baby but were unsuccessful. Chronologically, they are part of a cohort that is still capable of having a baby. But because they have a history of repeated failure and usually receive the diagnosis of premature ovarian failure, they often feel old despite the fact that they are not.

Friends and family continue to expect them to become pregnant and support them. But they feel that "I'll never get pregnant." They often turn to egg donation as yet another procedure with which they can fail. Because they have learned to feel helpless from their repeated failure with their own eggs and because they report that they are upset with themselves for being jealous of their friends' happy IVF successes or spontaneous pregnancies, Group 6 often reports that they are extraordinarily depressed.

Group 7. The Medically Infertile

Group 7 consists of people who knew before they got married, or for several years, that they could not have children of their own. Some women, for example, were born without ovaries; others had medical treatment for cancer or another deadly disease that left them without ovarian function. When they discussed their condition prior to their marriage or after they won the battle with their disease, they came to grips with their condition as a couple.

Prior to egg donation, this group's only option if they wanted children was to adopt. Egg donation opened up the possibility of pregnancy and passing on the husband's genes. This group usually has a tremendous amount of support from family and friends who are rooting for them to achieve what they thought they never could.

Group 8. The V-8s: "Oh, I Forgot to Have a Child!"

These couples have been married for many years, are in their mid- to late forties, and have never had children. They tend to be low risk takers. They are very careful and weigh every aspect of the decisions they make. For many years they considered the possibility of having children, but were never certain that it was the right thing for them to do. Now, at a rather late stage of their life, they've decided they should give it a try.

These people are motivated to undergo the procedure so that they can say they tried. But they continue to be ambivalent about the decision to try. Sometimes they engage in behaviors that reflect this ambivalence. For example, one such recipient who got pregnant went into the sauna every day and used Retin-A despite the fact that her gynecologist implored her not to do so. Inevitably, she lost the pregnancy.

Members of Group 8 are in no hurry to select a donor. They are very uncertain that they are doing the right thing. They want to wait to make sure they got exactly the "right" donor. In contrast to members of Group 5, who place more emphasis on the physical attractiveness of their donor, members of Group 8 place greater emphasis on the intellectual abilities of their donor. They say they would never consider adopting a child. They report that they get virtually no support from family and friends prior to the pregnancy and birth, but once the baby is born many of the family members rise to the occasion.

Group 9. The Single Woman

More and more single women are choosing to do egg donation. Most single women report that they have tired of waiting for the man of their dreams and want to have a child first and then hope to build a relationship with a man. Occasionally single women report that they considered using a man with whom they have been involved as the provider of sperm, but most times they report that ultimately they use an anonymous sperm donor.

Single women are typically "savvy shoppers." They usually ask good questions about donors, request more information than most recipients, yet have enormous difficulty making the final selection and getting through the process. Perhaps this difficulty comes from the fact that they have no partner to help provide emotional support, and single women, more than any other group, are keenly aware that the baby-making process usually does require two people.

Although many practices restrict their egg-donation programs to couples only, we think that single women can and should be mothers if they have been properly oriented to the complexities of the procedure and their feelings about it.

Group 10. The Lesbian Couple

Lesbian couples bring a unique situation to egg donation. Often many of these couples, through their demographic situation, really fall into one of the other groups. Yet almost universally lesbian couples report their willingness to disclose that the baby is an egg-donor baby and sperm-donor baby. Couples in Group 10 often report that they have the blessings of friends and family who support the couple.

CHOOSING A CLINIC

Finding the right clinic to carry out your egg donation is extremely important. As you look at your various choices, think about:

- *Experience.* You should ask how many egg-donor procedures the clinic has done and for how long they have been in practice. Although the egg-donation procedure can be thought of as each half of an IVF being done by each person in the pair, the more experience the doctors have had with medicating a donor, who is often younger and hopefully more fertile than a typical IVF patient, the less room there is for mistakes. Also, the recipient takes medications as well, so the doctors need to be familiar with these.
- *Cost.* As we go to press, the cost ranges from $15,000 to $25,000 for an unshared cycle (in contrast to a shared cycle in which two recipients each get half of all the eggs produced by a single donor), with the fee to the donor ranging from a low of $2,000 to a more typical $5,000. Some clinics allow you to share a cycle, that is you and another recipient pay around 60 percent of the complete cost (you still pay 100 percent of your own cycle and split the cost of the donor's medical costs and fee) and you and the other recipient split the eggs that the donor makes.
- *Wait for a donor.* The average wait is six months. For someone who has been trying to get pregnant for some time, a wait of more than six months seems forever. But, on the other hand, everyone wants a donor who will work out and is the "right" donor. Most clinics underestimate the time it will take to "match" you or to get you in a cycle.
- *Ease of working.* Some clinics are set up to deal with "long-distance" recipients. The donor does all her work at the clinic; the recipient makes only three visits to the center. The first is for the initial interview and to have all the necessary medical tests that must be performed at the clinic (like the practice transfer and providing a sperm

sample to be frozen), the second is to provide a fresh sample on the day of the retrieval, and the third is for the transfer itself (which is typically two to five days after the retrieval).

HOW CLINICS MATCH RECIPIENTS TO ANONYMOUS EGG DONORS: THREE MODELS

Clinics match you with a donor in three basic ways. Sometimes it's hard to know before the fact which one you prefer, but it helps to think about the three types of matching. As you read the three scenarios below, picture yourself involved in each situation. Each model is based on a different philosophy.

Clinic Donor List: The Sperm Bank Model

The first model, a clinic donor list, lets you choose an egg donor from a list the same way you would select a sperm donor from a sperm-bank list. Clinics using this model completely screen a donor before they even put her on the list. The advertisement "100 donors screened and ready" is in fact true. In the same manner as they do for a sperm-donor list, a clinic using this model fully screens the donors because they assume that the donors will be used in up to ten matches, so the cost of this screening will be absorbed by ten couples. The clinic publishes a list with information such as height, weight, ethnicity, eye color, hair color, number of years of college, and number of children. You can request longer forms with more information. Typically, then, you match yourself and select one or many donors you would like to match with. You can put yourself on the "waiting" list for that donor. The whole process can occur without much human intervention, although the clinic may have a nurse coordinator who can provide her opinion of the looks or intelligence of the donor.

Pros: You are in charge of the matching. You keep control. You can select as many potential donor candidates as you wish. You don't have to allow anyone else to make the match for you.

Cons: You may pass up a donor who is perfect for you because on paper she doesn't sound like a match. The human touch is missing from the process. The donor you select may be already selected and has six matches before you. The donor may be into another phase of her life. Although previously she was ready, now she's pregnant.

A Person or a Committee Does the Matching: The Matchmaker Model

The matchmaker model is loosely based on the dating-service model. When you come to visit a clinic using this model, a person screens you and that same person screens the donors. The interview is the critical piece in this model. Prior to this important interview, the clinic asks that you complete a form listing characteristics of both you and your husband, as well as your expectations about your donor's characteristics. During this interview, the donor coordinator uses this form as a starting-off point. From that list, the donor coordinator informs you what expectations are realistic and how long the wait for that particular donor might be. During the interview, the coordinator spends several hours observing you and your partner. Then all of you together draw up a working list of essential characteristics that are possessed by your donor-to-be. When an appropriate donor is recruited, the coordinator presents this match to you. Important to the success of this model is a donor coordinator who is able to listen and observe well, who is able to help you figure out what is really important to you, and who can carefully screen donors in an equally significant donor interview.

When we do our work, we use the matchmaker model. (Maybe we like this model because the two of us met through a personal ad in *The New York Review of Books*). After matching donors and recipients for almost ten years, we can say that this model is our favored modus operandi. Before we meet with our potential recipients, we ask them to summarize their physical characteristics, education, and interests on a form we provide. We also ask them to think about their "wish-list" characteristics and fill in a similarly detailed form. Filling out the form is an exercise in and of itself. Even if your clinic has its own form or has no form at all, we encourage you and your partner to complete the form separately and then use your responses to stimulate discussion between the two of you.

DONOR MATCHING FORM

Assign a weight from 1 (not important) to 10 (extremely important) to each of the following donor characteristics. Please add comments when applicable.

Egg-Donor Characteristics	Importance	Comments
Donor's age		
Donor's blood type		
Donor mom's race		
Donor dad's race		
Donor mom's ethnicity		
Donor dad's ethnicity		
Donor mom's religion		
Donor dad's religion		
Donor's height		
Donor's weight		
Donor's body type		
Donor's skin type		
Donor's eye color		
Donor's hair color		
Donor's hair texture		
Whether donor went to college		
Donor's major (if went to college)		
Donor's occupation		
Donor's hobbies and interests		
Donor's motivation to be a donor		
Whether donor has children and how many		

Many recipients tell us that they fill out the form separately from their partner and then come together and find out that they are shocked and surprised at their partner's responses. They also say that the form made them take stock of what really matters in a donor. We use the form as a starting point for a long and intensive discussion, during which time many recipients are made aware of what really matters in their quest for parenting. We review their ideas concerning ethnic and religious prejudices, the notion of heredity versus environment, what life skills they value, what they believe constitutes intelligence, what they consider beautiful, for example. Then, we share with them our own personal experiences and the experiences of other recipients with views similar to theirs.

Pros: A trained person who knows both you and the donors does the matching. You can have a realistic assessment of the time the process might take, based on your lists of essential characteristics. The donor coordinator can help you figure out what really matters to you. There is one person who has met all three of you and can talk about why the match is a good one.

Cons: Your coordinator may not match you with someone you find suitable. The matching process is controlled by someone else. The coordinator may have not correctly estimated the waiting time and you remain unmatched for months. You may be presented with a donor who has yet to be medically screened. You must accept the word and the judgment of the coordinator or others at the practice in terms of beauty of face and figure because the procedure is always anonymous.

Next in Line: The Medical Model

The medical model is based on the notion that egg donation is merely a medical procedure—the next step in your quest to have a baby. As recipients, you provide the clinic using this model with a short list of essential characteristics—yours and the potential donor's. The list of waiting recipients is dealt with fairly chronologically. If you are the next person on the list, you get the next available donor, who often may not match you physically or intellectually. If you refuse the donor, the clinic may present you with another donor but frown on your refusing. If you refuse, you go to the bottom of the list, or at least farther down the line. Implicit in this matching is that an egg is an egg is an egg.

At the clinic, you are encouraged to view your donor in much the same way adoption agencies ask you to think about your birth mother—as someone who facilitates the creation of a baby. If you adopt a baby, you may not know much about the characteristics of your birth mother. Physicians at the clinic view the donor as someone who will provide eggs to enable you to become pregnant and probably believe that environment plays a critical role in how the child turns out. And, of course, you do get to use your husband's sperm to provide half of your child's gene pool. And you get to provide the uterine environment in which your baby is nurtured.

Pros: Shorter wait, less complicated matching process.

Cons: You may be presented with a donor whom you feel is a less-than-ideal match; you may have to balance your desire to be matched soon with your feelings that the donor presented is less than ideal. You may develop a reputation as "difficult" if you reject a donor. Also implicit in this model is that, because the staff believes that the donor is merely facilitating the procedure, they may treat the donor as if she were not particularly important. You should view your visit as an audition; you are "trying out" how you would feel if you were to do your cycle here.

WHO ARE DONORS?:
TWO TYPICAL PROFILES

One of the first questions potential recipients ask us is "Who are the donors?" Many recipients cannot believe that anyone would willingly go through a drug cycle for someone else, because they themselves have endured so many Pergonal cycles. Others tell us that they are sure that the only reason donors go through the procedure is for the money. Consequently, they view donors as decidedly unsavory.

You too probably wonder who the donors are and why they undergo the procedure. You probably harbor some misconceptions about donors and would really like to get a sense of who your donor could be. We have interviewed about 2,000 potential donors. Although each donor is a unique person with a set of characteristics and experiences that are all her own, we can make some generalizations about donors:

- Many donors have family or close friends who have experienced infertility or adoption.
- Most donors have confidence that their bodies work right. In contrast to recipients, who often feel that their bodies "betray them," donors report that their bodies can withstand physical and emotional stress. Donors tell us that they are up and around the day after surgery or childbirth, that they never get sick and require little sleep. They don't worry about the drugs or the retrieval.
- Many donors are physical risk takers. They state that their hobbies are ones like skydiving or rock climbing. In contrast, recipients often tell us that they are risk takers in life (in business or career or finance or even emotionally) but would not say they are physical risk takers.
- Most donors report that they are content with their life and love their families. A typical population of college women scores about 11 on a widely used measure of depression, the Beck Depression Inventory—they are depressed.[2] College donors, in contrast, score under 5: They are not depressed. They report, for example, that they love their parents and are happy with their lives. Donors (ones who are accepted to be donors) are motivated only in part by the money they are paid. Donors are most often motivated by altruism or by healthy narcissism, or a little of both.

Jennifer: More than a Kmart Shopper

On paper, Jennifer seems pretty average. She's five-feet-six-inches tall, weighs 150 pounds—a little more than she should—and has brown eyes and brown hair. She's almost thirty years old, has never been to college, and is a full-time mom with two little girls, aged nine and seven. But Jennifer is far from "average." She has been a donor five times and each time she has made a pregnancy for the recipient. She calls herself a "Fertile Myrtle" and thinks of her "doning" (as she and so many other donors have termed it) as "the second most important thing in my life." The first, of course, is being a mother.

Jennifer came to a donor seminar in the mid-nineties. She knew nothing about the drugs or the injections and the number of visits it would take. When she found out all the information, she was not sure she could master all the drug mixing or the schedule or whether her husband could give her shots. Her husband's initial reaction was that it was too much to do: "It'll really change our lives—no more beer on the weekends, no more trips to the shore in the summer. I don't want my wife to work. I don't want it to screw up her fertility. What if we want to have another child?"

After thinking about whether she wanted to be a donor for over a month, Jennifer called the clinic and scheduled her psychological screening. She brought with her a list of her husband's concerns as well as her own. She talked a lot about her large and loving family. She explained that she learned a lot about giving growing up but how difficult it had been financially for her in a family of five sisters and two brothers. She wanted to explain how she always wished to go to college but there was no money. She said she thought she always wanted to be a decorator or maybe an architect—she told us how she was steaming wallpaper off the walls of her "incredibly old farmhouse" and each layer revealed a "different time and older and older styles of wallpaper—I got a glimpse of older and older generations of moms. I felt like I was reaching back over time." Jennifer seemed smart but was rough around the edges.

Liz: A Student on the Go

Liz is very typical of another sort of donor we meet at every seminar. Liz is a twenty-three-year-old college student extraordinaire. She's a double major: sports medicine and psychology; she's a member of the college soccer team; she belongs to many clubs and organizations; she's been to "twenty-six of the fifty states" and wants to get a graduate degree in health psychology when "I'm around thirty." She'd also like to get married someday, "but not now," and have at least "three kids." As well as being physically active—she works out and runs at least three times a week—and very busy socially, she holds down a part-time job at the local deli because she's paying her own way through school. At twenty-three, Liz has one more semester to earn a bachelor's degree at a major state university.

Liz describes her family as "good-looking and smart." Her father is a businessman and her mother is a full-time mom. Neither of them went to college, but Liz and her two brothers and one sister are "all headed for that bachelor's degree." Liz does have a steady boyfriend with whom she is sexually active. "He supports my decision; it's my body and I can do what I want with it. In fact, Nick will be my injector." Liz has told her mother about the donation: "She's okay with it and wishes she could be a donor—she's forty-five, but I think she looks like my sister." Liz hasn't told her father, who might "get upset about the Catholic stuff." Although Liz was raised Catholic, she says, "I got all the good stuff but none of the bad. I think what I am doing is really wonderful, not a sin at all. I won't burn in hell for this." When asked about what she would do if she found herself with an infertility problem when she was in her forties, Liz said, "I'd get a donor, what else?" Liz is clearly a risk taker and is a donor "in part for the money, but more for the experience and to learn about my own fertility and to help some couple along the way."

Like many other college-student donors, Liz is motivated in part by healthy narcissism, a high positive but realistic appreciation of herself. "My eggs should be out there. I am pretty and smart and so is my entire family. I'm not using these eggs now; I just flush 'em down the toilet. I'm ready, willing, and able." This confidence helps keep Liz motivated to do a good job and be compliant and dependable. Liz wants to use this activity as a line item on her résumé. "I get something and so does the couple. It's a positive deal for everyone."

USING A DONOR BROKER: WHAT YOU CAN EXPECT

Donor brokers always seem to make the news. Ads suggesting that all former donors are models, actresses, brain surgeons, or physicists seem very appealing to recipients in a hurry. Donor brokers run the gamut: from honest and reliable to despicable. Because of sensational ads promising everything under the sun, it's easy to see why these brokers have grabbed media attention. With notebooks filled with photos and bios, or attractive Web sites offering click-of-the-mouse matching, the donor broker enticingly seems to have what you want. But as you investigate what the broker has to offer, make sure you ask important questions, which are listed below.

- *Recruitment:* How are donors recruited? Where do they run their ads? How large is the operation of the donor broker firm? Does the recruiter work in one state and recruit donors in other states, never actually meeting the donor face to face?
- *Numbers:* For how many procedures have they provided donors? How many donors are currently available? Do they provide statistics in terms of numbers of pregnancies and/or success rates? (Remember that no bureau oversees statistical claims except those made by a medical practice.)
- *Screening:* How is the donor screened psychologically and medically? What tests or profiles are part of the typical screening package? Can you request additional tests over and above this package, and what is the charge? How much of the information is self-reported and how much of the information is verified by the broker? For example, when the donor provides a photo, who can vouch for the fact that the donor looks like her photograph or indeed even is the person in the photograph? Or if the donor says that she has achieved 1300 on her SATs, for example, does she supply an official notification of that result? When the donor takes a psychological test, like the Minnesota Multiphasic Personality Inventory (MMPI), is it administered by a psychologist who remains in the room or can the donor take it home and return it by mail?
- *Repeat Donors:* If the donor has been a donor before, can your medical facility get cycle notes and stimulation sheets from her previous cycles?
- *Degree of Anonymity:* Does the broker provide photographs of the donor and her immediate family? Who verifies that these photos are legitimate? Can the recipient talk to the donor? Can the recipient meet the donor?
- *Commitment:* How many donors have completed cycles? How many

donors have dropped out of cycles? Once a donor is selected, how is the cycle scheduled?

- *Ability to Travel:* Does the recipient need to travel to the location of the donor? If the donor must come to where the recipient is, how many times and for what length of time must the donor be at the recipient's practice?
- *Fees/Insurance/Travel Costs:* What are the fees paid to the broker? To the donor? What legal, insurance, travel, hotel, per diem fees are charged over and above the broker and donor fees?
- *Logistics and Responsibility:* Who administers the donor's injections if she must travel away from home? What protection do you have from the broker if something goes wrong with the donor? Or, after testing negative before being chosen, she tests positive for drugs during the cycle? Or if she doesn't respond to the medication?
- *Practice's Policy on Use of Donors Screened Elsewhere:* Will your practice consider using a donor screened elsewhere? Will they need to rescreen? Will the donor need to travel to the practice prior to starting the procedure? Can the donor start her cycle and be monitored near her home before coming to your area for the week prior to retrieval?

It is the main goal of a donor broker to sell their services to you. Rarely, if ever, do they have a "personal" relationship with you. They have a business relationship with you and want you to use a donor from their pool. Recipients tell us that they would never buy fertility medications over the Internet, yet they turn around and use the services of a donor broker who provides information on the Internet. Use caution if you decide to move to a donor broker.

Recently we had an experience with a donor broker who was working with Louisa, one of our clients. Louisa was looking for a donor who was very "WASP"y—someone tall and thin, with a family originating in England and Scotland and with a college degree. A representative from Broker Deluxe told Louisa that Alexis, a donor who fit the bill perfectly, had been "recruited" but not personally screened. Louisa could think only about the perfect match, not the question of screening. Even though Louisa had to fly the donor to New Jersey from Montana and pay for her hotel while she was being screened,

Louisa was certain that Alexis would pass all the physical and psychological screening.

We all loved Alexis; she passed the psychological screening and all the personal-interview phases of our practice's screening. It was only when Alexis filled out the detailed medical screening form and was in the process of discussing her answers with the nurse coordinator that it came up that Alexis's family had a history of Huntington's disease. Alexis's mother had only recently shown signs of it and Alexis herself was unwilling to be tested for that disease. Alexis could not be a donor under those circumstances. Of course we were sad for Louisa, who was disappointed that she needed to go back to the drawing board in her search for a suitable donor, but we were sadder for Alexis, who faced a 50 percent chance of contracting the disease herself. Prescreening the donor could have saved time, money, and heartache.

KNOWN VERSUS ANONYMOUS DONORS

Most of our recipients seem quite happy to use donors who remain anonymous. They feel that this anonymity protects them, in part, from the donor trying to become involved with them or with their child. They trust that the practice provides them with information essential for them to know. Donors, too, tell us that they are happy donating anonymously. Their concern is very different from the fears of the recipients. Donors fear that a child created from their eggs will grow up and try to meet them and enter their lives. Although we cannot assure any donor or any recipient that this meeting will never happen, we believe in the good-faith decisions of all parties involved and that the donation and all identities will remain anonymous.

Sometimes recipients want to use as their donor someone who is already known to them or even related to them. Sisters donate to sisters, nieces to aunts, and best friends to best friends. There are obvious plusses to this arrangement. The biggest plus, of course, is that the medical, psychological, and educational history of the donor is known in its entirety. If the donor and recipient are related, they share some of the same gene pool. Also, of course, a known donor is less likely not to comply with the protocol or to back out of being a donor. Since a known donor has been privy to much of the infertility quest of the recipient, she is extremely motivated to do a good job.

Unfortunately, there are also downsides to using a friend or relative. If the procedure doesn't work, for example, the donor may take it just as hard as the recipient. And this failure can permanently affect the relationship. Even though she was unsuccessful as a donor, we often see many cases where the donor goes on to have her own pregnancy a few months or even a few years later. The recipient, although outwardly happy for her donor, somehow feels, at least in part, that the baby to be born should have been hers. So many sisters in this situation tell us that they can't believe that their donor sister has gone on to have another successful pregnancy and birth and they remain childless.

DISCLOSURE: BEFORE, DURING, AND AFTER

One of the most riveting questions you may be grappling with is whether or not to disclose. Should we tell? Whom should we tell? When should we tell? How should we tell? Of course there are no right answers to these questions. Interestingly, the "classic medical" answer would be not to tell at all. Quite a few doctors would say that egg donation is merely a medical procedure and the nature of that procedure and its outcome is nobody's business.

On the other hand, certainly it may be the business of the child. You may take the "enlightened" approach and believe that all the world must know what you've done. One of our clients answered a simple question asked by someone in front of her in line in the grocery store—"Where did he get those blue eyes?"—with a long story beginning with the statement, "You know I'm forty-eight years old and never thought I'd have a baby until we got a donor with the most beautiful blue eyes." Our client could have answered with a ready retort like "Thanks, they are beautiful. We think they came from my husband's grandfather, who had lovely blue eyes." Deciding to disclose does not always mean that you have to tell even total strangers.

If you have not decided whether you wish to tell the potential child that he or she is the product of egg donation, you must not tell anyone.

At a recent initial screening meeting, the Jones couple said, "We've hardly told anyone. Just both our mothers and fathers and all our siblings. And some of our very closest friends." When we asked, in response, "Then you're planning to disclose to the baby?" And they answered, "No, we absolutely don't want the child to know." We then explained to them how difficult it might be to keep it from their child since everyone else knew about it.

Gwendolyn and James got married when Gwen was forty and James was thirty-four. Even before she was married, Gwen wanted to be a full-time mother with at least "four or five or six kids, running and playing." They had two children through IVF. After three subsequent failed IVF failures, it was clear that Gwen and James needed to use an egg donor if they wanted their big family.

When she came to see us, Gwen brought her three-year-old and her almost-two-year-old IVF babies. James obviously loved them but at this point in his life seemed less interested in having more, particularly since he worked long hours as an architect. He also felt that this procedure would produce children who looked substantially different from the two current children, who looked very much alike. "I think it would be bad for everyone: Gwen, my kids, me. Gwen is forty-five; she should just stop. I guess I'd do it if we didn't have to tell the new kids. Is it a requirement?"

We explained that disclosure wasn't a requirement, although we often felt it was harder not to tell than to tell. We also explained that we couldn't guarantee that the new child or children would look like the first two. Our discussions helped James understand what was driving Gwen and Gwen to understand how James was worried that their family wouldn't look right together. They decided to go ahead with the procedure; we matched them with a donor of the same height, weight, ethnicity, coloring, build, with a mother and father very similar in height, weight, coloring, and ethnicity to Gwen. The procedure was a success and they have their third child, Jimmy, who does in fact look very much like the first two. Interestingly, Gwen says, "This one is the best—the prettiest, the sweetest, the nicest disposition. Everyone tells me this baby is my most wonderful one so far, because we tried so extra long to have him. I'm glad I decided not to disclose to anyone, particularly since James was so adamant. And how could I ever admit that this perfect baby is not genetically mine? I don't ever think about that."

Disclosure was not the right choice for this couple. Clearly, to tell would have been perceived as undermining the nature of the family unit. Both Gwen and James did not want to bring babies into the world who they felt would be "poor relations, not really the brothers or sisters of Nick and Sarah, our first two." Gwen is about to embark on a transfer of frozen embryos created during the same donor cycle that produced Jimmy. James is happy that they have decided not to disclose. He is thrilled with little Jimmy. He supports Gwen on her quest for the "party of five."

Disclosure seemed right for our second couple, the Caplans. Eileen married young the first time. In less than a year, she had given birth to Barbara and a year after that divorced. Eileen was a single mother for sixteen years and worked and took care of Barbara. Eileen dreamed of having a different life—a loving husband and more children. When she was almost forty, Eileen met Aaron, a man just about her age who had never married. He adored Eileen and Barbara. After a whirlwind courtship, Eileen and Aaron married. Soon after, Aaron adopted Barbara. Soon after that, Eileen and Aaron began trying to have a baby. Aaron was thrilled to be Barbara's new father. He bragged about her all the time. Barbara was delighted that she might be a big sister. She loved her new father. Genetics didn't play a big part in making this family a family.

When Eileen found out that her Day 3 FSH was elevated, she felt sad for a time, but as soon as she got information on ovum donation, she knew that this procedure was right for them. It never occurred to Eileen that she wouldn't disclose. She was just happy that Aaron could be biologically connected to one of their children. It even seemed fair—she was genetically connected to Barbara and Aaron would be to this new baby.

Eileen was matched quickly. She believed strongly that environment plays a major part in how children turn out, so the characteristics of the donor were only of marginal importance to the couple. Eileen became pregnant during her first attempt at egg donation. David's birth announcement read: "Through the generosity of an anonymous woman and through the work of God, we announce that we are the proud parents of David Joshua, born to us on February 21st. Big sister Barbara shares with us in our joy. The four of us ask that you see us as the Caplan family, a family united by love."

MY EXPERIENCES: WORDS FROM
A RECIPIENT MOM

The first questions couples who are considering egg donation ask us are "What was it like?" and "What is it like now?" They want to know everything about the procedure: the pregnancy, the childbirth, and raising and telling the children. Although Helane doesn't consider herself the authority on egg donation, she feels that, having gone through the whole procedure as well as talking with so many donors and recipients, she can tell it like it is, at least for her. Here is Helane's view:

"Since I have not had children who are genetically my own, I cannot compare these children to children who don't exist. The image I had of the children who would have been genetically connected to me was of short, smart, dark-haired, funny children resembling the childhood pictures of myself. These images of my children-to-be did not include factoring in my husband's genes, because these images were created long before I knew my husband. My own real-life children look quite different from this fantasy picture, but look very much like my husband. They are smart; one is short and funny, the other is tall and quite serious. Both are more wonderful than I could ever have imagined. I also cannot imagine loving any children more than I love these two.

"I chose to do egg donation because I had experienced too many failures and disappointments. I had fifteen inseminations and five IVF failures and two miscarriages. Also, between my two pregnancies, an attempted egg-donor cycle, with a wonderful friend as donor, did not even get to retrieval because my friend did not stimulate on Pergonal. Although my doctor at the time thought I should try one more cycle with my own eggs, I felt that I could not face another failed cycle or, worse yet, another miscarriage.

"I actually talked the doctors at IVF New Jersey into doing the procedure. I was their first success and actually joke about how they were one page ahead of me in the medical textbook. But pregnant I was, and with twins!

"When I became pregnant with these babies, I did not know anyone who had given birth to a donor baby. I was absolutely terrified during the first few months of the pregnancy. What had I done? Who would these babies be? Why had I used this particular donor and not some other mythical donor? I tried my best to provide a wonderfully nurturing physical and emotional uterine environment for them to grow. My husband marveled as I focused all my energy on growing these babies and making them my own.

"The questions really subsided the moment I felt the babies kick. It was as if the psychological pressure had lifted. These babies were alive! (Although I had known they were from the ultrasound scans.) They existed as my children and it was now my job to continue to nurture them and to get to know them.

"Because they were twins, I could focus on both how they were similar and how they were different. I knew there had not been any studies on the effect of uterine environment as differentiated from genetics, but I wanted to begin to shape the developing babies. Even though I would never know if it had any effect, I felt that these nine months would be my contribution to their development prior to birth.

"The day my children were born, my husband videotaped me actually predicting what the children would be like. I felt I knew them so well. Nathaniel liked consistency. His heartbeat was regular; he moved at the same time every day. When I was cold, he seemed unhappy. "Make it like it was before," he seemed to say. My everyday diet of tofu and broccoli was fine with him. Nathaniel likes to eat the same thing every day and has trouble on the first day of a vacation and on the last. He likes everything to stay the same. I joke that he will fall in love in the second grade and remain faithful to his choice and ultimately marry her.

"Allegra, on the other hand, was my risk-taking-in-utero dancer. She flipped and flopped and kicked and was quiet whenever she pleased. She didn't care if it was cold or hot or what I ate. She kicked me so hard in one of my classes that my students at the back of the room saw her foot push at my upper abdomen. They all predicted, as did I, that she would never stop moving. And indeed she never has stopped. She was always hard to find in my uterus; she moved wildly and then slept whenever she wanted. She still does. She walked at 10½ months and hasn't stopped.

"When I saw the children at the moment of their birth, I was struck by how much they both looked like my husband. It almost seemed as if the donor provided the X chromosomes that enabled conception but my husband had contributed the lion's share. (And, interestingly, so many egg-donor babies look just like the daddies. And I know, since I have seen the donor and the daddy!) The inequality that so many couples talk about—that he contributed and I didn't—seemed a plus, not a minus, since the moment I saw my children I knew that they were like the man I married. I was happy that his genes were central.

"When people tell me how gorgeous my children are, I always say, 'Yes, aren't they?' It's as if doing this procedure allows me to be unnarcissistic because their appearance is not about me. I too can step away and marvel at their beauty. I must say that when I look into their eyes, I do not see my grandfather or my father or my mother or myself. The faces are not mine or anyone's in my family. Yet when I look deeper into their souls or when I see them move or hear them speak, I do see and hear myself.

"Our family started talking about donors when our children were two years old. Nathaniel always hears what he wants. He thought I had said "doughnut baby" and somehow must have believed he was made at Dunkin' Donuts, like the Munchkins he likes.

"Not much discussion happened until they were four. Occasionally, when the phone rang, Allegra would say, 'It must be a donor.' One day, when she was almost five, she turned to me and said, 'What exactly does a donor give you?' I told her that our donor gave Mommy a chance to have two babies: you and Nathaniel. At six, Allegra said, 'I know who my donor is. It's Auntie Susan' [Dr. Susan Treiser, one of the medical doctors at IVF New Jersey]. I explained that Auntie Susan had been one of the doctors but not the donor. I explained that the donor didn't want Allegra or Nathaniel to know her and that, because she had been so wonderful, we had to honor what she wanted. Allegra then said, 'But did she have yellow hair?' I said yes and that seemed to suffice.

"One of the most chilling incidents occurred the May that Allegra was five. One Sunday night I gave Allegra permission to watch the Tony Awards on television. I thought she would just fall asleep on the sofa and I could watch the program quietly. Instead, she was noisy and disruptive and wasn't about to watch the program or fall asleep. I told her that she needed to go upstairs to bed because Mommy wanted to watch the show. She turned to me and said, 'You're not my real

Mommy.' My heart fell. 'Why not?' I asked. 'Because my real Mommy would let me do exactly what I wanted.' 'No,' I said, 'a real mommy would teach you to be polite and to let someone else have a special moment. You go to bed now. I'm your real mommy and I insist.' She complied, but I have to say that, even though I know that what she said was a typical bratty five-year-old remark, it certainly made my heart stop for an instant. Now that I've had one of my worst fears realized—even though it came from an overtired five-year-old—that my children would someday reject me as Mommy, I'm certain I can deal with the real thing should it arise.

"We continue to prepare what we tell the children. We have established a weekly ritual during which all of us put money into a container to be given to a local charity anonymously. We explain to the children that the best way to give charity is without telling who we are so that the person receiving the charity doesn't feel indebted to us in particular. We hope that the children learn to embrace those principles of giving gifts without strings. We also hope that we will be good enough parents that they continue to be people who are givers. We also hope that they will honor the request of the donor and not try to find her.

"Each day brings new challenges. But I have what I have always wanted: a family. Our children are uniquely themselves—a combination of their daddy, their donor, and me, but primarily they are loving, happy, healthy, bright children, just as I had hoped they would be. When it comes right down to it, I suspect that's your dream, too."

CHAPTER 11

Using Third Parties to Help You Get Pregnant: Sperm Donation, Surrogacy, and Embryo Donation

he previous chapter was devoted to a discussion of egg donation. In this chapter we discuss the remaining third-party procedures: sperm donation, surrogacy, and embryo donation. Taken together, all of these third-party procedures augment other forms of assisted reproduction, giving couples the means to get pregnant when they thought they couldn't.

SPERM DONATION

The procedure of using sperm from a donor when your partner's sperm is not effective or if you do not have a male partner is called sperm donation. As you read through this and other books about sperm donation, you may find that the authors use a variety of other terms, including therapeutic donor insemination (TDI), which we ourselves used in the last edition but choose not to use in this edition. Because many people use donor sperm for IVF as well as for insemination, we believe that the term *sperm donation* more accurately describes what we discuss in this chapter. Other terms include *donor insemination*, *artificial insemination*, and *therapeutic insemination*.

Sperm donation has been used as a treatment for male infertility for almost 125 years.[1] An estimated 30,000 babies are born annually in the United States as a result of sperm donation. Of all the third-party procedures described in this chapter, sperm donation has the highest success rate and is the least expensive and simplest to accomplish, medically speaking.

One reason for the popularity of sperm donation is its versatility. Donor sperm can be used in cervical inseminations, intrauterine inseminations, during natural menstrual cycles, or during cycles stimulated by fertility drugs, either with an insemination or with an ART procedure. Your own medical situation will dictate how the donor sperm will be used and how it will affect your success. Women who have two healthy fallopian tubes, no endometriosis, need no medication to stimulate ovulation, and are under the age of thirty-five have an excellent chance of becoming pregnant within three to six cycles.

If you have one or more medical problems, your chances for success will be lessened. Before you begin making the decision to use donor sperm, it's important that you ask your physician for a realistic assessment of your chances for success in your particular situation. Obviously, costs for all your treatment will vary substantially, based on what you need to have done medically; one intracervical insemination will cost much less than a series of six IUIs. Sperm typically costs from $125 to $250 per vial. Typically, you will probably need one to three vials per procedure. If you feel confident that you have selected the sperm donor for you, you may wish to purchase a number of additional vials in case your first several procedures are not successful, or if you want to use the same donor for a subsequent pregnancy.

Donor Sperm or Partner's Sperm: A Decision-Making Activity

Couples come to see us to help them decide whether to use donor sperm or partner sperm. We advise them to use the decision-making procedure we introduced earlier in this book. If you are in the throes of making this decision, here is a table to help guide your thinking.

Factor	Weight (A)	Grade for Donor Sperm (B)	Grade for Partner's Sperm (C)	A x B	A x C
Cost of procedure					
Likelihood of success					
Invasiveness of technique for partner					
Concern about medications for woman					
Concerns about partner's genetic link to child					
Feelings of having a stranger's sperm inside woman					
Other factors					

If you are a single woman, a lesbian with a female partner, or if you have a male partner who carries a genetic defect and does not want to risk passing on that defect, you will probably go directly to donor sperm.

Finding the Sperm Bank for You

It's hard to know how to begin your search for a sperm donor. We encourage you to visit the Web sites of the leading sperm banks. To give you a sense of what you will find there, we have prepared the following table, which will help you get started.

Selecting a Sperm Bank

Sperm banks vary widely in terms of their number of available donors, the types of donors available (ethnically and educationally, for example), the completeness of information available, kinds of medical testing, profile types (long and short, for example), cost, identity release, specimen claims, availability of washed and unwashed sperm, and how, where, and to whom they will ship.

We recommend that you collect lists and information from at least five banks before you even begin to make a selection. In addition to the ones mentioned in the chart above, you can find information at http://www.ihr.com/infertility/provider/spermbank.html. You can also visit http://www.fertilitext.org/sbanks.html to review information about accreditation of banks. Make sure that you select from banks that are licensed. Any reputable sperm bank will be licensed in more that one state; many sperm banks are members of the American Association of Tissue Banks (http://www.aatb.org/), an organization that provides quality screening of the bank itself. Also make sure to find out if your doctor or clinic has one or two preferred banks. Often doctors have had successful experiences with several sperm banks and not such positive experiences with others.

More than anything else, your sperm donor needs to have fabulous sperm. Even if a donor has movie-star looks, genius brains, and is the right ethnicity for you, if his sperm is not of high quality, he's no good as a donor.

Selecting Your Sperm Donor

After you have narrowed your sperm-banks list to at least three preferred banks, start looking through the lists. As you read through the lists, you will need to start narrowing down your search. In order to do that, it's important to figure out what matters to you. You may want a donor who is a "duplicate" of your partner in terms of ethnicity, education, religion, blood type, height, weight, eye color, hair color, college major, career, hobbies and interests—the whole package. Or you may want to duplicate you, particularly if you don't have a partner. So if you are Irish and Italian, have type O-positive blood, Catholic, tall

Name of Bank	California Cryobank	Fairfax Cryobank	Xytex	Sperm Bank of California	New England Cryogenic Center (NECC)
Contact Info	http://www.cryobank.com Client Relations Manager, Melonee Evans 1019 Gayley Avenue Los Angeles, CA 90024 (310) 443-5244 Fax: (310) 443-5258 (800) 231-3373 E-mail: mevans @cryobank.com	http://www.fairfaxcryobank.com/ 3015 Williams Drive, Suite 110, Fairfax, VA 22031 (800) 338-8407 703-698-3976 Fax: (703) 698-3933 E-mail: cryobank @givf.com	http://www.xytex.com/ 1776 Peachtree St., NW, Suite 175 Atlanta, GA 30309 Phone: (404) 881-0426 Fax: (404) 881-6444 E-mail: info @xytex.com	http://www.the spermbankofca.org/ The Sperm Bank of California Reproductive Technologies, Inc. 2115 Milvia Street, 2nd Floor Berkeley, CA 94704-1112 (510) 841-1858 Fax: (510) 841-0332 E-mail: info@the spermbankofca.org	http://www.necryogenic.com Catherine R. Rizza, President and CEO, New England Cryogenic Center 665 Beacon St. Boston, MA 02215-3202 (617) 262-3311 Fax: (617) 262-1234 E-mail: necryo @necryogenic.com
Fees	DONOR SEMEN SERVICES ICI (intracervical insemination) Prepared donor specimen: $165.00 IUI (intrauterine insemination) with prepared donor specimen: $195.00	Fairfax Doctorate $208.00 (ICI) $248.00 (IUI) Fairfax (Regular) $168.00 (ICI); $198.00 (IUI) Family Solutions: $115.00 (ICI); $115.00 (IUI)	Complete Donor Profile without PhotoFile: $10.00 Complete Donor Profile with PhotoFile: $25.00 Six-month registration fee with unlimited access: $100.00	Donor Specimen Donor Specimen 0.8cc–1.0cc $150 Donor Specimen 0.5cc $95 Donor Specimen IUI ready: $185 Donor catalogue: Free Donor profile	Fee schedule not listed on Web site; Same day orders $25 extra Photo matching: $50 Characteristic matching (you fill out a form with characteristics you are looking for): $25 extra

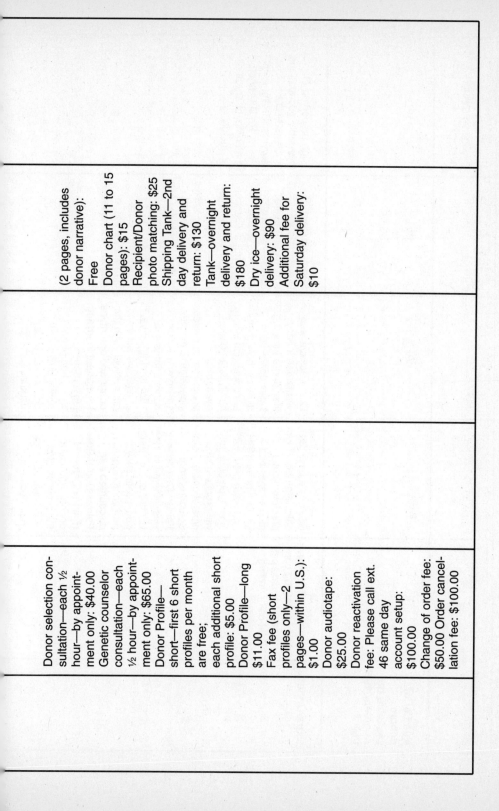

Donor selection consultation—each ½ hour—by appointment only: $40.00

Genetic counselor consultation—each ½ hour—by appointment only: $65.00

Donor Profile—short—first 6 short profiles per month are free; each additional short profile: $5.00

Donor Profile—long $11.00

Fax fee (short profiles only—2 pages—within U.S.): $1.00

Donor audiotape: $25.00

Donor reactivation fee: Please call ext. 46 same day account setup: $100.00

Change of order fee: $50.00 Order cancellation fee: $100.00

(2 pages, includes donor narrative): Free

Donor chart (11 to 15 pages): $15

Recipient/Donor photo matching: $25

Shipping Tank—2nd day delivery and return: $130

Tank—overnight delivery and return: $180

Dry ice—overnight delivery: $90

Additional fee for Saturday delivery: $10

Name of Bank	California Cryobank	Fairfax Cryobank	Xytex	Sperm Bank of California	New England Cryogenic Center (NECC)
Number of donors available on Aug/Sept 1999 List	169	114	76	40	87
Extra Options	Genetic counseling, donor matching consultation, audiotapes, racial color coding of specimens.	Site has a birth date calculator, blood-type predictor (enter mother type and father type and RH and table tells you what type of donor will produce what type of child); Family Solutions from Fairfax Cryobank was initiated in 1998 to offer donor sperm from pregnancy proven donors at a discounted rate; Fairfax Doctorate (Fairfax Cryobank donors who are in the process of or who have completed their doctorate	Donor essays, supplemental donor profiles (extra info, e.g., Does donor have dimples, how many people in donor's family have blue eyes, etc.), photofiles, babyfiles, videofiles; if the offspring of a Xytex donor contacts us after turning 18 years of age, we will try to get in touch with the donor and determine his interest in arranging a meeting; Xytex has permanently preserved donor cells to be used as genetic	Sperm storage; Directed donor screening (private donors); semen analysis; sperm washing; assistance with home insemination; will ship to patient if you register through a medical professional who can be a doctor, nurse practitioner, osteopath, physician's assistant, or certified nurse midwife.	High proportion of desirable occupations such as M.D.s, lawyers, CPA's, engineers, Ph.D.s; photo matching, characteristic matching.

degrees, these individuals include: chiropractic, dental, law [juris doctorate], medical, optometry, and Ph.D. students and graduates; Photo matching; Genetic counseling; 2nd child by same donor; Donor reactivation; Keirsey temperament sorter	records. This process is known as Patriarch Genetic Tracking.		No form available for searching.	
Search options	Form available; can specify following variables on which to search: Race, previous pregnancy made, availability of audiotape, ethnic origin, blood type, religion, height, weight, hair color, hair texture, eye color, skin tone, years of education, occupation.	Form has search options for height, eye color, college education, race, blood type, ethnic background, hair, race.	Form allows you to search on hair color, eye color, blood type, height.	No form available for selecting based on specific characteristics.
Hard-to-find donor ethnic availability	African American, Chinese, Latino, East Indian, Polynesian, Jewish	Asian Indian, Chinese, Filipino, Japanese, Jewish, Korean	Puerto Rican, Native American, Filipino, Taiwanese, African American, Jewish	African American, East Asian Indian, Asian Chinese, Latino, Jewish	Chinese, African American, American Indian, Hispanic, Jewish

and thin, and like camping and history, you might look for someone with these traits. That way you can help up the odds that your baby will look like you and maybe even prefer the same sorts of activities. (There are many experts who say that it is socialization and nurture, not nature, that determines whether your child will like, say, camping.) Or you may want to read the long profiles of several very different sorts of donors and then select a donor who has fabulous sperm and seems like a nice guy—someone you think you might like to spend time with, if you could. You and your partner might make your selections separately and then compare notes. Or you may wish to work together throughout the process. We have helped countless couples and single women make their choices, and we can say that no two conducted their search in exactly the same way.

Here is a form you can use to help you evaluate potential donors. Photocopy this form and make several copies to use for this activity. If you prefer, you can download this form from our Web site, http://www.gettingpregnantbook.com. Next to each characteristic assign a weight from 1 (not important) to 10 (extremely important) to each of the following donor characteristics. Then use a separate form to assess how well each donor measures up to these characteristics. Write some remarks in the "Comments" column next to each characteristic if you have something special to say about that characteristic for that particular donor.

How Gary and Sabrina Selected Their Donor

Gary and Sabrina, a married couple in their early thirties, came to see us to help them select a sperm donor. While in his twenties Gary had been treated for non-Hodgkins lymphoma and was essentially sterile. Just after he met Sabrina, Gary had explained his medical condition to her, so now Sabrina felt very comfortable with having a baby by donor insemination.

What we did to help Gary and Sabrina was to send them on a computer search, to visit the sperm banks at each bank's Web site, and to collect all the available information from these five banks. What really struck them was the wide variety of donors available across the five banks.

Donor # _____ Sperm Bank _____

Sperm Donor Characteristics	Importance	Comments
Donor's age		
Donor's blood type		
Donor mom's race		
Donor dad's race		
Donor mom's ethnicity		
Donor dad's ethnicity		
Donor mom's religion		
Donor dad's religion		
Donor's height		
Donor's weight		
Donor's body type		
Donor's skin type		
Donor's eye color		
Donor's hair color		
Donor's hair texture		
Donor's education		
If college, donor's major		
Donor's occupation (present or future)		
Donor's hobbies and interests		
Donor's intelligence		
Motivation to donate		
Has donor made pregnancies?		
Other		

At our second session, Gary and Sabrina seemed more relaxed: They knew they had some choices. They felt empowered because the decision seemed back in their hands. We then asked each member of the couple to make a list of from seven to ten characteristics important to each of them, listing from most to least important.

Gary's list: Healthy, smart, Jewish, no family history of cancer, no drug or alcohol abuse, family history of longevity: Grandparents lived until their eighties/parents still alive, O-positive or A-positive blood type, athletic, brown hair, light eyes.

Sabrina's list: Over five-ten, thin, handsome, brown curly or wavy hair, blue eyes, athletic, funny, smart in science, likes the outdoors, Jewish.

Understandably, Gary's list was primarily about health. "I want this kid not to go through what I did. I want this baby to be healthy and be smart and Jewish. I know that any baby born to us will be raised Jewish, but I'd feel more comfortable with a Jewish donor. And I hope that the blood type would be like ours. Then I'd hope for a donor who is athletic and has light eyes and brown hair like everybody in my family."

Sabrina was very much concerned about the looks of the donor. She wanted a donor who shared Gary's physical characteristics as well as his interests and abilities. "I love Gary. I know I'll love any baby we have together, but I'm sad that the baby won't look like Gary. I'll do anything I can to pick a donor who's the best 'stand-in' for Gary. For me, physical characteristics are a way to start. Then I want to read the long forms. I need to know the donor, and like him. I feel as if he were the uncle of our baby. Is that weird?"

We assured Sabrina that her feelings weren't weird, that it was important for her to feel connected to her donor. We asked her to understand that Gary needed to feel that the donor was healthy and came from a healthy family. We spent the session making a list of the characteristics that would shape our first search through the sperm donor lists at all five banks. The couple felt comfortable with using these characteristics as criteria for their donor: Jewish, at least four years of college (note that college doesn't necessarily mean that a donor is smart, but it was one objective way of determining the donor's intellectual potential), five-eight or taller, brown hair, blue eyes. Gary and Sabrina also decided that they didn't want current photos, baby pictures, videotapes, or audiotapes ("Too creepy" was what Sabrina said), but they knew that they wanted to read the long form on each donor they were considering. "The long forms are not so expensive and you learn so much. I also want to be able to give these forms to our OB-GYN and the pediatrician so that we can be prepared for everything medically," explained Gary. Sabrina felt she needed the long form so she could get to know the donor and his family.

Before the next session, we encouraged Sabrina and Gary to go through the banks and select those donors who met their criteria. We encouraged them to begin to get the long profiles of all donors who seemed like possibilities. Two weeks passed before we saw the couple. Then they walked in with a pile of forms. Both Gary and Sabrina were smiling. "You were right. You said that the long forms would help. We really only had six donors who met our criteria. Two of them had cancer and heart attacks in their family. One said he had absolutely no athletic ability. One more said theater was his major—we wanted science. So two seemed really perfect. Then I saw that Donor 751 at Fairfax shared Gary's birthday and even had a dimple. We ordered his sperm that's IUI-ready and hope to have an insemination next cycle. In fact, we ordered enough for three inseminations and have vials in storage for our second pregnancy. We're ready."

Gary and Sabrina got pregnant on their second insemination. Sabrina is carrying a singleton baby and the couple is very happy with their decision.

How Teresa and Janelle Selected Their Donor

Teresa and Janelle came to see us because the practice where they were having their treatment required, based on ASRM (American Society for Reproductive Medicine) guidelines, that all couples seeking the use of donor sperm receive counsel on the implications of their decision. Teresa and Janelle had been together for over three years. Since they hoped to have children together, the couple planned first for Teresa to bear a child and then Janelle. Teresa, who was now thirty-six, had been trying to become pregnant for almost a year through home inseminations. Her partner, Janelle, was just twenty-five. "I hate to go to Plan B already. I wanted to have the first baby and then Janelle the second.

It didn't seem to be working. I just found out my tubes are blocked. I'll go through at least one in vitro, but we'll see how it goes before I decide if I want to do another. I'm really sorry we didn't buy more vials of our donor's sperm. We liked him a lot, but he's been retired."

Both Teresa and Janelle were aware of the implications of their decision to use donor sperm. They had several friends who had achieved pregnancy through donor sperm. Both their families supported their decision. Their employers also knew what they intended to do. They felt comfortable that they had a strong support system. What they were unsure of was what to do in terms of selecting a second donor.

The couple had been using donor sperm from the Sperm Bank of California for a number of reasons. They liked the fact that the bank worked with all individuals, including lesbian couples and single women. The Sperm Bank of California had worked with them to arrange shipping to Teresa's office (where somebody is available between nine and five to receive the shipment), had given them detailed directions for self-insemination, and had supported them through their pregnancy quest. They decided to continue working with this bank.

When they made their lists of three, both Janelle and Teresa had placed Donor 1019 on their lists. When they read his long form, they liked everything about him, most specifically that he had a one-year-old egg-donor brother. They were sure that the whole family was open-minded. That characteristic, plus the fact that the donor was working on a law degree, made him the couple's choice.

SURROGACY

Surrogacy is the oldest infertility procedure; it has been used and written about since biblical times. Yet even in the Bible surrogacy has been fraught with difficulty:

"Now Sarai Abram's wife bore him no children; and she had a handmaid, an Egyptian, whose name was Hagar. And Sarai said unto Abram, 'Behold now the Lord hath restrained me from bearing; go in, I pray thee, unto my handmaid; it may be that I shall be builded up through her.' And Abram hearkened to the voice of Sarai." (Genesis 16:1–2).

Hagar was the first but not the last surrogate for a matriarch. Sarai's grandson, Jacob, married Rachel, who was also infertile. Rachel said to Jacob, "Behold my maid Bilhah, go in unto her; that she may bear upon my knees, and I also may be builded up through her." (Genesis: 30:3). Not to be outdone by her sister-in-law, Leah, dealing with secondary infertility, demanded a surrogate for herself. "When Leah saw that she had left off bearing she took Zilpah her handmaid, and gave her to Jacob to wife. And Zilpah Leah's handmaid bore Jacob a son." (Genesis 30: 9–10). Surrogacy was clearly a widely used, and evidently, according to biblical statistics, a highly successful infertility treatment as far back as several thousand years ago.

Despite the fact that the matriarchal surrogates produced children, the matriarchal families experienced considerable emotional turmoil and familial upheaval. Currently, surrogacy is less successful but equally stressful. In this section we will discuss the many complexities of modern-day surrogacy.

Who Needs a Surrogate

A woman considering surrogacy typically selects this option for any of the following medical reasons:

- She has no uterus.
- She has been diagnosed with cancer and is about to undergo chemotherapy that will destroy her ovarian function.
- She has structural problems of the uterus or severe uterine scarring.
- She has been advised not to attempt pregnancy for medical reasons.
- She has failed IVF despite the fact that she and her partner produced embryos and her uterus appears to be normal.

Two Types of Surrogates

A surrogate mother is a woman who is artificially inseminated with the sperm of a man whose wife is infertile or otherwise unable to carry a pregnancy. In this procedure, now called *traditional surrogacy*, both the egg and the uterus are provided by the surrogate. After the child is born, the surrogate gives the child to the husband and wife, who legally adopts the child either before or after its birth. In the traditional surrogacy procedure, the child is the genetic child of the woman who carries it. Although the procedure is fairly simple medically (with the surrogate typically getting pregnant without fertility drugs and after one to three months of inseminations), the psychological issues—primarily a mother giving up her child—are extraordinarily complex. In fact, it is this form of surrogacy procedure that created Baby M, who was at the center of a bitter custody battle between the couple and the surrogate, who described an "unexpected bond" to the child.

A second type of surrogacy, growing in numbers, involves an IVF procedure during which an egg is aspirated from the wife (or even from an egg donor) and fertilized by the sperm of the husband in a petri dish. The resulting embryo is placed into the uterus of the *surrogate gestational mother*, also called the *gestational carrier*, who carries the baby for nine months and then gives birth. Although this form of surrogacy procedure involves complex medical intervention—fertility drugs, egg retrievals, and gamete manipulation in the lab—psychological reports suggest that it is less complex psychologically than the more traditional type of surrogacy procedure.

Emotional Aspects of Surrogacy

Opinion polls suggest that the general public takes a dimmer view of surrogate mothering than it does of other third-party procedures. Talk shows featuring surrogates lamenting how they have been exploited and couples describing their decision to use a surrogate as a decision of convenience don't really reflect the majority of how surrogacy is practiced but do much to shape the negative connotation of surrogacy. Couples considering surrogacy tell us that their friends and family fear that their surrogate will be the one in a hundred who refuses to give up the baby.

Participating in a surrogacy procedure is something that no couple can do without exploring all the emotional issues involved. Infertility itself can put a tremendous strain on a marriage. But unlike the other third-party procedures, surrogacy demands that an outsider become part of your life for at least nine months. Working as a Team, therefore, is critical to keeping your marriage on solid ground. Often the relationship with your surrogate doesn't end at the time of birth. Particularly when the surrogate is a friend, she may become part of your extended family. People opposed to surrogacy fear its potential to destroy or undermine a marital bond. On the other hand, pro-surrogacy organizations report that couples who have used a surrogate rarely divorce (only 1 percent as compared to the 49 percent divorce rate in the general population).

Women seeking a surrogate often have personal issues about the procedure, including unresolved feelings about their own infertility, their sense of failure as a woman, their fear that their husband may have "feelings" for the surrogate, their worry that the child may reject them when he or she understands the nature of the conception, and even concern about how others will view the way in which their family-building occurred. A professional counselor can help you explore what you are feeling prior to making the decision, during the pregnancy, and as you raise your child.

The Financial Strain of a Surrogacy Procedure

Financial issues are also difficult ones; surrogacy procedures are very expensive. The table below presents the various expenses you are likely to incur. (The information was provided by Melissa Brisman, an attorney who practices reproductive law at Melissa B. Brisman, Esq., L.L.C., in Montvale, New Jersey.)

Item	Cost
I. Initial attorney's fees	$7,000
II. Carrier's reimbursement for monthly living expenses including food, rent, utilities and telephone:	
a. Single fetus	$1,444/month ($13,000 total)
b. Multiple birth	$1,888/month ($17,000 total)

Item	Cost
III. Carrier's possible reimbursements	
a. Term life insurance	$200
b. Maternity clothing	$500
c. Carrier's reimbursement for an unsuccessful transfer	$500
d. Transportation allowance	$500
e. Attorney's fee for carrier's representation	$500–$1,500
f. Medical expenses not covered by carrier's insurance for doctor's visits, delivery, labwork, etc.	Depends on carrier's insurance
g. Psychological counseling	$600
h. Criminal background check	$200
i. Child care when performing duties under contract	$3–6/hour
IV. Court order for birth certificate	$2,000–$4,000
V. Other possible expenses	
a. Health insurance for carrier per month	$150–$200
b. Lost wages	$2,000 cap
c. Housekeeping if carrier is confined to bed	$50/week
d. Child care if carrier is confined to bed	$3–6/hour
e. Advertising	$2,000
Total expenses for above items	$25,000–$35,000
Additional costs for IVF procedure	$12,000–$15,000
Estimated total costs*	$37,000–$50,000

*Costs for the medical procedure are not included in the estimated expenses. Many couples' insurance policies will cover these expenses. As a result, these costs are highly variable. The medical facility and the attorney's office can help obtain more detailed information upon request. In addition, this represents an estimate of the actual costs incurred. In some circumstances costs may be less that those estimated and in some cases costs may be greater. Couples should use this sheet as a guide. Due to the unusual nature of these types of arrangements, this sheet should in no way be interpreted as a guarantee of costs.

Legal Concerns About Surrogacy

Laws relating to surrogacy are very complex and vary from state to state. Even within one state, laws can be quite complex. What's critical here is that both you and the surrogate secure separate legal counsel and that each of you understands the nature of the contract you are signing. Obviously, any contract is only as good as the people who sign it, but there are many aspects in terms of decision-making during the pregnancy (such as whether or not to continue carrying triplets), clinical intervention (such as amniocentesis), and management of the pregnancy, and provisions for medical problems (the birth of a handicapped infant) and life changes (the death of a member of the couple or a divorce) occurring during the pregnancy.

A Success Story to Help You Through It All: A Surrogate Mother's Tale

Much of this section has been filled with disclaimers and negatives. Yet we need to share with you a happy story. We must stress that most stories about surrogacy are happy ones. Most procedures have a positive end; couples and surrogates report that the procedure and its outcome are primarily positive. We asked Melissa Brisman, a surrogate mother herself and an attorney who aids couples in their search for surrogates, to write her story. Her life and her profession, like ours, have been shaped by her personal experience with infertility.

"After many years wondering if I would ever have a child, my husband and I decided to embark upon a long journey. We decided to pursue gestational surrogacy. Although I could not myself carry a child, I produced healthy viable eggs that could be fertilized with my husband's sperm and placed in a gestational host who would carry the baby to term.

"The journey began with our first visit to the doctor's office on Christmas Eve. My husband and I sat in the office as the doctor explained the medical procedure. The science, he told us, was the easy part. Our chances were over 50 percent each cycle; however, we would need to find a carrier who was both medically and psychologically suitable. As I left the doctor's office my head was spinning. There was so much to digest in one sitting. I began to do research in the area. As a lawyer, I knew there were serious considerations when it came to selecting a carrier. The laws in each state where a carrier might be obtained had to be examined. Each state's law was different with respect to the legality of surrogacy and the legal rights of the intended parents.

"The carrier we eventually found met our expectations and more. She had a family of her own with three children. She had a loving relationship with her husband, who was supportive. She passed the psychological and the medical screening that involved extensive testing for sexually transmitted diseases.

"Even though I was an attorney, I retained a lawyer to assist me with the contract and other complex legal issues that concerned me. By way of example I worried: Could the carrier change her mind? Who had control over the medical decisions once the carrier was pregnant? Whose insurance policy would cover the pregnancy? Whose policy would cover the babies after they were born? Whose decision would it be to reduce the number of fetuses if our carrier became pregnant with more than two fetuses or if one was malformed? Would the provisions in any contract be enforceable? What if the carrier decided she wanted to keep the babies? Could we legally pay our carrier for carrying the babies? All these questions needed to be answered before our carrier became pregnant.

"After all these issues were resolved and the paperwork was done, we were ready to begin. We were lucky and produced nine healthy embryos, three of which were implanted in our carrier's uterus. All three of them stuck initially but by the sixth week of pregnancy only two remained—one had miscarried. We were so excited to be having children after we never thought we could. We prayed the remaining two fetuses would develop into healthy babies.

"The ultrasound at the twentieth week was one of the highlights of the pregnancy. We drove up to Maine to observe and there they were on the ultrasound screen—two healthy boys kicking away in our carrier's uterus. I will never forget the day. After all the hard work it finally seemed like our dreams would become reality. As the birth approached, I tried to see if there was a way to get what is called a parentage order from the local court. This would allow the biological parents, myself and my husband, to be placed on the birth certificate of the children, and would not force my husband and myself to adopt our biological children. I was told that had never been done in Maine and was not possible. I decided to petition the court to see if the court would entertain the possibility. After much hard work I was successful. My law degree was one of my biggest assets in this process, not only with the birth certificate, but also with the many small battles along the way. Our carrier's health insurance refused to cover the carrier's pregnancy when they found out she was carrying the babies for another couple, a legally impermissible tactic that took many painstaking hours to resolve.

"Once all these battles were over, the birth was approaching and we were so excited. Everyone in our family was busy buying two of everything. Then when our carrier was thirty-seven weeks pregnant, the doctor told us that he thought the babies should be delivered shortly. We packed our bags and drove to Maine immediately. After we arrived, our carrier was induced. The room was like a circus with two teams of doctors, my husband, myself, and my carrier's husband. The birth came and went before we knew it. She delivered both little guys fifteen minutes apart. I was able to cut the cord on my firstborn son. The room was filled with joy and our two sons, Andrew and Benjamin, had finally arrived.

"Andrew and Benjamin are healthy and our greatest joy. They are now twenty months old. We wish anyone embarking on this journey all the success and happiness we have enjoyed."

Who Is Your Surrogate?

Couples often wonder what kind of woman would be a surrogate, either a traditional one or a gestational carrier. It seems a difficult thing to do—to carry a baby for nine months knowing that it must be given up. In general, people believe that at worst surrogates become surrogates because they need the money and at best they become surrogates because they want somehow to be the ultimate do-gooder and/or represent altruism extraordinaire. In fact, surrogates often become surrogates for a combination of reasons: altruism, the need to help, and to make restitution perhaps for an abortion or for placing a baby up for adoption in the past.

The Center for Surrogate Parenting (CSP) (www.creatingfamilies. com) describes the typical surrogate mother as a woman who is between the ages of twenty-one and thirty-seven, has two children, and thirteen years of education. Seventy-five percent of CSP's surrogates are married, and one-third have full-time jobs outside the home. The majority of these surrogates are raised in a Christian home; 25 percent are Catholic. The Center for Surrogate Parenting describes these women as responsible and empathetic, and as looking forward to the experience of helping an infertile couple have a child.

Motivations to become a surrogate mother include a positive pregnancy experience of one's own, a history of uncomplicated pregnancies, an opportunity to feel special, empathy for childless couples, importance of one's own children in one's life, financial gain, and a chance to make restitution for a terminated pregnancy or miscarriage. The Center for Surrogate Parenting requires that each of their candidates be between the ages of twenty-one and thirty-seven, have a child of her own, and be financially secure.

How to Get Started

Unless you already know a woman willing to carry your child, you'll probably want to work with a surrogate agency or a specialized law firm. While most agencies do all the legal work and medical arrangements, they charge the recipients a large fee, which is not covered by insurance. In selecting an agency, look for one that carefully screens surrogates and is willing to tell you its screening procedure. If its rejection rate of surrogate applicants seems too small (under 20 percent), go elsewhere no matter how charming its director is. We stress this point because many agencies are notorious for scrimping in this area, a situation that can lead to emotionally and financially devastating custody fights. So Educate Yourself by interviewing several agencies, and Make a Plan by talking to others who have participated in a surrogacy arrangement and by developing personal guidelines for surrogacy selection. A good agency will provide several references and offer guidance in making your selection.

Once you choose your surrogate, the agency should:

- facilitate and coordinate meetings;
- arrange and coordinate a schedule of medical and psychological evaluations;
- recommend legal counsel for both parties involved and provide a model contract:
- coordinate medical procedures;
- act as intermediary between the couple and the surrogate;
- provide ongoing psychological support for both parties and their families;
- monitor the pregnancy; and
- counsel couples on the impact of surrogacy on their social interactions.

To Know or Not to Know Your Surrogate

Most couples select their surrogate, so the issue of anonymous versus identified surrogacy is usually not a factor. What does become a factor, however, is whether you should meet, talk with, and have a relationship with your surrogate or have as little contact as possible. Some couples end up establishing a relationship that is somewhere in between.

The more involved you are with the surrogate prior to the birth, the more likely you are to have a continuing relationship with her after the baby is born. Be aware that some surrogates have difficulty breaking the bond with the baby, especially if they contributed half of its genetic material.

EMBRYO DONATION OR ADOPTION

When embryologists became able to freeze embryos successfully, couples became able to make an additional attempt at pregnancy without undergoing another stimulation cycle. The majority of couples use their embryos to keep trying, if they are unsuccessful, or to have more children if they have been successful. There are, however, couples who decide against another attempt or a second or third pregnancy (particularly if they have had a higher-order multiple pregnancy the first time). These frozen embryos are potentially available to be used by infertile couples who have not been successful with their own eggs or sperm.

Presently, there are no easy ways to locate embryos available for adoption. We suggest that you consult the list of clinics in the "Clinic Resources" section at the end of this book. Choose a clinic located in your geographic area and contact them about the availability of donated embryos. Some clinics are beginning to create lists of couples waiting for embryos.

Few centers or banks have actually made available their stored embryos, for a number of reasons. Many IVF couples, for example, find it difficult to donate a "potential sibling" of the child or children who were successfully conceived. Since their own child stands before them, couples prefer not to "give away" a potential child, but rather would prefer to destroy them or donate them to research. Even couples who initially believed that they would donate prior to undergoing the procedure may have changed their mind afterward. Also, agreements signed in the late eighties and early nineties were vague about time limits and about how to dispose of embryos once the clinic and the couple lost contact. Many clinics report that they are unable to contact the couples who have frozen embryos because the couples have moved and left no forwarding addresses. Even though registered letters and other repeated attempts remain unanswered, clinics are unwilling to donate embryos unless a specific agreement is on record.

Additionally, clinics are freezing fewer and fewer embryos, far fewer than they did even ten years ago. Ironically, the advances in freezing techniques have not increased the number of frozen embryos per treatment cycle, but rather decreased the number of embryos. The reason is simple: Embryologists are more able to determine before they freeze whether they believe that an embryo will survive the freeze and thaw. Even though techniques are more refined, embryologists don't want to freeze embryos that they believe will not thaw to make a successful pregnancy.

Researchers at the Alta Bates IVF program in California investigated what happened to the frozen embryos in their practice. They found that the couples who are most likely to donate their frozen embryos after they have achieved a successful pregnancy and delivery are the ones who used a donor egg, not those who used their own eggs.[2]

The results of this study found that less than 20 percent of regular IVF couples donated their frozen embryos to other couples, in contrast with almost 70 percent of those couples who achieved pregnancy through the use of an egg donor and the husband's sperm. The authors suggest that this willingness to donate may be because of the greater genetic distance between the couple and the embryo, or perhaps because the couple wishes to perpetuate the altruistic impulse. We believe that an additional factor is attributable to the fact that most egg recipients at Alta Bates were involved in *shared* cycles—cycles where two recipients split the cohort of eggs retrieved from the same donor. Since they knew that some other couple already may be parenting a child conceived from the same group of eggs they used, these couples may have been more willing to donate their unused embryos to yet another couple.

As we wrote this new edition, we struggled with the appropriate term: *embryo adoption* or *embryo donation*. When we considered the term *adoption*, we were thinking about it in the social sense, not really in the legal sense. Yet there are centers who think about the procedure of *embryo adoption* almost in a legal sense, with home studies and decisions about open arrangements. One particular program, for example, the Snowflake Embryo Adoption Program of the Christian Adoption & Family Services Organization (www.snowflakes.org), does re-create the traditional adoption model and views embryos as pre-born children. They screen couples through an application process and ask them to write letters to "Dear Genetic Mother": Couples with frozen embryos select a couple to adopt their embryos. Families are encouraged to have open communication, with information being shared on an as-needed basis. Fees include a $4,500 agency fee, a $200 out-of-pocket fee, and, of course, the medical costs of the frozen-embryo transfer and medications.

The more "typical" approach is the one handled by clinics who have had embryos donated by couples who no longer wish to use them. We term this type of procedure *embryo donation*. Embryo donation typically describes a procedure where couples donate their frozen embryos to a clinic, who matches the characteristics of the gamete providers in some way to the couple receiving the embryos. There are typically no agency fees, although the receiving couple pays for the medical aspects of their own treatment as well as often being asked to pay for the recent lab storage fee of the frozen embryos. Embryo donation is almost always anonymous: Recipient couples know only as much information as clinics can provide them (usually about as much as can be gleaned from short forms of sperm banks); couples who donate their embryos do not decide who gets their embryos, but rather trust the donation process of the clinic, which is typically overseen by the egg donor coordinator or psychologist on staff.

Interestingly, a procedure we have termed *double donor* in this book is also sometimes described as embryo adoption or donation. In this procedure, a couple or a single woman uses an egg donor as well as donor sperm to create embryos, which are then transferred into the woman's uterus. In some ways, we could term this an *embryo creation* procedure, during which a couple can combine their choices of gametes and have a greater sense of control, as well as the illusion that they are creating an ideal child. Mental-health practitioners Susan Cooper and Ellen Glazer, in their chapter on embryo donation in *Choosing Assisted Reproduction*[3] term this kind of embryo creation a sort of cosmic accident because the "sources of the gametes who produced her did not ever have a human connection of relationship to each other." Children born via embryo creation may need some help in developing a sense of their identity, but we believe that disclosure at a young age can help start the process.

Emotional Issues

Embryo donation is a complex procedure. As we researched this chapter, we read many essays voicing ethical concerns about the donation of embryos. It seems that the rights of many must be considered: the rights of childless couples to seek out embryos that have been donated, the rights of children born from donated frozen embryos to have knowledge of and acquaintance with their siblings born from the initial IVF procedure, and the rights of children born from this procedure to have a mother and father who are theirs genetically, socially, and gestationally.

Despite these ethical concerns, we support couples who choose to adopt embryos. We encourage them to learn as much as possible about the genetic background of the embryos they may bear. We also encourage them to accept embryos from only one couple at a time to enable them to know as much as possible about their potential child or children. (Obviously, to transfer frozen embryos from more than one couple for any single transfer has the potential of creating "twins" who are not genetically related to each other—a true parenting nightmare!) We also encourage couples to talk openly with each other about the various issues, including disclosure, genetic disconnectedness, and family-member reactions to embryo donation.

FINAL WORDS

The three procedures discussed in this chapter, sperm donation, surrogacy, and embryo donation, are all quite dissimilar despite the fact that each is a third-party procedure. Two are relatively inexpensive, and one is extremely expensive. One involves no genetic connection to your child, while the others offer some genetic connection.

Having worked in reproductive endocrinology practices for the past decade, we have become familiar with many physicians' views about third-party procedures. To medical doctors, these procedures are "just another medical treatment for infertility." This view is 180 degrees removed from the view of many mental-health professionals, who write about the monumental psychological and emotional issues posed by these treatments. As with most things in life, the truth probably lies somewhere in the middle.

These procedures are more than just medical choices. Obviously, a sperm is not a sperm is not a sperm. True, they may all have the same likelihood of getting you pregnant. But one sperm is more likely to bring you a child who will look like you. One embryo is more likely to enable you to have a child of the same ethnicity as you. And one gestational carrier may make you feel more confident that she will take better care of herself for her nine-month pregnancy than will another. These are not trivial issues, and you need to give them careful consideration. But don't weigh them so heavily that you get mired in endless ruminations about the implications and consequences of each decision you make. To do so will stymie you. By the time you emerge with a clear head, the opportunity to use these procedures will have passed you by.

CHAPTER 12

Secondary Infertility: The Loneliest Kind

arrie, a thirty-two-year-old homemaker and mother of one, was on the verge of tears. She had never before sought the help of a psychotherapist, but her problem was growing unbearable.

"I'm sort of embarrassed to say he was an accident because of what's happening now, but he was," Carrie said of her five-year-old son, Bobby, who was conceived shortly after she married Chuck. "We thought we'd get pregnant just as quickly this time. We started trying when Bobby was two. A year later when I wasn't pregnant, I went to my doctor, who told me we should just relax. We did relax, but I knew something was wrong."

Like tens of thousands of parents, Carrie and Chuck suffer from *secondary infertility*—the inability to conceive or carry a second child to term and live birth after bearing a first child.[1] There are two types of secondary infertility: One where pregnancy came easily the first time but is elusive the second time; the other where primary infertility plagued the first pregnancy and is resurfacing as the couple tries to conceive again. In the latter case, the couple is actually experiencing primary infertility the second time around.

As many as 70 percent of all couples who are infertile already have at least one child, according to a 1988 national survey, the most recent one available.[2] Women with secondary infertility, however, are only *half as likely* to seek medical treatment as women with primary infertility, the researcher who conducted the survey discovered. Because these couples already have at least one child, they may believe either that nothing can be done to help them or that they shouldn't tamper with nature.

But the urge to enlarge one's family can be just as compelling as the urge to have one's first child. And the inability to have more children can be just as psychologically and socially devastating as being childless against one's will. Despite the enormous problems it can cause for couples, secondary infertility is arguably the least explored aspect of infertility—medically, psychologically, and socially.[3]

The lack of research in this area leads many busy OB-GYNs to view the secondary infertility patient as a "pain" or "impatient." So many of their patients have second or even third pregnancies that they assume this patient will also conceive. They tend to postpone diagnostic testing that might uncover the problem, or they neglect to prescribe therapy that might solve it.

Outside of the doctor's office, your problem is even less visible. Acquaintances, friends, and even some family members might assume you don't want any more children or that you're simply waiting for the "right time" to get pregnant again. In the throes of raising two or more youngsters themselves, some friends may be unable to empathize with your plight; they might even envy your relative freedom.

People with secondary infertility often tell us that they have trouble fitting in with any group. They don't feel they're part of the infertile world because evidence of their earlier fertility is scampering around the house. Yet they don't feel they're part of the fertile world, either, because they can't get pregnant again. It's not unusual for people with secondary infertility to avoid women with children, pregnant women, and babies because these others make them feel blue. The only person you may feel comfortable talking with at this point is another woman with secondary infertility, if you can find and befriend one. One place to find understanding others is in an Internet-based forum. You can find a newsgroup on secondary infertility at alt.infertility.secondary. You can join a mailing list devoted to secondary infertility by sending e-mail to listserv@maelstrom.stjohns.edu. Finally, you can find an active discussion group on the Web site of the International Council on Infertility Information Dissemination (http://www.inciid.org).

If you feel misunderstood and different from others, you are what social psychologists define as a "marginal woman," someone who "stands on the boundary between two groups." You do not belong to either group, or you are uncertain of your "belongingness."[4] You have lost membership in the primary infertility group by attaining the dream that these women still long for. How can you ask them to understand the anguish you feel at not having a second child? Yet you feel you do not really belong to the world of the fertile. They can choose the size of their family, whereas you cannot increase the size of yours.

Many of our clients describe superstitious thoughts and behavior patterns that are fairly unique to secondary infertility. For example, couples may even try to re-create the conditions of the first conception by revisiting the romantic restaurant they ate in the night they conceived, by listening to the same music, or even by traveling to a distant hotel. Many people with secondary infertility also begin to wonder whether their first child was a fluke. They may even feel they are somehow being punished for not raising that child properly.

Others view secondary infertility as an omen: "Stop trying." "Be satisfied with the child you have." "Don't tempt fate, or you'll give birth to a defective baby," are some of the notions that wander through their minds. Yet it's perfectly reasonable to want to expand the size of your family. Perhaps you came from a large family and desperately want your child to grow up in a similar environment.

Women suffering from secondary infertility grow extremely jealous of fertile women. They also grow angry with themselves. Secondary infertility makes them feel like second-class citizens.

While these feelings are common and perfectly understandable, it's important to move beyond them so they don't stand in the way of your treatment and ultimate success. Through this chapter, we will try to help you help yourself out of this rut.

A COUPLE'S PROBLEM

Like primary infertility, secondary infertility is a couple's problem, not an individual's problem. Yet, more likely than not, the woman struggles alone. The most common reason: In general, men and women have diverging needs with respect to parenthood. Both want to be parents because parenting confers adult status, among other reasons. And both want to be able to pass on their genetic lineage to the next generation. So when a couple is childless, both the husband and the wife feel equally invested in conquering the fertility problem. In most cases, the childless husband is fully supportive of his wife's efforts, needs, and concerns.

After their first child is born, however, most men's parenting needs are fulfilled. Women, on the other hand, may have an entirely different and more enduring image of what a family should be with regard to size. Usually, it is an image of two parents and two or more children. The inability to have a second child can distort that image and leaves a gaping hole in a woman's emotional life.

Not so with many men. For them, a second child is desirable but not critical. Women with secondary infertility, therefore, are more likely to lose their husband's support and are at higher risk for marital conflict.

If that weren't enough, women yearning for more children also may lose the support of friends, relatives, physicians, and women with primary infertility. Friends and relatives often say the wrong things because they cannot comprehend that you have a medical problem. In contrast to the woman grappling with primary fertility who can elicit sympathy because she has repeatedly failed to conceive despite heroic medical efforts, the woman with secondary infertility appears to have living evidence that her infertility problem is "all in her head." The most common, and for many the most exasperating, advice women hear is: "Relax, and you can do again what you did before."

THE MEDICAL FACTS

Carrie and Chuck both came from large families and wanted their son, Bobby, to grow up in a large family as well. After a year of secondary infertility, Carrie changed doctors. This new physician put her on Clomid and "told me to have sex a lot when I was ovulating," she related. "I wasn't sure I was even ovulating, but the doctor told me I just had to look at Bobby to know I was fertile."

It didn't work. Looking at Bobby with no brothers and sisters only made Carrie cry. "My mother told me I was ruining my marriage and upsetting Bobby because I cried so much," Carrie said. "My younger sister, who has three kids, told me how grateful I should be that I only had to buy one pair of shoes and one load of toys instead of three."

After Carrie failed to conceive after several months on Clomid, her doctor performed some tests, which revealed a fibroid in Carrie's uterus. Since a fibroid may prevent an embryo from implanting, the tissue was removed surgically. Now three years had passed since Carrie and Chuck began trying to have their second child.

Diagnosis had been delayed because Carrie's first two doctors assumed that the possibility of a medical problem was remote. As Carrie's case proves, that assumption is not always correct. Most specialists we know agree that there is no one problem typical in the secondary-infertility population. In fact, the breakdown of problems mirrors that of the primary-infertility population.

It's also important to realize that people's bodies are not static. Couples get older. Their health may have deteriorated. Adhesions and fibroids can develop after a first pregnancy, but not necessarily as a result of that pregnancy. Environmental contaminants, leisure activities, and medications all can contribute to a change in fertility status. If your doctor is still pooh-poohing your infertility a year or more since you began trying for a second baby, it's definitely time to find a specialist who cares.

Even if nothing else in her life has changed, a woman's fertility declines as she ages. The 1988 survey cited previously showed that 8.3 percent of women between ages twenty-five and thirty-four and 8.8 percent of women between ages thirty-five and forty-four had secondary infertility.[5] While the difference between 8.3 and 8.8 may seem small, it actually represents nearly 100,000 additional infertile women.

Their problems may include:

- poor ovulatory function;
- an increased number of eggs with genetic abnormalities that prevent fertilization;
- decreased implantation rate caused by these genetic abnormalities or by a poor endometrium caused by hormonal problems;
- increased pregnancy loss.

Life experiences that occurred since your last conception also may have diminished your fertility. Both men and women may be exposed to environmental toxins in their jobs, have illnesses that affect their fertility, or may have taken prescription or even illicit drugs that can hurt their ability to produce a baby.

While researching this book, we met two people experiencing secondary infertility. Mandy had contracted Hodgkins disease after her first pregnancy. Even though her medical team tried to modify the radiation therapy to protect her fertility, Mandy's ovaries were damaged by the treatment. We also met Jack, who was treated for Crohn's disease with medications that reduced his sperm count.

Other life experiences can affect fertility temporarily. As already described, men and women who engage in too much exercise or who are under too much stress can have difficulty conceiving until they reduce their activity or stress level. For men, taking too many hot baths or spending long periods in a Jacuzzi can temporarily reduce sperm production. Riding a bicycle or a motorcycle for extended periods can similarly diminish sperm count.

Often these changes are subtle or so integrated into a person's lifestyle that they may be missed as a factor contributing to infertility. Unless they've suffered a devastating illness or a trauma, most people expect their bodies to work as well now as they did three, five, or even seven years ago.

For those in their second bout with infertility, being familiar with treatment doesn't make things easier. In fact, sticking to your treatment protocol while rearing a child can be more difficult than ever. Try taking your temperature religiously every morning when your child is screaming for you in the next room. Or try keeping your five-year-old out of the bedroom when your husband is giving you a Humegon shot. These are tough challenges. And don't expect much sympathy. People who supported you emotionally during your first round of fertility treatment may find it hard to believe you're doing it all again.

COPING WITH YOUR NEGATIVE EMOTIONS

Why aren't I pregnant? Definitive answers to this question are rare. The best most of us can do is guess. A primary infertile person "guesses" that the reason is medical. But a woman with secondary infertility is more likely to resort to nonmedical "guesses" to explain why it "worked" the first time but not now. Often she will invoke a superstitious or other bizarre explanation.

Primitive cultures feel compelled to use symbols and potions in an attempt to cure childlessness. At the beginning of the twentieth century, infertile women spit to deter the "evil eye," slept with an egg under their bed, or kept a child's photograph under their pillow. The same psychology can propel modern-day infertile people to seek out a magic cure. People will believe in anything—fertility earrings and herbs, astrologers, psychics, fortune cookies, magic nighties, making love on the anniversary of their last conception, or sleeping on the same bedsheets—purported to make a difference.

We know one couple who bought three "fertility dolls," two pairs of "fertility earrings," one bottle of fertility-inducing mineral water, went to several fortune-tellers, and saved fifty fortune cookie fortunes. If you act on these impulses, relax. You are not going crazy. You are just trying to find a greater truth or appeal to a greater power, whatever that may be. Quests for a "magic cure" can help ease the gnawing fear that maybe a second pregnancy will never happen.

Women with secondary infertility can experience other alien feelings, such as being repulsed by an infant or by pregnant women. While such aversions seem logical for those battling primary infertility, it seems less logical (to the outside world) that someone who once had a pregnancy and a newborn can no longer tolerate them in others.

To further explore this phenomenon, we asked a woman in our secondary infertility support group to write down her feelings about fertile women with several children. She wrote: "I *am* a member of your club, but I'm not a member. I *am a parent* (like you) but *I can't have another baby* (so I'm not like you). I want to be like you and I can't, so I hate you for having what I don't. But I can't take responsibility for that hatred without ambivalence because I do have what you have, in part at least." In contrast, the primary infertile woman can hate another's pregnancy unequivocally because she completely lacks what the other person has.

Another set of contradictory emotions that can plague a woman with secondary infertility is resenting her only child because the child impedes her ability to have a second one. She has difficulty justifying treatment when it means finding a baby-sitter and spending time away from her child. She can afford artificial inseminations but feels angry when her parents say she should be saving the money for her existing child's college education instead. She dreams of a "family" vacation in Disney World but resents her child's asking for it now when her family is not yet complete. Some women wish their son or daughter would disappear long enough for them to finish their infertility treatments. The guilt, as you might already know, can be debilitating.

As we counseled Carrie and Chuck, the couple experiencing secondary infertility, many emotions—ones neither ever expected to feel—came out. Carrie admitted that she often felt guilty about wanting another child. Few couples experiencing primary infertility feel that their desire to have a child is inappropriate. They may feel guilty about their behavior prior to their diagnosis of infertility, but rarely do they feel that their wish for a child is unjustified. On the other hand, couples with secondary infertility often feel that "one should be enough." Like Carrie and Chuck, you may feel that you are being "greedy." Looking at the childless women in your doctor's office, you may feel that they are more deserving than you of becoming pregnant. In situations like these, try to remind yourself that there is no pregnancy quota or lottery. One woman's pregnancy has nothing to do with another's. You are not in a game show with just one winner. Whether you are trying for your first, second, third or fourth child, each person's desire is as important as any other's.

When we asked Carrie why she felt guilty for wanting another child, she pointed to the torment her childless neighbor was going through. We helped Carrie change her thinking patterns in order to believe that she is *entitled* to have as many children as she wants. So are you.

It is irrational to believe, like Carrie and Chuck do, that "nature is trying to tell you something" because you are not yet pregnant. While subscribing to this notion may help you accept your predicament, there is no reason to believe that you are trapped in it, considering all the medical means available to help. If technology does not foster your pregnancy, it is you who will decide when or if to stop trying—not some greater power.

USING GPST TO DISPUTE IRRATIONAL BELIEFS

Getting Pregnant Self-Talk is particularly helpful for secondary infertility because so many of the statements you are making to yourself are probably irrational or superstitious.

GPST for Secondary Infertility: An Activity

Directions: Make a list of all the negative statements you are making to yourself about your infertility. These statements could be about the medical procedures, your state of mind, or your relationship with your husband, your child, or other family members. On the second grid below, write these statements in the left-hand column. To give you an idea of what we mean, we have printed some of the negative statements members of our secondary infertility group have generated.

NEGATIVE STATEMENT	COUNTERARGUMENT
I don't think I can take my temperature one more time.	
I don't think I can handle being infertile much longer.	
I don't think I can keep going for these high-tech procedures forever.	

NEGATIVE STATEMENT	COUNTERARGUMENT
I don't think I can get pregnant.	
I don't think I can manage much more disappointment.	
I'm afraid I will never carry a baby to term.	
I'm afraid I will never have a second child.	
I'm afraid I will never get pregnant.	
I don't want to get my hopes up just to have them dashed.	
I don't want not to have another baby.	
I don't want to mix with fertile people.	
I think that a miscarriage will happen again.	
I seem to always view my self-worth by the number of children I have.	
I don't want to ruin my son's childhood over something that may never be.	
I don't want my son to be an only child.	
This can't be happening.	
I'm scared of what the future holds.	

Now use the chart that follows to fill in your own statements. Just fill in the negative statements. Later, we'll talk about disputing these statements with counterarguments.

NEGATIVE STATEMENT	COUNTERARGUMENT

Now it's time to dispute these statements. Again, we provide what our group members said to help you create counterarguments to your own negative statements.

NEGATIVE STATEMENT	COUNTERARGUMENT
I don't think I can take my temperature one more time.	By taking my temperature I up the odds of getting pregnant.
I don't think I can handle being infertile much longer.	I'll be as strong as I need to be.
I don't think I can keep going for these high-tech procedures forever.	I think I can psych myself up for three more tries.
I don't think I can get pregnant.	I can get pregnant when I take charge of my treatment.
I don't think I can manage much more disappointment.	Every disappointment is a step closer to success.

NEGATIVE STATEMENT	COUNTERARGUMENT
I'm afraid I will never carry a baby to term.	I know I will find the answer to this puzzle of miscarriage.
I'm afraid I will never have a second child.	At least I was able to have one child.
I'm afraid I will never get pregnant.	By pursuing treatment, I'll be satisfied that I tried everything humanly possible to get pregnant again. Anyway, research shows that only children often are more secure and have higher IQs. We can make our daughter's life rich and full.
I don't want to get my hopes up just to have them dashed.	Perhaps getting my hopes up will help me get through the next procedure.
I don't want not to have another baby.	I will be happy with my family.
I don't want to mix with fertile people.	The future is bright. I have a loving husband and a wonderful child. Technology is developing at such a rapid rate that the chances are I'll get pregnant eventually.
I think that a miscarriage will happen again.	I am strong enough to deal with another disappointment.
I seem to always view my self-worth by the number of children I have.	I am a worthwhile person in my own right.
I don't want to ruin my son's childhood over something that may never be.	I'm doing this because I want my son to have a sibling. Maybe he'll understand someday.
I don't want my son to be an only child.	If my son is an only child, he'll be happy and well adjusted anyway.

NEGATIVE STATEMENT	COUNTERARGUMENT
This can't be happening.	This is not a punishment or a curse but a fact of life.
I'm scared of what the future holds.	This experience, in a bizarre way, has made me a stronger person.

Now, in the right-hand column of your chart, fill in your counter-arguments.

COMMUNICATING WITH YOUR SPOUSE: GETTING PREGNANT LISTENING AND LEVELING

As we mentioned earlier in this chapter, staying united in the face of secondary infertility is often more difficult than uniting to combat primary infertility. While a husband and wife are generally equally committed to having a first child, one member—usually the husband—is apt to feel less strongly about the importance of the second.

Certainly, if this second child came easily, your husband would happily participate in the pregnancy. But since pregnancy is not happening quickly, your husband probably does not share your pain. Your long-held images of motherhood—two sons fishing together, a brother and sister sharing friends in high school, everyone piling into a minivan for a family vacation—are shattered. Since these images are so hard to surrender, you are driven to make them a reality.

Your husband's notion of family, meanwhile, has probably been more vague. His desire for children probably isn't as strongly tied to number and age spread. Having one child made him a father, so he may wonder: Why all the fuss to have another child?

Chuck's sadness is triggered by Carrie's sadness, not by the secondary infertility. Sure, he fantasizes about taking two sons fishing, and how nice it would be to cuddle a little girl. But, he says, "I figure we don't have a six-figure income; we don't have a five-bedroom house;

we don't have a Mercedes or even a van, so a second baby is just one more thing we don't have."

This is not to say men are neutral toward secondary infertility. It's just that the lack of a second child does not contradict long-held fantasies of ideal family size, nor does it suggest a lack of sexuality to the outside world. As long as your husband has proved that he can father at least one child, the world thinks he could still do it but he has decided not to have any more children. The wife, on the other hand, typically endures comments such as: "When is the next baby coming?" Men generally are not asked these kinds of questions.

The discrepancies can be a recipe for marriage problems.

"I love Carrie and I want to be supportive," Chuck says. "I've gone along with all of her requests for treatment. We've been through all kinds of treatments for many years. But at some point you just have to say enough is enough. I think we've given it a fair chance. It hasn't worked. It's time to quit."

Carrie vehemently disagrees. "I refuse to give up," she says. "I'll do this until I've tried everything. As long as I have strength and we have money, I'll keep trying."

HUSBAND-WIFE NEGOTIATION ACTIVITY

In order to keep your marriage happy, you and your husband must find a way to negotiate a consensus on whether to begin or to continue infertility treatments. Negotiation is an important skill in building a good working team.[6] It is built on Listening and Leveling and Asserting Yourself—two Getting Pregnant Workout skills introduced in Chapter 2. Negotiation requires that each of you understands how the other person's desires are reasonable for him or her; *even if you have a different set of wishes*. You then must strive to be flexible in your demands, by using trade-offs, for example. Remember to be as honest and specific as possible when telling your spouse what you want.

It is a mistaken assumption that your desires are not legitimate because your husband refuses to abide by your requests. And it is human nature to believe that if he doesn't value your wishes, he doesn't value you as a person. To help avoid these traps, begin by communicating your love and respect for each other.

No matter how long you two have been together and how well you think you know each other, neither of you can crawl into the other's head and experience his or her emotions firsthand. Your job, therefore, is to try to explain the reasons behind your wishes, such as why it makes sense to you to continue treatment rather than give up. Your husband's job is to listen carefully and to ask himself, Do I really understand why she feels this way? By asking you questions and sharing his reactions with you, he can come closer to understanding your needs from *your point of view.*

At this stage, he should *not* try to convince you to adopt his point of view. You will know he has completed his tasks successfully when his words indicate that he believes your wishes are reasonable. The following example addresses disagreement over continuing treatment, but the exercise can be adapted to any issue about which you and your husband disagree.

Part I: Statements of Wishes and Reasons

For the wife: Write down why you feel it's important to continue treatment and how you would feel if treatment were to be stopped. Since you will be giving this statement to your husband, write it in a way that will lead him to conclude: Now I understand why my wife wants to keep trying. Her wishes are reasonable. She's not off the wall for wanting to go on.

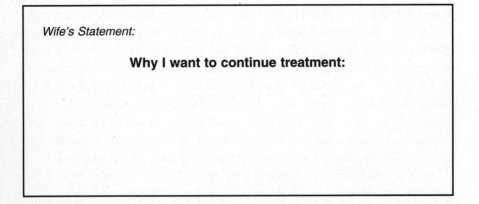

Wife's Statement:

Why I want to continue treatment:

For the husband: Write down why you wish to stop treatment and how continuing treatment would make you feel. When your wife reads what you have written, she should be able to conclude: Now I understand why my husband wants to stop. His wishes are reasonable. He's not off the wall for wanting to stop.

Husband's Statement:

Why I want to stop treatment:

Part II: Communicating Mutual Understanding

Now comes the difficult part. After reading each other's statements, reiterate to your partner what you understand his or her position to be. Try to convince your husband that you believe his position is a reasonable one, and he should do the same for you. As you move through this part of the exercise, remember that *you don't necessarily have to agree with what the other person wants.* All you have to do is to try to see things through the other's eyes, from his or her perspective.

To evaluate whether you've achieved full communication, both of you should be able to sign the statement below comfortably. It might help to read the statement aloud.

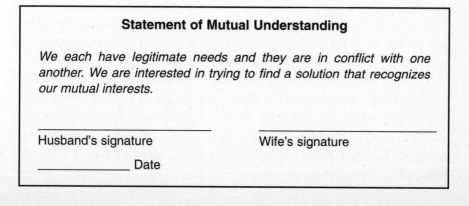

Statement of Mutual Understanding

We each have legitimate needs and they are in conflict with one another. We are interested in trying to find a solution that recognizes our mutual interests.

_____   _____
Husband's signature   Wife's signature

_____ Date

Part III: Brainstorming Different Solutions to the Problem

Brainstorming means coming up with creative compromise solutions in a nonjudgmental atmosphere. Come up with as many ideas as you can, but don't hammer them back with a barrage of criticism. Your ideas should focus on four primary concerns: time, money, family, and your child. Here is an example of what we mean:

TIME: How many months or years should be set aside trying to solve the problem?

MONEY: How much out-of-pocket money should be allocated to the effort? If money must be diverted from other expenses to pay for treatment, where should it be taken from?

FAMILY: What family activities are you willing to sacrifice (i.e., traveling out of town for the holidays) to meet the demands of treatment?

CHILD: You each have an image of the kind of parent you want to be to your son or daughter. But your effort may require some sacrifices in your parenting. What are you willing to give up to pursue this effort (such as being unable to chaperon a class trip)?

Keeping these four concerns in mind, continue to brainstorm more solutions to the problem. Write down all ideas. Ideally, you will end up with a laundry list of possibilities.

Part IV: Creating an Acceptable "Package"

The next step is to hammer out a proposal to solve your problem. The key words here are "compromise" and "trade-off." For instance, you might want to try low- and high-tech treatments for two more years and spend $15,000 out of pocket. Your husband might want to try only low-tech treatments for three months and spend $5,000. One acceptable trade-off might be trying for six months but spending $15,000 on high-tech treatments only. Another compromise might be to try various treatments for a year but spend no more than $7,500 of your own money.

Part V: Creating the Final Agreement and Signing It

Once you've negotiated an acceptable compromise, make it official. Write it as though it were a legal document, being as specific as possible. Use the form below. At the end, write: *This agreement was made in good faith. We are both committed to making it work.* After you both sign and date your document, put it in a safe place. If you get into arguments later about the same issue, take out your "contract" and review it.

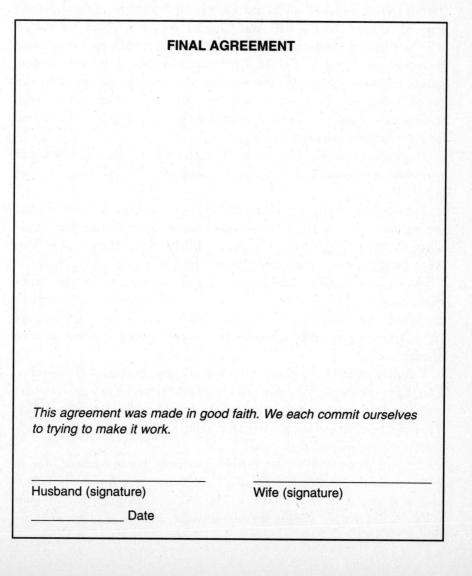

FINAL AGREEMENT

This agreement was made in good faith. We each commit ourselves to trying to make it work.

_____   _____
Husband (signature)   Wife (signature)

_____ Date

DEALING WITH YOUR FAMILY

If families were perfect, your parents, aunts, uncles, and cousins would give you undying support as you grapple with secondary infertility. Unfortunately, it is not always easy to know what to say and what *not* to say to infertile couples, particularly those who already have a child. Carrie and Chuck's relatives think the pregnancy quest is disrupting their family and putting unnecessary stress on their marriage and on their son, Bobby, who has begun acting out in school. Bobby, like his grandparents, thinks Carrie and Chuck are somehow unhappy with what they have. Like Carrie and Chuck's relatives, yours too might wish you would focus on your marriage, or get on with your career and be happy parenting your child, particularly if your child is in kindergarten or grade school. We have provided a resource on our Web site called A *Family's Guide to Secondary Infertility*. Print it out, personalize it, and give it to members of your family to help them understand better what you are experiencing.

It may seem impossible, but by Managing Your Social Life, you can turn your family around and win their support. To do this, you must Assert Yourself.

How your family reacts depends largely on whether you are experiencing primary infertility the second time around or secondary infertility. People in the former category are likely to hear: "Not again. You went through this torture once. Stop. Don't put yourself through it." These relatives may be speaking out of genuine concern for your emotional health, or they might be speaking out of selfishness; perhaps they think they will see your existing child less often while you engage in treatment or be called upon for baby-sitting services if you do have another child.

Couples battling secondary infertility might hear: "Just relax. You'll get pregnant. You just need to give it time." They can't understand how someone who had a baby can suddenly lose that ability. They can be even less supportive than relatives of couples with primary infertility the second time around.

As you grapple with secondary infertility, we encourage you to make copies of "A Family's Guide," which you will find on our Web site, and give it to your relatives. The guide is designed to give your relatives the insight they need to empathize with your plight.

YOUR CHILD'S VIEW OF INFERTILITY

You carry the heavy burden of your secondary infertility in your heart as well as in your head. But your child cannot possibly comprehend the depth of your pain and worry. Your youngster may observe behavioral changes in you that are *consequences* of your inner turmoil. Without a hint as to what's wrong, your child is apt to draw erroneous and potentially damaging conclusions.

A little boy or girl who sees his mother with a sad face or a low energy level may worry that Mommy is sick. Your child might think Mommy and Daddy don't love each other any more if they're arguing over some aspect of the infertility. And a youngster could conclude that babies are despicable creatures because Mommy has begun to recoil in their presence.

If you are spending a lot of your own money on infertility treatments, you may no longer be able to buy your child certain items or take a family vacation. Your child might begin to feel deprived or unloved. Compounding your guilt over this trade-off is the feeling that perhaps you should be saving the money for your child's college education or spending it on him or her instead.

Perhaps the most blatant example is when an insemination or an IVF retrieval conflicts with an activity you planned with your child. Say you promise to attend a school play or a birthday party and then leave early or fail to show up. Lacking an understanding that some procedures cannot be delayed, your child may feel confused. Your son or daughter might conclude that Mommy cannot be trusted or depended upon anymore. Children learn ethics and values from what you do as well as from what you say. So by shying away from infants and pregnant women in the presence of your child, the youngster might think something is wrong with him or her. How should you handle this situation?

As a mother combating infertility, you are left with two difficult options. One, you must monitor your behavior in the presence of your child as much as possible. The goal is to avoid communicating the wrong nonverbal messages, such as "Babies are bad." Or you must explain your actions to your child. This second option is by no means an easy task, especially if you are having trouble justifying your actions to yourself. Also, your child might be too young to understand how babies are made in the first place.

Talking with Your Child

Unlike the woman with primary infertility, you have to deal with a child's questions—or lack of them—about your family size, your treatment schedule, and your feelings about both. It's important to be truthful without burdening your child with too much information. Obviously, you can't describe IVF or even IUI to a five-year-old, but you can explain that you need to take medicine and visit a special doctor to help you have a baby.

You know your own child better than anyone else does. You are best suited to ferret out the concerns behind your child's questions, and you know how much he or she can grasp. Many children who seem to be asking about the details of IVF really only want to know when their little brother or sister will be born. It's important to answer questions with facts that are appropriate for your child's developmental level and in language that can be understood.

Answering Questions About Treatment

Depending on your child's age and powers of perception, it is possible that he or she already is aware that something is wrong. You get up earlier; you frequent the doctor's office; Mommy and Daddy go into their bedroom at odd hours and lock the door. Such changes in routine might make your child feel angry, and rightfully so. If this happens, it is important that you acknowledge his feelings and explain to him what's going on.

Hearing pieces of conversations about "doctors," "blood tests," and "shots," meanwhile, can evoke fear in a child. Many children will imagine the worst: that you are dying, that you and your husband are divorcing, or even that you and your husband want a new baby instead of their existing child.

Assure your child that:

- no one is going to die;
- you're taking medicine and visiting the doctor to try to have a baby;
- you love him or her just like before and want another baby *because* you love him or her so much;
- you may sometimes act sad or disappointed because things aren't working out the way you hoped;
- he or she will have to try extra hard to cope with any changes in routine;
- some people have more trouble than others when they want to have a baby; and
- this information is private so they shouldn't tell their friends or teacher what is happening.

Answering Questions About Your Feelings

Most children are acutely aware of their parents' moods. The rigors of treatment schedules, hormonal shifts caused by medications, and the many losses associated with infertility can all trigger unusual mood swings. When this occurs, assure your child that he or she is *not* the source of your unhappiness. At the same time, *do not* make your child your confidant or give the impression that you need to be taken care of. While it is reasonable to expect your child to be sympathetic, it is inappropriate to let your child bear the responsibility of making you feel better. The only way you should let your child help you is indirectly. You can remind yourself that the joy this child has given you is one of the reasons you want another child in the first place.

When you have trouble hiding your disappointment when you get your period, give your child a basis for your mood change. When your child asks, "Why are you sad, Mommy?" say, "I am sad because I am disappointed that I didn't get what I wanted: a baby growing in my belly." If you are feeling harried, tell your child: "Mommy is going to see a special doctor. I have to go to the doctor very early in the morning, and it's hard for me to get up that early. So I'm tired and sometimes I'm grumpy. Even though you didn't do anything, sometimes I yell at you. I'm sorry."

Answering Questions About Family Size

Most older children are perfectly satisfied with the size of their family. Being an only child has its advantages: They don't have to share toys or their parents' attention. Still, it's important to explain to them why you want more children while pointing out the positive aspects of being an older sibling.

By contrast, most younger children are upset about not having a sibling. "Bobby's first mention of my infertility came out of the blue," Carrie recalled. "I was feeling very generous one day, and I asked him what he wanted most in the world. I thought he'd say a tricycle or a Nintendo game, but he looked at me with his earnest blue eyes and said, 'I want to be a brother.' It just broke my heart."

Young children, usually between the ages of four and six, typically ask why they have no brothers or sisters. Such questions can arise in social situations, such as when a friend or neighbor shows up with a baby carriage and other kids in tow. Your immediate response needs only be: "We're trying" or "We want a new baby, too." Later, in the privacy of your home, you can give your child additional information if he wants to know more.

In cases where your child is clearly perplexed by the changes in your lives but lacks the language to ask you about your fertility problems, it may help to offer information in the form of a fairy tale. We've written one called "Maybe Next Year," which is appropriate for three-to-six-year-olds. (Some older children like it too.) After reading it to your child, you can follow up with a discussion.

MAYBE NEXT YEAR: A SECONDARY INFERTILITY STORY TO TELL YOUR CHILD

The little boy in the blue striped polo shirt was very sad. His friend with the red hair had a new tricycle. His friend who lived in the green house had a new bicycle. The little boy waited and waited for his mommy to get him a bicycle too. But no bicycle came. He said,

"Mommy, I'm so sad. My friend with the red hair has a tricycle. And my friend who lives in the green house has a bicycle. When will I have a bicycle?" His mommy said, "I'd like to get you a bicycle, but I can't this year. Maybe next year."

The little boy in the blue striped polo shirt was sad but also mad. He said, "Everybody gets what they want. But not me." His mommy said, "That's not true. Just ask the seal who lives in the zoo who balances the ball on her nose." The boy in the blue striped polo shirt loved the seal in the zoo who balanced the ball on her nose. He went to visit the seal. "Seal, I'm very sad. I want a bicycle and my mommy can't get me one this year. Did you ever want something that you didn't get?" Seal said, "My little ones love sardines. When we lived in the ocean, I used to catch sardines and give them to my little ones. But here in the zoo I don't have any. My little ones are sad. I told them maybe next year I'd get to the ocean and bring them some sardines."

The little boy in the blue striped polo shirt felt bad for the little seals. He went home and said, "Mommy, I feel sad. The little seals and I can't get what we want. But everybody else gets what they want." Mommy said, "That's not so. Ask Squirrel who lives in the tree who wiggles his tail." Squirrel lived in the tree in front of the little boy's house. The little boy used to talk to Squirrel. So he went outside and by and by he saw Squirrel. "Squirrel, I'm so sad. I want a bicycle and Mommy can't get it for me this year." Squirrel said, "That's sad. My little ones want acorns. I used to collect acorns from the oak tree across the street. Then last year there was a big storm and the tree was knocked down. Now we have no acorns. I told my little ones that maybe the town fathers will plant a new tree so that in a few years we'll have more acorns."

The little boy in the blue striped polo shirt was sad. He went home and said, "Mommy, I'm so sad. The little seals don't get sardines and the little squirrels don't get any acorns and I can't get a bicycle. Everybody but us gets the things they want." Mommy said, "That's not true. You never even knew that the little seals wanted something that they didn't get. And you never even knew that the little squirrels wanted something that they didn't get. Everybody wants things they don't get."

The little boy in the blue striped polo shirt said, "Mommy, is there anything that you want that you didn't get?" Mommy said, "Yes. I want a baby to be your brother. Daddy and I have been trying to have a baby but we haven't gotten one yet. But maybe we'll get one next year." The little boy in the blue striped polo shirt said, "Maybe next year Seal and her little ones will get the fish they want. Maybe next year Squirrel and her little ones will get the acorns they want. And maybe next year you and Daddy and I will get the baby brother we all want."

CHAPTER 13

Pregnancy Loss After Infertility

or most women, losing a pregnancy is a tragedy. But losing a pregnancy after months or years of infertility treatments seems the cruelest loss of all. Unfortunately, the same problem that made it difficult for you to become pregnant in the first place may contribute to an increased risk of miscarriage. In this chapter we will address some of the causes of miscarriage and possible preventions, and offer suggestions aimed at minimizing the potentially devastating psychological impact of losing a pregnancy after infertility.

Miscarriage, sometimes referred to as *spontaneous abortion,* is technically defined as the loss of a pregnancy up to twenty weeks after conception.[1] A woman who loses two or more pregnancies in the first twenty weeks has suffered what doctors call *recurrent pregnancy loss.* After the twentieth week, the loss is called *premature labor.*

WHAT CAUSED THIS MISCARRIAGE?

The most important thing to remember after suffering a miscarriage after infertility is this: Probably nothing you did—either in the past or in the present—had anything to do with your misfortune. If you find this hard to accept, you are not alone. Many people we talk with believe that the miscarriage, like their infertility, is some kind of punishment for past behaviors. "As a kid I used to misbehave," one woman told us. "My mother used to say to me, 'You'll be sorry. You'll pay for this when you grow up.' My miscarriage is my payment for being a bad girl."

Other people—a much larger group—describe a different source of guilt. They believe the miscarriage is the result of something they did or didn't do during their pregnancy, such as sitting too close to a computer screen or taking an airplane trip. They truly believe that if they had done things differently they would still be pregnant.

If you are locked into this kind of mind-set, let yourself off the hook. Recognize and accept the fact that some causes of miscarriage, particularly genetic causes, are beyond your or anyone else's control. To keep from worrying about future miscarriages, know what medical steps you can take that might prevent a miscarriage in the future.

The Likelihood of Miscarriage

Dr. James Wheeler, a researcher specializing in the causes of recurrent pregnancy loss, describes what he terms "the natural history of spontaneous abortion." He points out that very few of the many sperm and eggs a couple produce are actually used for procreation. Some 10 percent to 15 percent of all *normal* eggs will fail to fertilize. Another 10 percent to 15 percent of the eggs that do fertilize fail to divide or implant. And of those that do divide and implant, 15 percent to 20 percent (up to one in five) are spontaneously aborted before twenty weeks of pregnancy. "Thus a fertilized egg has, at best, a 60 percent chance of reaching 20 weeks of gestation,"[2] Wheeler concludes.

For the infertile population, the miscarriage rate is even higher, although researchers aren't sure exactly why. Here are some of the medical reasons that do have a scientific basis.

Hormonal Causes

Hormonal problems are a possible cause of recurrent miscarriage. A lack of sufficient progesterone is associated with luteal phase defects. Doctors don't know precisely how a luteal phase defect contributes to miscarriage.[3] They do know, however, that patients with this defect have a high incidence of miscarriage—anywhere from 23 percent to 60 percent. One way to supplement progesterone levels is by giving the woman injections or vaginal suppositories of natural progesterone (the synthetic form must be avoided during pregnancy). If you have had one or more miscarriages, ask your doctor whether progesterone supplementation might be helpful in your case.

Infection

It has recently been discovered that certain types of bacterial infections can cause miscarriage, just as they cause infertility, by hurting the quality of your eggs as well as their ability to be fertilized and implant in the uterus, according to Dr. Niels H. Lauersen, co-author of *Getting Pregnant: What You Need to Know Right Now.* The most common bacteria linked to pregnancy loss are those usually associated with sexually transmitted diseases, including chlamydia, T-mycoplasma, gonorrhea, and syphilis.[4] Dr. Lauersen says that the use of erythromycin, an antibiotic, is "one of the most beneficial treatments in preventing miscarriage."[5]

Having undergone infertility diagnosis, you probably have been tested for bacterial infections already. If you haven't been tested, or if it's been a long time since your initial workup, it cannot hurt to be tested again.

Many doctors do not believe that these infections can cause miscarriage. But being tested and taking antibiotics if indicated, at the very least, *will give you the feeling* that you are improving your future pregnancy outlook.[6]

Anatomic Causes in the Cervix and Uterus

Certain anatomic problems have a high probability for causing miscarriage. A weakness in the cervix, which can be natural or caused by a "cone" biopsy, surgical removal of a cone-shaped portion of the cervix, usually as a treatment for a pre-cancerous condition, is a major cause of miscarriage, particularly after the first trimester. You may have heard that repeated dilation and curettage (D&C) procedures can increase the risk of cervical incompetence. We realize this is certainly not something you want to hear right after you've had a D&C for your miscarriage. The good news is that modern D&C techniques use instruments that don't weaken the cervix. The other good news is that *any time before you are about twenty weeks pregnant* doctors can put temporary stitches in the cervix to tighten it, thereby preventing this cause of miscarriage.

Another cause of miscarriage is a wall, or septum, in the uterus. Because you've probably had diagnostic testing that included an HSG or a hysteroscopy in order to get pregnant, this problem would have been detected and remedied prior to pregnancy. But if you are still worried, talk to your doctor.

Women who were exposed to DES (diethylstilbestrol) while in utero also have an increased miscarriage risk. A study that compared DES-exposed women with non-DES-exposed women found that only 54 percent of the DES daughters had live births compared with 82 percent of non-DES-exposed daughters.[7] If you are a DES daughter, insist that your doctor take all steps possible to best manage your pregnancy. Some possible steps include careful monitoring throughout your pregnancy, early ultrasound scans, more than usual bed rest, avoidance of strenuous activities, and frequent cervical examinations.

Immunological Factors

The mechanism by which immunological factors may contribute to miscarriage is not clearly understood. The most reasonable explanation is based on the notion that our immune system protects us from invasion by foreign bodies. When the immune system perceives something as "foreign," it mobilizes special cells to attack and destroy it.

It's important to understand that immunological factors can contribute to repeated spontaneous abortions (RSAs) in three ways: through immune system attacks against the cells of your own body, of your husband's body, and of those of the developing fetus. In the several years since our last edition, the treatment of these various responses has grown enormously and is perhaps one of the most controversial treatment areas in reproductive medicine. Treatments range from one as simple as a woman taking a daily baby aspirin before and during treatment and pregnancy to one as expensive and controversial as injecting her with a substance made up of pooled donated blood cells monthly for several months prior and during pregnancy. Treatments vary greatly in terms of cost, safety, effectiveness, and success rate.

But the embryo contains cells that are foreign to the mother's body. A reasonable question to ask is: Why doesn't the woman's immune system perceive an embryo as a foreign body and destroy it?

One proposed answer is that the woman's body produces "blocking antibodies," which prevent the immune system's killer cells from destroying the embryo. How these blocking antibodies are mobilized is a mystery.

Perhaps the developing embryo itself sends a chemical message triggering this protection. The special mix of two very different genetic materials, each contributed by one of the spouses, may trigger a "hold-your-fire" signal. On occasions when the embryo fails to signal the body to "hold your fire," miscarriage will ensue, according to this theory.

Some experts speculate that an immunological response against an embryo or fetus occurs when there are too many genetic similarities between the husband and wife. Without enough genetic dissimilarity, the stimulus to produce the hold-your-fire signal is perhaps not triggered.

Lymphocyte Immune Therapy (LIT)

One controversial treatment involves injecting the wife with her husband's white blood cells. The procedure is called LIT, lymphocyte immune therapy. Doctors who prescribe this treatment claim it stimulates the blocking antibodies or at least prevents the attacking antibodies from destroying the fetus.

The American Society of Reproductive Immunology sponsored a worldwide collaborative study to determine how effective LIT is. The investigators studied 456 women who were randomly assigned either to a group treated with LIT or a group receiving no treatment. The study found that among women who had three or more previous miscarriages, LIT reduced the miscarriage rate, but:

- the extent to which it prevented miscarriage was small. Only one out of every eleven women who would not otherwise have given birth went on to conceive when treated with LIT;
- LIT did not significantly reduce miscarriage rates for women who had already carried a pregnancy past twenty weeks; and
- LIT actually *increased miscarriage rates* for women who had autoimmune problems.

Intravenous Immunoglobin (IVIg) Therapy

IVIg therapy is another controversial treatment to prevent a rejection of the embryo by the mother's immune system. This treatment involves the use of gamma globulin obtained from purified serum of a pool of blood donors, which somehow suppresses immune rejection of the embryo.

Even the most favorable results of research studies can offer only modest support for IVIg therapy. The most favorable results indicated a 28 percent reduction in miscarriage rate. On the one hand, approximately one out of four women who would not have become mothers were able to take home babies after their IVIg treatment. The other three women who did not give birth, also had to undergo strenuous treatment that included the risks involved in using donated blood as well as financial burden of this treatment (often exceeding $50,000 per attempt). Ask your doctor whether he or she believes in the theory and whether immunological treatment might prevent future miscarriages for you.[8]

A different type of immune-system deficiency causes a blood-clotting disorder that prohibits the growing fetus from getting enough blood flow to grow and develop. The problem occurs when certain antibodies, most specifically *anticardiolipin* or *cold lupus anticoagulant*, cause your body to develop blood clots in the vessels leading to the placenta. The clots prevent the baby from getting the vital nutrients it needs. To overcome this problem, you can take baby aspirin and injections of heparin, an anticoagulant. Again, ask your doctor whether this approach is appropriate for you.

Chromosomal and Genetic Causes

Chromosomal abnormalities are the most common causes of first miscarriages or isolated miscarriages. Sadly, there is nothing you can do to remedy a chromosomal defect during pregnancy. Dr. Wheeler reports that 40 percent to 60 percent of all first-trimester miscarriages show evidence of chromosomal abnormalities. Many of these abnormalities are *random* (chance) errors that occur during *meiosis* (when gametes lose half their chromosomes before fertilization) or during *mitosis* (when cells divide in half as the embryo grows). Defective genetic material in your eggs or in your partner's sperm can create embryos that are too weak or too deformed to survive. *Genetic* defects (in contrast to chromosomal abnormalities), however, are very rare.

Sometimes this genetic abnormality may be a statistically uncommon occurrence that will never again happen to you. In other cases, you or your partner may have a chromosomal problem that will cause repeated miscarriages. To find out, you and your husband can have your blood cells tested for chromosomal abnormalities.

Finally, if you are thirty-five or older, your chances of having an embryo with genetic problems, some of which are serious enough to cause a miscarriage, rise substantially. We've included the chart below[9] not to terrify you, but to apprise you realistically of the odds.

RISK OF SPONTANEOUS ABORTION WITH INCREASED AGE	
Maternal Age in Years	**Percentage of Spontaneous Abortions**
15–19	9.9%
20–24	9.5%
25–29	10.0%
30–34	11.7%
35–39	17.7%
40–44	33.8%
Over 45	53.2%

COPING WITH MISCARRIAGE AFTER INFERTILITY: LONG-AWAITED FANTASIES

Infertile couples tend to fantasize about being pregnant beginning with the first Clomid pill or Humegon shot. As time goes on, however, some couples begin to fight back such fantasies because the treatments have failed so many times. So when pregnancy finally occurs, the fantasy floodgates tend to swing wide open, and justifiably so.

Like pregnant women everywhere, you began to think ahead—to the last months of the pregnancy, to the moment when you'll first cradle this long-awaited baby in your arms. You make plans to borrow your sister's maternity clothes and circle your due date on every calendar in the house. You gleefully walk into baby-furniture stores and infantwear departments—venues you previously avoided because they were too depressing. You begin to picture yourself playing with your child in the nursery of your dreams. Everything seems to be falling into place.

Then—suddenly, or slowly—you're not pregnant anymore. The baby, who may already have been given a name, no longer exists.

If you have miscarried once or several times after infertility, the loss can be overwhelming. Each pregnancy, no matter how brief, gave you permission to believe that this pregnancy would be successful. Each pregnancy, no matter how brief, causes physical, hormonal, and emotional changes that are very real.

In his book *Preventing Miscarriage*, Dr. Jonathan Scher states that "the major changes in a woman's hormonal makeup take place *early* in pregnancy, almost just after conception."[10] So when you lose the pregnancy, it can feel as though you gave birth and lost that child. And, in fact, you *have* lost that child.

We lost our first pregnancy in the eighth week—but not until after rejoicing in a positive pregnancy test and the sight of our fetus's heartbeat on a sonogram. April 6 was our due date. We shared our joy with other couples whose pregnancies had occurred around the same time as ours. We allowed ourselves to fantasize with sheer abandon.

In addition to suffering the sadness associated with miscarriage in general, we were further saddened because we realized that not only had we had trouble conceiving, but we also would have trouble maintaining a pregnancy. As we recovered physically and emotionally from the pregnancy loss, we developed many coping activities, which we describe later in this chapter. Many of our clients also found these activities extremely helpful.

Then we got pregnant a second time with a Pergonal/IUI cycle. It was our first attempt after the miscarriage, no less. We charted this second pregnancy, just as we had the first. We calculated a due date: August 27. But this time we were less inclined to talk freely about our pregnancy, although we did confide in a small number of trusted friends, family, and associates.

In the ninth week, we were no longer able to detect a fetal heartbeat. Our recovery from the second miscarriage was slower and more difficult for us. Unlike the shock we felt with the first miscarriage, this miscarriage was characterized by a deadness we both felt inside. We talked to each other about how unfair it all seemed. We had thought we were on the brink of winning our war against infertility, but we had conquered only one battle.

Despite all the emotional pain, enduring two miscarriages gave us more knowledge and insight to help ourselves and others through this horrible ordeal. The information contained in the following section summarizes what we have learned through our literature research and from numerous doctors and couples we have talked to.

GETTING IN TOUCH WITH GRIEF AND LOSS: AN ACTIVITY

If you've experienced a miscarriage after trying so hard to get pregnant, it can be difficult to allow yourself to feel the pain because the loss is so utterly devastating. Another reason the grieving process is especially difficult is that you've worked so hard to stay optimistic for so long. In fact, your pregnancy reinforced the importance of Not Giving Up, because you did get pregnant. You'd learned to move past the devastation of a failed IUI or IVF and steel yourself for the next treatment. You taught yourself to view the period after a failed cycle as one more step toward your goal. Even as you grieved with your period, you reminded yourself that it was also Day 1 of your new cycle: one when a pregnancy could occur.

A miscarriage is far more profound and overwhelming because it is more closely associated with a real death. The probability of pregnancy had become a possibility and, in so many ways, the baby had seemed a reality-to-be. You had a positive pregnancy test and saw a gestational sac on the ultrasound; you may even have seen a fetal heartbeat. Then the bleeding started. Or maybe there was no bleeding and you got the unforeseen news during an ultrasound scan. The news might have come from a radiologist you'd never met before, and maybe you had no one else around to support you emotionally. To make matters worse, your body may still have felt pregnant, but there was no longer a life growing inside you.

When you are *trying* to get pregnant, the odds, for any given attempt, are *not* in your favor. Even a couple having no fertility problem has only a 20 percent chance of conception for each attempt. The situation is beyond your control. Therefore, although you *hope* you will succeed, you know that the odds are against you, and you don't spend mental energy trying to "make it happen."

But once you do get pregnant, the odds of staying pregnant (unless you are over forty-five) *are* in your favor. And for certain conditions, there *are* steps you can take to prevent miscarriage. Therefore, you *hope* you will stay pregnant and you *try to exert control* to make sure that you stay pregnant. Then, when a miscarriage occurs, you feel as though your sense of control was just an illusion. This sudden realization that you have no control over your pregnancy can plunge you into a dark depression. In order to get past this experience, you must allow yourself to experience your emotions, to express them to each other, and to ask for what you need from those around you.

Our society has many rituals for mourning death. Wakes, burials, sitting shiva, and condolence calls are all mechanisms for helping people come to terms with loss. Tombstones, remembrance plaques, and photographs all serve as memorials to the life of the deceased. Unfortunately, society has created no comparable rituals for mourning and remembering fetuses who died. To rectify this problem, registered nurse Pat Schweibert and Dr. Paul Kirk have written a book called *When Hello Means Goodbye*,[11] in which they discuss mechanisms for dealing with the loss of a fetus. We recommend this book as a supplement to the ideas we discuss in this chapter.

Difficult Dates

Couples who have suffered miscarriage typically describe difficult dates and encounters that seem to halt recovery just as healing begins. The day your baby had been due or the anniversary of the day you conceived can be extraordinarily difficult to get through. Equally difficult is seeing women who got pregnant around the same time you did but are still carrying or have already given birth. Be aware that these circumstances can signal trouble for your emotional well-being. Making a Plan can help you cope with painful thoughts triggered by these dates and encounters.

Here is what some of our miscarriage clients listed as difficult dates. At the bottom is space for you to list dates you anticipate to be a problem.

DIFFICULT DATES

Dates our clients found difficult:

- Day your baby was due to be born

- Anniversary of your miscarriage

- Anniversary of a positive pregnancy test

- Milestone for a baby born around the time your baby was supposed to have been born (e.g., christening, bris, baby naming, etc.)

- First day of school

Fill in your difficult dates:

-

-

-

Steps to take:

- *Get in Touch with Your Feelings.* In advance, think about these difficult dates and give yourself time to grieve and mourn the tragedy of your loss.
- *Make a Plan.* These dates will undoubtedly be difficult for you and your partner. Use Listening and Leveling skills from Chapter 2 to help him or her understand why you expect to be upset.
- *Work as a Team.* Plan some activities you can do together on these dates. You might see a movie, go to a museum, take a walk in the country, go skating, or go out to dinner.

MANAGING YOUR SOCIAL LIFE: SOME ACTIVITIES

It's very difficult for friends to know what to say and what to do after you've suffered a miscarriage. You can help yourself by coaching them about what to say and what not to say. *Don't write people off for their initial insensitive remarks.* Few people are professionally trained to respond to someone in pain. Some of your friends may have better instincts than others.

One client's friends told her: "Sally, we're so sorry about your miscarriage. We can't know the grief you are experiencing. We can only imagine how painful it is. You're in our prayers." Warmed and uplifted by those words, Sally decided that she would tell other friends about the statement and encourage them to take a similar tack should the miscarriage come up in conversation.

Lisa, another client, told us about a particularly disturbing remark made by a colleague who was trying to be helpful: "You're young and healthy," the colleague told her. "You'll have a baby, and then you won't even remember this miscarriage." To alleviate the threat of hearing hurtful comments in the future, we helped Lisa develop a way to teach her friend more helpful "lines." Although Lisa initially felt uncomfortable about coaching her friend, she agreed to try. She told her friend: "Yvonne, I know you were trying to be kind, but what you said made me very upset. It's hard for me to imagine that I'll ever forget this miscarriage. So when you say that to me, it makes me very angry."

Hindsight—What You Wish You Had Said

If people make unsympathetic or otherwise hurtful remarks to you, you cannot change what they actually said. But you can diminish the pain that lingers with the memory of their words. By using mental imagery techniques, you can relive these scenes putting more helpful words into their mouths. The following Hindsight activity helps you do just that.

Directions: First list the hurtful statements that were made to you. Then create your response to those statements using 20-20 hindsight. Your response is what you wish you had said. Here are some examples:

REMARK: Did you hear about Carol's pregnancy? She's going to have twins.

HINDSIGHT RESPONSE: I'm glad that Carol's pregnancy is going so well, but it's very hard for me to hear about it at this time. Please don't talk to me about people's pregnancies. I'll let you know when I'm ready for that.

REMARK: I'm sorry you lost the pregnancy. But at least you can have fun trying to get pregnant again.

HINDSIGHT RESPONSE: Thank you for your concern about my loss. I'm sorry that you didn't realize that I've been undergoing infertility treatment for a long time. In our case, getting pregnant isn't fun, it's work.

REMARK: I heard about your miscarriage. I'm so sorry. But I guess it was just God's will.

HINDSIGHT RESPONSE: I appreciate your support and concern. I don't like to think about my pregnancy in those terms. I like to believe that God is on my side. If it helps you to think about tragedies in your life this way, then that's right for you. But it doesn't help me.

Now it's your turn. Recall a situation that happened after your miscarriage that was particularly painful or difficult to endure. Allow yourself to go back to that time and place. Try to experience the situation in as much detail as possible. Hear the hurtful statement made by your friend or acquaintance. Take as much time as you need to experience the scene fully. When you have a clear picture in your mind, allow yourself to come back to the here and now. Write down what you found so difficult to hear. Don't be surprised if much of the pain returns as this memory becomes more vivid. Just breathe deeply and let yourself go with it.

Using hindsight, construct a retort. Your retort should let the person know how much what he or she said hurt your feelings. Take care to construct a statement you would be comfortable making—one that is assertive and that communicates your feelings.

Now return to the difficult scene in your mind's eye. Recall that scene in as much detail as possible. Hear your friend making the hurtful statement. This time, instead of responding in the way you did, or instead of not responding at all, make the statement you just scripted. See your friend's face when you make that statement. Feel better now that you've communicated what you needed to.

Once you've reexperienced the scene on your own terms, return to the here and now. Armed with the language to deal with a similar situation should it arise in the future, you can let go of the pain and move on, putting the hurtful incident behind you.

Should We Try Again?: A Husband-Wife Communication Activity

One of the most difficult aspects of your miscarriage can be how differently men and women perceive the experience. Many of the women we talk with focus on the "emptiness" they feel. But more women describe the pain of waiting—waiting for a menstrual period and the chance to try again. Because infertile women who have experienced miscarriage have been actively involved each month in getting pregnant, this waiting time seems like a punishment for failing rather than a time to recover. Getting a period, which is the important first step in trying again, can take up to eight weeks.

To husbands, the loss is altogether different. One male client likened the miscarriage to climbing a rope, almost reaching the top, and then sliding to the bottom again. Another man described how he and his wife had worked so hard to build an elaborate sand castle, then stood back to admire it, only to watch the sand castle be carried away by the tide. They feel that all their efforts to overcome great odds against pregnancy were in vain. Perceiving the miscarriage as a failure, many husbands are loath to risk another defeat. As their wives anxiously wait for the opportunity to try again, these husbands want to discontinue infertility treatments.

It is at this impasse that couples come to see us after suffering miscarriage in the wake of extended treatments. Couples who once had no problem Working as a Team now have trouble understanding each other's perceptions and feelings. As you and your husband struggle over whether to give up or try again, we urge you to call upon the communication skills you acquired in the Getting Pregnant Workout. Remember, both of you are:

- trying to understand your partner's world of experience;
- conveying information about your own world of experience; and, as a by-product of the first two processes;
- commenting on the relationship.

Mindy and Stefan, both in their late thirties, came to see us shortly after Mindy's second miscarriage. As described above, Mindy was caught up in the interminable wait. Stefan was demoralized and frustrated. She wanted to try IVF again; he wanted to quit. Their dilemma was threatening their marriage.

The discussion in our consulting room began with an air of great tension. This couple, who had been through so much infertility treatment together and had comforted and supported one another for years, were now fuming at each other. Each regarded the other as "stubborn and irrational." We spent a great deal of time coaching them in Listening and Leveling skills. Despite this coaching, they repeatedly fell back upon former habits of assuming they knew what their partner was thinking and feeling. Their dialogue was merely a recitation of what each wanted, with neither party paying much attention to what their partner was saying:

MINDY: I want to try again.

STEFAN: Enough is enough. We tried so many times. We had two pregnancies and two miscarriages. I'd say that's giving it a reasonable shot.

MINDY: I just want to try one more time. I think it'll work next time.

STEFAN: And then if that doesn't work, you'll want to try again. How long will it go on?

MINDY: Why are you being so unreasonable? You used to be so supportive.

At this stage in the dialogue, all that was being communicated was desperation and accusations. We urged Stefan and Mindy to share their worlds of experience with one another. After much work, they were finally able to have the following productive dialogue:

STEFAN: Let me tell you what I'm feeling. I'm so frustrated. I feel like we've done everything in our power. We've spent tons of money. We've devoted four years to this quest. We're getting older. We still have time and money to adopt. Two years from now, we might be too old and too poor to adopt. Let's get on with it.

MINDY: Your points are valid. I know it seems like we've been doing this forever. And I appreciate all the support you've given me. I love you for what you've done. But I need one more chance.

STEFAN: Why is having one more chance so important to you?

MINDY: Because I feel like a failure, and I need one more time before I can allow myself to give up the idea that I can be a biological mother. It's hard to explain, I know, but one more try will make all the difference in how I see myself.

STEFAN: Well, I can't say I understand your reasons, but I'm willing to accept what you say. The thing that's worrying me, though, is that if we try and you miscarry again, you'll come back with the same statement again that "I need just one more time." Then we're right back on the merry-go-round.

MINDY: But there's one difference. We still have one more IVF attempt that insurance will cover. Please, let's just try that one last time, and if it doesn't work, we'll quit.

Now they were making some progress. They understood one another, but they still were unable to resolve their differences. As a result of their discussion, however, they understood the issues that were dividing them.

Our next step was to help them develop an agreement they could both live with. With our assistance, Mindy and Stefan wrote an agreement that they signed and dated. Here is what they wrote:

AGREEMENT

We agree to try one more IVF attempt. We are hopeful that it will succeed and that a resulting pregnancy will go to term. However, should we fail to get pregnant, or get pregnant and have a miscarriage, we agree that we will end our efforts to have our own biological child. Instead, we will begin to explore adoption as a way to expand our family.

_____   _____
Mindy Mateja (wife)   Stefan Mateja (husband)

_____   _____
Helane S. Rosenberg (witness)   Yakov N. Epstein (witness)

Date _____

Like Mindy and Stefan, you may resolve your pregnancy quest with a decision to adopt if your next attempt does not succeed. Most importantly, you must find a way to deal with your infertility as a strong, loving team.

CHAPTER 14

The Internet and Infertility

he origins of today's Internet go back only about a quarter of a century. Yet within the last decade the Internet has grown enormously. Computer experts estimate that the number of users in the year 2000 is over 300 million. You can up your odds of getting pregnant by joining their ranks.

Initially, you may think it's strange to have a chapter in a book titled *Getting Pregnant When You Thought You Couldn't* on how to use the Internet to help you get pregnant. Obviously, *Getting Pregnant When You Thought You Couldn't* is meant to stand on its own and to be a complete and up-to-date guide on everything you could possibly need to know. Yet we would be foolish if we believed that nothing would change in the treatment of infertility, and maybe even in the treatment of your own particular infertility problem. Getting through treatment means that you have to take an active part in finding the support and information you need.

One of the best ways to find out about the newest advances in infertility and to locate people who can provide you with support and encouragement is through the Internet. We're not saying that you must race out and buy a computer and start e-mailing up a storm. But you may find that a particular answer to your medical question is not found in *Getting Pregnant When You Thought You Couldn't*. You may want to arm yourself with the very latest information about your diagnosis in order to Be a Partner in Your Treatment. In order to Educate Yourself About Infertility, you may want to get the very latest statistics about a particular practice. Or, as you start feeling down about your situation, you may need the support of others facing similar problems to help you Get in Touch with Your Feelings. If you are having difficulty Getting Organized, you might want to supplement the Cycle Log detailed in this book with an Internet spreadsheet where you can keep records of your basal body temperature. It's hard to say what will change in the course of your treatment, but knowing about it might make a difference.

We believe so strongly in the value of the Internet in your pregnancy quest that we ourselves have become moderators of several Internet-based infertility forums and members of the advisory board of the International Council on Infertility Information Dissemination (INCIID), an Internet-based non-profit organization dealing exclusively with infertility. This chapter is a guide for you to use the Internet to help you up your odds even more.

COMMUNICATING VIA THE INTERNET

The Internet will neither provide the magic answer to all your infertility problems nor signal the end to human communication as we know it. Becoming involved with the Internet has both pluses and minuses. We think you should know something about what the experts say are the pros and the cons of communicating via the Internet.

The Positives

The biggest plus in terms of communicating on the Internet is that you have immediate access to the newest information concerning the treatment of your particular medical problem. And you have this access twenty-four/seven, as they say, meaning twenty-four hours a day, seven days a week, right from your own computer at home or at work. This information is available to you free or at low cost. Most people pay about $20 a month for unlimited dial-up telephone access to the Internet.

As well as being able to have access to information, the Internet provides you with access to people. These are people who can share their experiences with you: what medications they took, what physicians they saw, how their partner felt, how their families responded, and what social situations they encountered, for example. You can have a non-face-to-face relationship with others in a situation similar to yours. You can interact in as intense or as casual a manner as you like and not worry about how that interaction might jeopardize your daily life. Through e-mail you can meet people with your specific medical and social problem when in "real life" you might never come across anyone with the same medical condition as yours. You can gain and give support for a major part of your day or just a small part of your day and feel validated and understood.

Linda was thirty years old. She and her husband, Gordon, had been trying to get pregnant for over two years. Linda had taken Clomid for nine cycles. She was extraordinarily proactive in every aspect of her life, but Linda felt unable to handle the situation of her infertility. She kept going to see Dr. Z, the only gynecologist she had ever been to since she was thirteen. Linda felt that he really wasn't helping. As soon as Linda got on the Internet, her decision to seek the opinion of a doctor specializing in infertility was supported by over thirty postings in under a week. Linda felt elated!

Linda began visiting Web sites of clinics in her area. She even posted queries about a certain clinic and read lots of favorable opinions. Within a month Linda had an appointment at the one she chose. After just a few weeks of testing, one of the doctors at the clinic informed her that the probable reason for her failure to get pregnant was that both of her tubes were blocked and her fimbria were damaged. She never would have become pregnant the regular way, with or without Clomid. Although she was not happy to know that her tubes were "virtually useless," Linda was pleased that she had gained the strength to leave her gynecologist and she was eager to try IVF. After one cycle of IVF, Linda was pregnant. She called herself "Another Infertility Internet Success Story."

The Negatives

The negatives are equally compelling. You can, for example, find an enormous amount of information on the Internet that is faulty or misleading. It may be hard for you and for many others to sort through this barrage of misinformation and figure out what is wrong or right; its presentation can seem so scientific. Similarly, you can participate in an on-line support group and feel so powerfully linked to those members that you listen to their advice and forgo the advice of your doctor.

Also, participation on the Internet can be addicting. You've probably read stories of high school and college students who spend more than ten hours a day on the Internet and never get their schoolwork done. We have also come into contact with clients who report that they spend a similar amount of time on the Internet getting and giving advice, visiting Web sites, reading articles, and not dealing with the world at large. Being on the Internet does take you away from face-to-face contact. If your situation is so terrible and you have difficulty being in the real world, Internet communication can provide relief for a time. But at some point we all need to reenter the world.

Jill's story is one of the many unfortunate tales we hear about almost daily. Jill was an Internet whiz. She visited Web sites, participated in newsgroups, and attended countless auditoriums. She prided herself on "knowing everything about everything." She and her husband had two failed IVF attempts. Through visiting countless Web sites, Jill selected a new clinic. As she prepared to do an egg-donor procedure, Jill spent hours e-mailing everyone about the selection of her donor. As the group suggested, Jill chose a repeater who had made many eggs in her last cycle.

From the beginning, the doctors at her carefully selected clinic suggested that they try an intracytoplasmic sperm injection (ICSI) procedure to fertilize her eggs because her husband's sperm had not "behaved consistently" in their two prior attempts, but Jill would not consider it. Since Jill ran the show, James, Jill's husband, always deferred to her. Everyone in her groups encouraged Jill not to use ICSI. In the archives of her e-mails, it's hard to tell whether the group members did not encourage her because of their misguided medical knowledge or because she herself was not keen on the whole ICSI procedure.

Jill held firm. Even at the eleventh hour, the doctors asked her to consider at least dividing the eggs into two groups: one to be fertilized in the regular way and the other to be ICSI'd. Jill refused. The next day, there was no fertilization.

After five frantic hours on the Internet, Jill agreed to second-day ICSI. Although five of the eggs did fertilize, Jill did not get pregnant. Suddenly, her fertility on-line buddies stopped e-mailing her, started to write more positively about the ICSI procedure, or told Jill what a crummy donor she had chosen. Jill felt abandoned and alone. After carefully selecting a clinic, one with a wonderful reputation and a high success rate, Jill listened to her well-meaning Internet friends and not to her experienced doctors.

The lesson to be learned from this story is that despite the bad press doctors often get, it's important at least to listen to their advice, particularly over the advice of Internet buddies. We hear so many stories of couples who make this mistake. We encourage you to gather information, to gain support, and to Be a Partner with your doctor, but not to run the cycle yourself.

NEWSGROUPS

What Is a Newsgroup?

Newsgroups are Internet discussion forums. There were over 30,000 newsgroups in 2000.[1] As we write this section, we have located more than one dozen newsgroups devoted to some aspect of infertility. But additional newsgroups are added every day. So a year from now there may well be several additional newsgroups devoted to infertility and some of the current ones may no longer exist.

Messages sent to newsgroups are sometimes referred to as *articles*. This term is misleading because it connotes a level of authoritativeness you might expect to find in a journal article. In fact, many of these "articles" are simply biased opinions or sometimes factually incorrect material. Anyone belonging to one of the infertility-related newsgroups can post an "article." News servers remove "old" articles after they "expire." You can locate many "expired" articles. A service called *dejanews* (http://www.dejanews.com/) archives expired articles. To attempt to find what you are seeking, you can search by the name of the author or under a given topic.

How Do You Access a Newsgroup?

In order to read articles posted to newsgroups, you have to *subscribe* to the newsgroup. You select from a list of available newsgroups; *not all news servers carry all 30,000 newsgroups.* Once you have subscribed to a newsgroup, you can see a list of the articles that have been posted. In order to see these articles and read them, you need a newsreader program. Most browsers include such a program.

An Example of Newsgroup Communication

The list of posted articles resembles the list of e-mail messages you will find in your inbox. Many newsreaders display the messages in a *threaded hierarchy.* This *threading* allows you to follow the thread of a discussion from an original article, to a reply to that article, to reply to that reply, and so on. Each article header displays a title, the name of the sender, and the date sent. If you want to read an article, you click on the heading and the body of the article is displayed.

To get a flavor for newsgroup communication, consider this example. Jane Polya has just had her first-ever intrauterine insemination (IUI). She is now in the difficult two-week time frame where she waits to find out if she is pregnant. To cope with her anxiety, she wishes to communicate with others who can understand what she is experiencing. So Jane posts an "article" to alt.infertility asking if anyone has ever gotten pregnant after her first IUI. Nan Jones, a woman who got pregnant after her second IUI, reads Jane's post and replies to the newsgroup telling Jane that she, Nan, succeeded this way. Jane's original post and Nan's reply to it begin a "thread." The thread is just the list of *message headers.* The header gives a taste of what the post concerns. If you are interested in the topic and want to read the post itself, you click on the header to open the entire message.

Others perusing threads on alt.infertility can read this interchange between Jane and Nan. If they wish to, they can add to the thread.

Newsgroups Devoted to Infertility

Our search of the Internet revealed the following newsgroups devoted to some aspect of infertility:

alt.infertility The largest newsgroup devoted to discussions of infertility. Its articles are often copied to other newsgroups.

alt.infertility.primary This is a subset of alt.infertility that tries to cater only to people with primary infertility. Some people get easily upset by things you might not have anticipated. One such "hot button" is a person talking about getting pregnant or a person discussing her wish for a child because she wants her son or daughter to have a sibling. Alt.infertility.primary is an attempt to create a safe haven where women won't have to hear complaints from others blessed with a child.

alt.infertility.secondary For women with secondary infertility.

alt.infertility.pregnancy A safe haven where you can discuss your pregnancy experience after having battled infertility.

alt.infertility.surrogacy For women contemplating the use of a surrogate or a gestational carrier.

misc.health.infertility Similar to alt.infertility.

sci.med.obgyn General discussions of women's medical issues.

alt.support.pco Discussion of issues of concern to women diagnosed with polycystic ovary syndrome disease. Some discussion relates to infertility and some to PCOS, but unrelated to infertility.

alt.support.des Discussion of issues of concern to women who are daughters of women who took diethylstilbestrol (DES). Some discussion relates to infertility and some to DES, but unrelated to infertility.

alt.support.endometriosis Discussion of issues concerning women diagnosed with endometriosis. Some discussion relates to infertility and some to endometriosis but unrelated to infertility.

alt.adoption Adoption discussions.

alt.adoption.agency Adoption discussions.

soc.support.pregnancy.loss Support for women who have experienced a pregnancy loss.

alt.med.endometriosis Medical information on endometriosis.

alt.support.endometriosis Support group for women with endometriosis.

Pro and Cons of Newsgroup Communication

Nowadays, newsgroups are being supplanted by bulletin board discussion groups associated with Web sites. The Web site of the International Council on Infertility Information Dissemination (INCIID), for example, has more than a dozen topic-specific medical-discussion groups moderated by physicians. It also has more than a dozen topic-specific discussion support groups. Each of these discussion groups has its messages archived frequently. You can easily locate old archived threads and search the entire archive for discussions of topics of interest to you.

MAILING LISTS

What Is a Mailing List?

Mailing lists are a special form of e-mail. In mailing lists' original incarnation, people located others who shared their interests and created a list of e-mail addresses. Rather than sending e-mail to an individual, a person would send mail to the list of individuals. Hence the term *mailing list*. Typically, one person would take on the role of "owning" the list. She would establish a "home" for the list on some computer. She would also be responsible for enrolling new members, adding their addresses to the list, and sending newly received messages to the entire list.

Mailing lists can change their location. If you are a member of several mailing lists, you may find your e-mail inbox filling up rapidly under these circumstances. One solution some mailing lists have adopted is to prepare a digest of all the e-mail received in a given day. This way you receive a single e-mail that summarizes multiple messages instead of a large number of individual messages. Some of the lists described in this section will automatically send your e-mail as a digest while others will give you a choice of getting individual messages or the digest.

Mailing Lists About Infertility

ACTL: A Child to Love For those trying to conceive and experiencing infertility. Contact Sonya Hill mailto:autonet@surfsouth.com or Krista Wolf at mailto:dkwolf@parrett.net with any questions.

BabyOne For people experiencing primary infertility. To sign on, go to http://www.onelist.com/subscribe.cgi/BabyOne.

B2: BabyTwo The BabyTwo list is an unmoderated support for secondary infertility. mailto:listserv@maelstrom.stjohns.edu. Type in message body: subscribe babytwo firstname lastname.

Bereaved Moms Share Christian-oriented list for support about miscarriage, stillbirth, or early infant death. You are asked not to subscribe unless you have had at least one miscarriage and share the Christian orientation. mailto:majordomo@List-Server.net. Type in message body: subscribebereavemomsshare for single messages or subscribebereavemomsshare-digest for digest.

Childfree Living: majordomo@teleport.com message: subscribe childfree yourmailname@yourmailaddress.

CPL: Christian Pregnancy Loss Support Support group composed primarily of committed Christian women (Catholic, Eastern Orthodox, and Protestant) who are struggling with infertility and/or have lost babies due to miscarriage, stillbirth, or neonatal death. CPLS opposes "genetic termination," "therapeutic termination," "interrupted pregnancy," "selective reduction." mailto:cpls@iname.com. Type in message body: your name and a short bio.

Cross Cultural Adoption hctahnee@umich.edu message: join yourlastname, yourfirstname.

DES Daughters A forum exclusively for women whose mothers took DES (diethylstilbestrol) while pregnant with them. mailto:tasc@surrogacy.com. Type in subject line: send des application.

Domestic Adoption: listserve@sjuvm.stjohns.edu message: subscribe adoption yourlastname, yourfirstname.

Donor Insemination Support mailto:external-majordomo@ postofc.corp.sgi.com. Type in message body: subscribe di-support.

Egg Donors A forum open only to egg donors. mailto: tasc@surrogacy.com. Type in subject line: send ed application.

Endometriosis (witsendo) message: subscribe witsendo yourname. mailto:listserv@listserv.dartmouth.edu.

Fitness for Fertility An offshoot of WAC for secondary infertility. mailto:fff-subscribe@makelist.com. Type in the body of the message: subscribe.

Fortility For women over forty. message: subscribe. mailto: fortility-request@columbia.edu.

A Heartbreaking Choice For those who have chosen to terminate a pregnancy due to severe fetal health problems. Include your name and story in the message. mailto:FGCK08D@prodigy.com.

IF-Adopt Adoption during or after fertility treatments. To sign on, go to http://www.onna.org/community/sisterlists.html.

Infertility (the "ilist") message: subscribe ilist. mailto: majordomo@plusnet.org.

Infertility2 Secondary infertility. To sign on, go to http://www.onelist.com/subscribe.cgi/Infertility2.

Klinefelter's Syndrome Provides support for sex chromosome variations 47XXY, 48XXYY, 48XXXY, 49XXXXY, 46XY/47XXY mosaic and other sex chromosome variants. mailto:listserv@home. ease.lsoft.com. Type in message body: subscribe XXY+Adults first-name lastname.

Ladies in Waiting Infertility support for married Christian women. message: subscribe. mailto:ladenwaitn@aol.com.

LA-ONNA For ONNA.org members in the Los Angeles area. Send e-mail to laonna-owner@onelist.com requesting subscription.

LIL: Lesbian Infertility List mailto:majordomo@queernet.org. Type in message body: subscribe LIL.

LIMBO: Loss in Multiple Births Outreach mailto: listguru@fatcity.com. Type in message body: sub limbo-1.

Loss of All in Multiple Birth (LAMB) Go to: http://LAMB. listbot.com/.

MAI: Miscarriage after Infertility mailto:listserv@listserv. acsu.buffalo.edu. Type in message body: subscribe mai.

MFI: Male Factor Infertility MFI is an unmoderated list for the discussion of issues pertaining specifically to male factor infertility. To sign on, go to http://www.onna.org/community/sisterlists.html.

Mothers Via Egg Donation A forum open only to women who have been, or are attempting to become, mothers through egg donation. mailto:tasc@surrogacy.com. Type in subject line: send mved application.

Multiple Miscarriages A forum open only to women who have had multiple miscarriages. mailto:tasc@surrogacy.com. Type in subject line: send mm application.

OASIS: Overweight and Seeking Infertility Support subject: OASIS message: include name, e-mail address, and a short description of why you want to join. mailto:oasis@fertilityplus.org. (OASIS now has a Web site: http://www.fertilityplus.org/bbw/oasis.html)

ONNA Oh No Not (my period) Again ONNA is for anyone seeking or wishing to share information about methods of conception. message: subscribe ONNA Firstname Lastname mailto: listserv@listserv.acsu.buffalo.edu.

OPSS: Overweight & Pregnant Support OASIS graduate group, but open to non-infertiles. mailto: Bake4me@aol.com. Subject: send questionnaire.

OYIP: Oh Yippee! I'm Pregnant! To sign on, go to http://www.onna.org/oyip/. OYIPAL OYIPAL is a pregnancy list for graduates of BabyOne and BabyTwo who have succeeded in overcoming infertility. To sign on, go to http://www.onna.org/community/sisterlists.html.

OYIM: Oh, Yippee, I'm a Mommy! To sign on, go to http://www.onna.org/community/sisterlists.htm.

PAM: Pregnancy after Miscarriage mailto:pam-request@fensende.com. Type in message body: subscribe.

Parents Pursuing Surrogacy mailto:tasc@surrogacy.com. Type in subject line: send pps application.

Parents Through ART For people who have successfully had a child through assisted reproduction techniques. mailto: tasc@surrogacy.com. Type in subject line: send pta application.

PANFERT: Pregnancy after Infertility mailto:external-majordomo@postofc.corp.sgi.com. Type in message body: subscribe panfert.

PCO mailing list message: subscribe. mailto:pco-request@lists.best.com.

PCO Mailing List mailto:pco-request@lists.best.com. Type in message body: subscribe.

PCONatural For those wishing to treat PCO without drugs. mailto:pconatural-request@lists.best.com. Type in message body: subsingle (for individual messages) or subscribe (for digest).

PCO Pregnancy List mailto:pcopreg-request@lists.best.com. Type in message body: subsingle (for individual messages) or subscribe (for digest).

Pregnancy after Infertility mailto:pal-list-request@cyberclick.com. Type in message body: subscribe. To sign on, go to http://www.onelist.com/subscribe.cgi/PAI.

Pregnancy after Miscarriage message: subscribe. mailto:pam-request@fensende.com.

Pregnancy & Infant Loss Mailing List mailto:majordomo@taex001.tamu.edu. Type in message body: subscribe infanlos.

Premature Ovarian Failure Support Group Go to http://www.capaccess.org/capbin/pof/subscribe. to sign on. Contact mailto:POF2@aol.com with any questions.

Russian Adoption listproc@list.serve.com message: a.parent.russ yourlastname, yourfirstname.

SPALS: Subsequent Pregnancy after Loss Support mailto:listmanager@lists.iSTAR.ca. Type in message body: subscribe SPALS.

Surrogate Mothers mailto:tasc@surrogacy.com. Type in subject line: send sm application.

SV-ONNA support group Both on-line and face-to-face support for ONNA sisters who live in the Silicon Valley. Send an e-mail to svonna-owner@onelist.com requesting subscription.

Triplets For persons with a triplet pregnancy. message: subscribe triplets. mailto:majordono@tripcom.com

UK Buddies Infertility in the United Kingdom. To sign on, go to http://www.onelist.com/subscribe.cgi/uk-buddies.

WAC: Wanting Another Child Secondary infertility or just trying again. mailto:wac-subscribe@makelist.com. Type in message body: subscribe.

WAW: Wanting and Waiting Open to all people who are trying to conceive. The list exists both for emotional support and for sharing of information. mailto:wantingandwaiting-subscribe@makelist.com.

WEB SITES

Commercial Infertility Web Sites

There are two types of Web sites dealing with infertility. One is the commercial Web site, and the other is an informational resource not connected with a specific commercial practice.

The most common type of commercial Web site is the medical practice site. Other commercial sites include sperm banks, egg-donor brokers, pharmacies, drug manufacturers, adoption agencies, infertility-related law practices, and counseling services.

Medical practice Web sites are, for all intents and purposes, advertisements for the practice. They provide information about the physicians and staff connected with the practice. You can often learn about the credentials of these individuals. Sometimes you can see photographs of these individuals. Sometimes you can see photos of the facility.

Medical practice Web sites have begun to post the latest success rates for their IVF and other assisted reproductive technology procedures. Reproductive endocrinologists have become frustrated by delay of three years between the time they obtain the results of a cycle and when the Society for Assisted Reproductive Technology (SART) and the Centers for Disease Control (CDC) post these results. The time gap is the result of the procedures used by SART to collect the information, have it audited, and prepare the report of the results. During this three-year hiatus, new techniques have been developed and embryologists have gained valuable experience. So the results obtained three years ago often do not reflect the current level of success of a practice. In a few minutes, you can "visit" a practice on-line and determine what is happening with that practice today, not three years ago.

We suggest that in educating yourself about infertility, you visit the Web site of a clinic you think you might work with and view their claims of current success rates. To help get you started, we have listed the Web addresses of all clinics whose address we could locate in "Clinic Resources" at the end of this book. As you read about each clinic on the Web, bear in mind that the information should be viewed as an advertisement. Success-rate claims, for example, are not yet audited by an outside agency. If you feel worried, try e-mailing others about their experiences with this clinic. Use newsgroups, mailing lists, or discussion groups on non-profit infertility-information Web sites to post queries. Conducting your own Internet investigation can help you make an informed choice among several possible clinics.

Medical practice Web sites try to make it easier for you to become a patient at that clinic. They often provide forms you can fill out on-line to register with the practice. Many contain contact forms that enable you to send e-mail to the practice. By the time you come to the clinic for a first visit, you can really have a sense of the practice and get right to your face-to-face questions.

The name of the Web site game is to get you to the site and entice you to come back often. To do so, a really active site provides incentives. One incentive is to offer you education and new information. Many sites will include brief articles about topics on the cutting edge of infertility. Another incentive might be a collection of useful links such as a link to a database of medical journals maintained at the National Library of Medicine. By visiting these sites frequently, you can learn about new advances in the field and read the best journal articles.

In "Clinic Resources" and throughout this book we have provided the Web addresses not only of medical clinics but also of other services and centers specializing in infertility. We encourage you to visit sites that can help you with your specific treatment. Sperm banks, for example, now allow you to visit their site on-line and get a current list of donors. What used to take days and entail many phone calls can now be accomplished in a few hours. Chapter 11 shows you how to use the Internet to select a donor from an on-line sperm bank. Similar Web sites exist for finding egg donors and surrogates.

Non-Profit Infertility Web Sites

There are a number of excellent non-profit infertility Web sites. Here are some of the most important ones:

The American Society for Reproductive Medicine (www.asrm.org) This is the Web site of the non-profit medical society to which most reproductive endocrinologists belong. The site contains an area devoted specifically to the concerns and questions of patients.

The American Infertility Association (AIA) (http://www.americaninfertility.org/) AIA is an information and advocacy organization headquartered in New York City. It includes discussion forums and fact sheets.

RESOLVE Inc. (www.resolve.org) RESOLVE is the largest and oldest consumer infertility advocacy and information organization. From the Web site of the national headquarters listed here, you can find the Web addresses of local chapters. When you visit a local chapter Web site you can learn how to join and find schedules of chapter events.

The American Surrogacy Center Inc. (www.surrogacy.com/) This site contains an extensive collection of information about surrogacy and egg donation. Use it to participate in discussion groups, to read professionally prepared articles, and to locate the services of surrogacy agencies and egg-donor brokers.

Fertile Thoughts (www.fertilethoughts.com) This Web site offers discussion groups and information on ways of building families through infertility treatment, adoption, and surrogacy.

FertilityPlus (www.fertilityplus.org) A non-profit site that has a good listing of egg-donor brokers as well as sources for embryo adoption, sperm banks, surrogacy, and adoption.

ConceivingConcepts (www.conceivingconcepts.com/index.html) Another community site with discussion groups, infertility news, and one novel addition: a fertility store that sells herbal remedies, ovulation-predictor kits, fertility books and tapes, guided imagery tapes, and Kokopelli fertility jewelry.

The International Council on Infertility Information Dissemination (INCIID) (www.inciid.org) We must admit our favorable bias toward INCIID. Almost from its inception, we have been actively involved with the organization. We both serve as members of its advisory board and have also moderated the INCIID donor discussion group and the INCIID emotional issues discussion group. In 1997, we were awarded the Heather Bruce Thiermann Online Angel Award for our work with these discussion groups. We also developed an on-line survey of how visitors to INCIID used its interactive features and what impact these features had on them. That said, we consider this site to be the most useful infertility-related resource on the Internet. Some of what this site contains can also be found on other Web sites. But none of the other Web sites has the breadth of coverage offered by INCIID.

Recently, many Internet Web sites have started to act as "portals" to the Internet. This portal serves as a single location for you to visit and accomplish all of the necessary tasks on the Internet. By having a single location to work with, you can work more efficiently. The INCIID Web site offers an efficient jumping-off point for successful use of the Internet.

The INCIID Survey

Despite some of the "scare stories" about how Web sites keep track of all sorts of information about their visitors, the truth is that most sites know precious little about the people who visit. For an organization such as INCIID, it is particularly important to know who is visiting and what they are getting out of their visits. Unlike commercial sites, INCIID exists to provide a service to a population in need. Knowing who these people are and what impact the site has can help INCIID modify its offerings so they are of greatest value to its clientele.

To obtain this information, in the spring of 1998 we, with the assistance of INCIID founders Theresa Venet Grant and Nancy Hemenway, designed a comprehensive survey and offered it on-line on the INCIID Web site. You can find a slide-show presentation of the results of this survey on our Web site at www.gettingpregnantbook.com. This survey of more than 600 respondents from most of the United States and many foreign countries showed that: infertility is stressful, and most respondents were moderately depressed. Respondents completed the Getting Pregnant Quiz. Those who were doing better at following our Pointers were less depressed than those who were not following them. Many women indicated that the Internet forums helped them Educate Themselves About Infertility, Be a Partner in Their Treatment, and get the support they needed.

The Downside of Internet Participation

In 1998, researchers at Carnegie Mellon University published an important study on the effects of participating in Internet activities. Their conclusion: "Greater use of the Internet was associated with declines in participants' communication with family members in the household, declines in the size of their social circle, and increases in their depression and loneliness." We found a similar downside for a substantial group of respondents to our INCIID survey. This special group consisted of people who agreed with the statement "Internet forums are my *only* outlet for talking about or listening to people talk about infertility." In our survey, 44 percent of those responding endorsed this statement.

How do these "only-outleters" compare with people with alternate outlets? By all measures, they fare more poorly. They are significantly more depressed, they get significantly less support from family and friends, and they are significantly less likely to talk about infertility with their spouses. Also, they worry more about their relationship with their spouse, they are less satisfied with their marital relationship, they are less satisfied with their relationship with friends, and they are more likely to agree with the statement "I am less happy nowadays than I was in the past."

CONCLUSION

The list of features on the INCIID Web site is enormous. This site, as well as the other resources available on the Internet, has great potential to help you as you struggle with your infertility. Make this resource one of the *many* tools you use in your pregnancy quest. But don't use it exclusively. Infertility can be a lonely journey. You need to have real interactions as well as electronic ones. Used appropriately, the Internet can provide you with the information and support that might just up your odds enough to enable you to get pregnant when you thought you couldn't.

CHAPTER 15

Questions and Answers

hroughout this new edition, we have presented the most up-to-date medical information on infertility. We have also given you new ways to cope with the rigors of twenty-first-century infertility treatment so that you can up your odds of getting pregnant.

Even though we've tried to make the new edition as complete as possible, we find that our clients ask us the very same questions over and over. Because our goal is to help you up your odds, we asked experts to answer these questions. We've grouped the questions into the following categories: legal and insurance issues, genetics, what goes on in the lab, and everything medical you always wanted to know but were afraid to ask your doctor.

INSURANCE QUESTIONS

Answers are provided by Andrew W. Vorzimer, Esq.; Lori S. Meyers, Esq.; and Milena D. O'Hara, Esq. of Vorzimer, Masserman, Ecoff & Chapman, tel. (323) 782-1400.

Biographical Notes: Mr. Vorzimer is admitted to the State Bar of California; United States District Court, Central, Eastern, Southern and Northern Districts of California; and the United States Court of

Appeals, Ninth Circuit. Mr. Vorzimer attended Harvard University; University of Miami (B.B.A.); and Whittier College School of Law (J.D., Magna Cum Laude). Mr. Vorzimer also was the executive editor of the *Whittier Law Review*. In addition, he was a teaching assistant at the Whittier College School of Law. Mr. Vorzimer is the legal moderator for the International Council on Infertility Information Dissemination (INCIID).

Ms. Meyers attended the University of California, Santa Barbara (B.A., Political Science) and Loyola Law School (J.D.). She practices in the firm's reproductive law division.

Ms. O'Hara attended the University of California, Los Angeles (B.A., English Literature) and Whittier College (J.D.). She works in the firm's reproductive law section focusing on gestational surrogacy and embryo donation.

1. *Do you think that when you call your insurance company prior to making a decision about the course of your treatment you are raising a "red flag" or are you getting information that will help you make your decision?*

It is important to exercise extreme caution when contacting insurance companies directly to request specific information about your policy. Whenever possible, confine your inquiry to a confidential "cold call" wherein you do not otherwise disclose your personal identification number, account number, legal names, or any other identifying information about the parties involved in your assisted reproductive arrangement. Perhaps most importantly, do not refer to the fact that you are inquiring specifically about surrogacy or any other fertility-coverage issues. Confine your call to a general request about maternity coverage and related exclusions and limitations that might apply. While you should *never* withhold information from your insurer, for purposes of obtaining a copy of your policy coverage in order to assess the applicability of coverage, there is no reason to disclose your particular circumstances at this stage. Clearly, upon commencement of the medical procedures, this information will be provided to your insurer.

2. *What is COBRA?*

COBRA was initiated through the Consolidated Omnibus Budget Reconciliation Act and the Tax Reform Act of 1986 and is commonly referred to as "continuation coverage." These acts permit individuals receiving medical benefits, generally from an employer, to obtain benefits after major-medical insurance benefits have formally ceased. Coverage may also be elected in the event of divorce, legal separation, and/or death of a subscriber. COBRA may not be awarded in the event that a particular subscriber loses coverage due to gross misconduct, negligence, or malpractice. This type of coverage is often offered at an increased cost to the employee in the event that insurance benefits are lost due to termination or a reduction of hours of employment. The increase in cost will vary from policy to policy, and in some cases it is quite substantial. Thus, it is worthwhile to investigate obtaining an alternative policy before coverage ceases prior to assuming COBRA benefits in order to ensure maximum benefits at the most reasonable price.

Employers with more than twenty employees are federally obligated to offer COBRA insurance to employees. This refers to the number of employees employed, not the number of employees covered by a health plan, and includes full-time and part-time employees. Employees are generally offered COBRA benefits only if they have been employed in the same position for a specific period of time (often twenty-four continuous months). Some policies offer COBRA coverage only if the member is disabled and unable to perform daily work activities and must remain under a doctor's care.

COBRA may also apply in the event that an employee qualifies for an approved family or medical leave of absence (as defined in the Family Medical Leave Act of 1993) if insurance contributions continue by the member. The employer must provide the member with prior written notice of the terms and conditions under which such contributions are made. In most cases, COBRA benefits will cease if the member fails to make payments within thirty days of the due date established by the employer. Subject to certain exceptions, if the member fails to return to work after the leave of absence, the employer has the right to recover from the member any contributions toward the cost of coverage made on your behalf during the leave or the employer may retroactively terminate coverage to the date the premium was last received.

In the event that COBRA coverage is elected by a member participating in an assisted reproductive arrangement, it is important to be cognizant of the amount of time extended through the COBRA policy.

Many COBRA policies are offered only for a limited period of time. COBRA coverage must be offered by such employers for a minimum of twelve months, with many policies allowing for COBRA coverage up to thirty-six months. If a COBRA member becomes eligible for Medicare, the COBRA period expires, or any other group insurance is obtained, the member will not be eligible for further COBRA coverage. Thus, it becomes critical to remain sensitive to the timing of individual cycles to attempt a pregnancy and carefully calculate the number of months required for coverage to ensure that COBRA coverage will continue throughout the desired dates required for an individual assisted reproductive matter.

3. Are there any generalizations you can make about insurance coverage or is each policy unique?

Insurance policies vary considerably in the type and extent of coverage offered, in addition to the price of the premium itself. More expensive insurance does not necessarily equate to better or increased coverage, especially when it refers to maternity and/or infertility benefits. Some policies continue to offer coverage (or a percentage of coverage) for expensive infertility drugs and procedures, while others will completely exclude all infertility benefits. Thus, there is no substitute for a careful policy-by-policy review of individual benefits prior to beginning any medications or initiating any medical procedures with respect to an assisted reproductive arrangement.

Insurance policies also vary state to state. California remains the most progressive state with respect to the legality of assisted reproductive technologies, both in their application as well as in the number of cases completed each year. The number of cases has increased dramatically as the technology advances. As a result, California insurance companies have also been the most aggressive with respect to using surrogacy and egg donation as a reason to exclude coverage. It is important to remember that without a written exclusion provided to an individual member, the insurance company has no legal basis for excluding coverage.

Some generalizations can be made with respect to group versus individual insurance coverage, as well as to some characteristics unique to California insurers. In recent years, California HMOs were the first to begin issuing written exclusions with respect to surrogacy, egg donation, and other infertility treatments. In general terms, California group-insurance policies frequently exclude infertility benefits, as California does not mandate infertility coverage. California is one of the few states to offer a large number of individual insurance policies. The proliferation of individual policies has been prompted by the needs of a large population of entrepreneurs in California, a population that is strongly on the rise. Entrepreneurial businesses are frequently sole practitioners or small businesses that will not otherwise qualify for group policies. In addition, individual policies are also secured by members opting out of a particular employer's group coverage (often an HMO) in order to secure more extensive benefits (i.e., paying a small increase to secure a PPO).

In states other than California, the opposite situation frequently presents itself. Fewer individual policies are available outside of California, with most coverage extended through HMOs or other group insurance secured through employment. However, insurers outside of California may not issue exclusions with respect to infertility treatments as readily out of a lack of sophistication or knowledge regarding the complex field of assisted reproductive technologies. In addition, there are currently fewer infertility specialists and clinics outside of California to bring large numbers of cases to the attention of insurers. Yet more and more insurance carriers are using assisted reproductive technologies, as well as their related services and procedures, to provide a basis for exclusions in coverage. Thus, there is simply no substitute for examining individual policies with insurance professionals in order to determine which coverage is best suited for you and your desired treatments.

4. If your company offers a variety of choices in terms of insurance-company coverage, how do you go about finding out which coverage is best for you?

The best way to determine the coverage that is best for you is to request copies and carefully analyze the "Summary of Benefits" booklets, which outline the various types of benefits that are included in specific policies. It is critical to compare and contrast the maternity benefits of individual policies in relation to their respective cost. It is equally critical to determine whether there are any written exclusions or limitations with respect to assisted reproductive technologies. These exclusions are often found in the "fine print" of your summary booklet or are otherwise hidden among the literature provided by the insurer. It may also be important to determine whether desired physicians are covered by your plan, as well as whether a physician has privileges at a hospital appropriate and convenient for you (or your surrogate or egg donor) to complete the desired medical procedures and/or deliver a child born pursuant to the provisions in the policy. You may also want to determine whether hospital care covers neonatal care, and the level of neonatal care provided by that hospital.

If you are considering working with an egg donor, it is important not only that the egg donor obtain and/or maintain major medical insurance but also that the insurance policy is reviewed to determine whether the unique complications that may result from the aspiration of eggs is specifically covered by the policy. Many insurance policies will *not* cover such expenses, notably hyperstimulation, for egg donors. Check with your attending physician in order to determine whether special supplemental insurance may be obtained to protect you and your donor from liability and expensive hospital bills in the event that she is admitted to the hospital for hormone monitoring after an unforeseen hyperstimulation occurs.

Ultimately, couples must review their own policies to determine what portion of a desired treatment and/or pregnancy might be covered under their policy. In addition, a surrogate and/or egg donor's insurance must also be examined to evaluate the adequacy of the respective policy. Such policies must be screened *prior* to beginning any medical procedures or medical treatments, including drug therapy.

5. *What advice can you give about the best way to go about reading and understanding my policy? If I have questions after reading it, whom can I turn to for help and advice?*

There is simply no substitute for completing an extensive "due diligence" prior to the initiation of any medical treatments. Couples are understandably anxious and frustrated when their own attempts to create a pregnancy have been unsuccessful, and they frequently overlook important insurance issues in their effort to focus on particular treatments or working with reputable fertility specialists. A careful and complete review of your assisted reproductive arrangement through an objective third party could save thousands of dollars as well as maintaining "peace of mind" throughout a difficult and emotional process.

Utilize the advice of experienced lawyers and agency representatives to assist you in obtaining insurance information. It is important to work with attorneys and agencies who have a clear track record and expertise with assisted reproductive technology arrangements. Such professionals should be capable of advising you with respect to "global" insurance issues and potential pitfalls in addition to reviewing your particular desired policy in detail. Experienced attorneys should possess repositories of insurance policies and have considerable actual and/or anecdotal experience with the various carriers and HMOs. At the same time, be wary of relying too heavily on professionals with respect to insurance issues. While infertility professionals have more experience dealing with insurers, only the individual parties can properly monitor changes in coverage and the timely processing of individual claims for services rendered. Moreover, there are attorneys who specialize solely in the complex field of insurance-coverage law, and they should be consulted when difficulties arise.

6. *What is a pre-existing condition and how does that affect insurance coverage for you?*

A *pre-existing condition* is generally referred to as an illness or injury for which medical advice, diagnosis, care, or treatment (including prescribed drugs or medicines) was recommended or received from a physician or practitioner prior to the enrollment date of the insurance policy. Expenses related to pre-existing conditions are often not covered if they are incurred within approximately one year from the enrollment date of the policy. In some cases, a pre-existing-condition limitation may be reduced by "credible coverage" determined to exist under a previous health plan, or by the operation of a law that prohibits enforcement of a pre-existing-condition exclusion. The determination regarding the length of any pre-existing limitation period that applies to you is often calculated within a "reasonable time" (varying from policy to policy) following the receipt of accurate and reliable information relating to prior credible coverage.

A key question in reviewing insurance policies is whether the policy determines that pregnancy is deemed a pre-existing condition. Some policies will exclude pregnancy as a pre-existing condition, while others will not provide maternity benefits if the applying member is already pregnant. Pre-existing conditions become especially important when a change in coverage or benefits is requested. In most states, it is possible to change benefits once pregnant only through an employment change (i.e., a new employer, if hiring a pregnant woman, cannot deny her maternity benefits for her pregnancy). Insurers may be reluctant to extend coverage in the event that a pre-existing condition is identified in the course of the initial application process, and rarely will expenses related to that exclusion be subsequently covered even if insurance is offered. Pre-existing conditions such as diabetes may also result in an increased insurance premium. Thus, it becomes critical to disclose any pre-existing conditions accurately from the outset of the policy to ensure eligibility, while at the same time discerning the particulars of the insurer's application and payment schedules in order to assure that payments are not wrongfully denied.

7. If I am advised to consult my human resources department but want to keep private the fact that I am doing infertility treatments, what can I do?

A human resources department (HRD) is a good place to obtain general insurance benefit information and request copies of applicable "Summary of Benefits" booklets for specific policies that are available to you. An HRD representative may also be helpful in analyzing payment plans and unique maternity riders in order to obtain your best possible coverage. You will need to coordinate benefits, submit applications, and discuss your selected policy with an HRD representative in order to secure coverage, but there is no reason to otherwise disclose potential assisted reproductive arrangements with your employers. In fact, it would be prudent to discuss general maternity benefits as opposed to specific treatments. Your personal medical information is best kept private and confidential between you and your physician. Once the medical procedures begin, the receipts will be submitted directly to the insurer by the attending physician, allowing for privacy and confidentiality at your place of employment. Maintaining this level of confidentiality may be helpful for your own emotional well-being, allowing you to begin medical procedures and attempt several cycles of treatment beyond the curious eyes of your employer or fellow employees. Again, there is no reason to disclose to HRD representatives the fact that you are involved in infertility treatments.

8. *Are there circumstances under which you would be advised not to call your insurance company before beginning a procedure?*

Due to the unique and costly treatments involved in infertility, insurance companies frequently look for a basis to deny benefits in accordance with written exclusions and limitations presented in the "Summary of Benefits" booklet and other information forwarded to you by the insured. In some cases, insurance claims are denied based on extremely general exclusions in which it is arguable whether the specific treatment would be included in the coverage. For instance, some claims are excluded based on "services not specifically listed in the [insurance] agreement as covered," or "exclusion for services that are not medically necessary."

In order to avoid any possible future claims of insurance fraud, it is critical that you as an insured openly disclose any and all relevant information to your insurer upon request, including the types of desired or necessary treatments. However, it may not be useful to you to inform your insurer in advance of desired medical procedures and treatment unless pre-approval by the insured is a prerequisite in initiating the treatment. The effect of early disclosure may result in the claim suddenly failing under one of the more generalized exclusions discussed above in order to provide the insurer with a vehicle to deny the claim. A more prudent approach would be to analyze the policy carefully on an anonymous basis prior to initiating treatment and then submit the claim to the insurer for payment. When you conduct any inquiry, it is imperative that you memorialize it in written form and transmit the confirmation to your insurance carrier. Also, keep copies of everything! Be aware, however, that willful ignorance will not serve as a defense should you become involved in an insurance dispute with your carrier as to the applicability of coverage.

9. *How can I appeal a claim that has been turned down?*

The appeal process for challenging insurance denials will vary from policy to policy. Your first step will be to contact the customer services department anonymously and determine whether there is a formal procedure for appealing the claim. Keep detailed notes and files with respect to the name and telephone number of any and all agency representatives you speak with throughout the appeal process. Many insurance companies offer formalized "grievance reviews," including an invitation for a grievance committee hearing in order to urge the insurer to reverse its decision. Such reviews are regulated by specific time periods that must be strictly adhered to by *both* the insured and the insurer. For instance, a grievance committee must generally provide a written notice to the member challenging a claim within fifteen days of receipt of the grievance to inform the insured of the method the committee will use to analyze the denial.

The most important step in initiating your challenge is to force the insurance company to memorialize the denial in writing. A written denial of a claim should include a complete explanation of the reason the insurer is denying the claim. Without a written denial, neither you nor any professional will be able to analyze properly whether the denial is valid. For example, most hospitals will require pre-approval of insurance prior to admitting a patient into a maternity ward. Surrogate mothers are sometimes informed at the time of their pre-admission interview at the hospital that the insurance company has verbally denied their insurance for the pregnancy. In such cases, it is critical to remain calm and demand a written denial from the insurer. In many cases, pressing the insurer in this way will force the company to focus on the written exclusions and limitations sections of your specific policy. Insurers may then be averse to expose themselves to liability for the issuance of a wrongful exclusion if there is no basis for the denial in your particular policy.

In the event that the appeal is denied after your efforts to challenge the exclusion have failed, contact agency representatives and an experienced insurance litigator if you wish to utilize the legal process to challenge the denial further. The success of your claim may depend on whether the insurer has relied on a general or specific exclusion in the policy. In recent years, insurance litigators have begun to analyze insurance denials for infertility treatments and the claims of surrogate mothers and egg donors under constitutional principles of equal protection and discrimination. It is possible that your denial may fall within a series of denials currently being investigated for purposes of a class action against your individual insurer. Legislators have been reluctant to pass statutes related to infertility due to the rapid growth of technology in this area and issues of personal privacy and confidentiality. At the same time, insurers are increasingly under legislative scrutiny for the issuance of denials related to women's health, especially in the context of HMO coverage. It may further be helpful to contact the office of your state insurance commissioner and/or state department of insurance to investigate the procedures for lodging a formal complaint against your insurance carrier or filing a petition to initiate the investigation of your denial via state statutes. Finally, in the event that your denial is upheld after all formalized appeal procedures are exhausted, contact experienced professionals and insurance litigators to determine whether your claim is ripe for legal review.

10. *Even though I believed that a certain procedure was not covered, I submitted the claim anyway in the hope that some part of it would be covered. To my delight, the insurance company paid most of it. Now I am worried they will figure out that they should not have paid for it and will ask me for the money. Can they demand that I repay money for a procedure they were not required to cover?*

The laws with respect to the payment of insurance claims vary from state to state based on specific insurance codes. First, it is important that an insured *never* provide information to an insurer that is misleading in any manner. If it is determined that the claim was paid based on misleading information provided by the insured, the insurance company will have a valid claim to seek reimbursement from the claimant to offset the amount wrongfully paid. Applicable state statues of limitations will govern the time period the insurance company has to seek this method reimbursement.

If the insured has justly submitted the claim with the expectation that the treatment or therapy will be covered under applicable insurance benefits, and the insured subsequently reasonably relies on the payment and/or assurances made by the insurer, then the insurance company will likely be prevented from seeking an offset or reimbursement if the insurer later determines that the payment should not have been made. These equitable principles should protect an insured from an insurance company wrongfully seeking repayment many months or years after expensive treatments were covered by the insurer.

11. *My husband and I work for different companies but each company provides us with the same insurance carrier. How do we coordinate benefits? If I have reached my lifetime cap through the policy I hold with my company, do I get to start again with the policy from my husband's policy?*

Most insurance policies provide for annual deductible amounts both for individuals and families, as well as maximum "out-of-pocket" limitations and lifetime caps. With respect to maternity and/or infertility benefits, it may be possible to reach the maximum allowance for an individual covered under the policy but still seek reimbursement under applicable "family" expense allowances. Due to this important distinction, it may be prudent to begin insurance submissions for a female member's drug therapies or other individual treatments to her own policy while submitting claims for benefits that affect the family and/or couple (i.e., costs associated with in vitro fertilization, if covered under the specific policy) under the spouse's policy in order to balance the amounts submitted. In this case, where the female member's lifetime cap has been met, it may be possible to seek reimbursement only under the spouse's insurance for specific infertility treatments that otherwise directly affect and involve his treatment as well. This will be especially true where the family and/or couple maintain coverage with the same insurer due to the likelihood that the insured will have easy access to all claims previously submitted to that individual insurance company.

12. *Can I purchase my own policy that will cover infertility?*

Unfortunately, insurers are not currently offering supplemental coverage to provide benefits for most infertility services and/or treatments. Hopefully in future years a policy will emerge from a progressive insurance company, likely at a high premium, to cover the cost of infertility- and/or surrogacy-related costs. Until then, the most prudent way to obtain the maximum benefit at the most efficient cost is simply to examine your own individual policy with respect to maternity benefits. Review in detail the type and extent of maternity coverage provided, including their related exclusions and limitations as outlined in the "Summary of Benefits" booklet and additional documentation from the insurer. It may also be helpful to call an insurance broker to identify smaller companies that may not otherwise be familiar to you in order to determine if there is a policy with greater coverage you may have overlooked. Discuss your findings with an experienced attorney and agency representative in order to determine whether a change in coverage would provide you with increased benefits. Only after this detailed process is completed should any treatments or drug therapies begin.

You may benefit from initiating your medical procedures through an established agency or infertility specialist for purposes of egg-donation procedures. It is possible that your agency or doctor carries a unique insurance rider, at a cost of approximately $350.00, that will cover complications resulting directly from the aspiration and transfer of donor eggs up to $150,000.00 for the egg donor *and* the recipient mother. Such coverage is generally a required expense when you are working with an agency and/or medical team offering the egg-donation insurance rider, and is the best possible protection from liability and exorbitant medical costs in the event of hyperstimulation of an egg donor or any other complications directly tied to the aspiration of eggs and their transfer. Thus, before you choose your agency or attending physician, investigate whether there are appropriate professionals in your area who carry such insurance prior to initiating treatment to ensure the best possible insurance coverage.

GENETIC COUNSELING

Answers are provided by William H. Sofer, Ph.D.

Biographical Notes: William H. Sofer is a professor in the Department of Molecular Biology and Biochemistry at Rutgers University, New Brunswick, New Jersey. He is a member of the Waksman Institute of Microbiology. Dr. Sofer earned a Ph.D. in cell and molecular biology from the University of Miami, Coral Gables. His research interests focus on the molecular mechanisms of the regulation of tissue-specific gene control in higher organisms. Dr. Sofer was a member of the Genetics Study Section of the National Institutes of Health and has served as an editorial board member for *Mutation Research-Reviews in Genetic Toxicology* and as associate editor for *Developmental Genetics.*

1. *What can you find out through genetic testing and what can you find out through chromosomal testing?*

Chromosomal testing will tell you if there are any gross chromosomal abnormalities, for example, trisomy 21, or Turner's syndrome (X/O), or whether one chromosome has translocated (broken and gotten attached) to another.

Genetic testing often (more and more) gives us information about specific genes. It answers questions such as: Do you have a mutation associated with the gene for breast cancer or beta globin (giving you sickle-cell anemia)? Sometimes genetic testing yields a correlation between some mutation and a genetic disorder. This might occur when the scientific community doesn't know which specific gene is involved in a disease but does know that there is a genetic component.

2. Please explain the various types of inheritance (things determined by single genes, things determined by chromosomes, things determined multifactorially).

Genes are sections of chromosomes, and they carry information to make proteins. Since proteins do nearly everything in organisms, it's important to have genes that aren't defective.

Chromosomes by themselves don't do anything but carry genes. When there are too few or too many of a chromosome, this changes the number of genes you get, which may cause abnormalities.

Most characteristics humans inherit involve the participation of many proteins working together. For that reason, most characteristics are determined by many genes.

3. What does it mean to say that someone is the carrier of a genetic disorder?

We all carry two copies of each chromosome (males carry only one copy of the X chromosome). It often happens that one copy carries a gene that is defective and one copy that's normal. Having only one good copy of a gene usually is sufficient; often there is no disorder connected with this situation. But since you pass on one of your two genes to the next generation, you may pass on either the good or the defective copy. In this sense, you are a carrier of a bad gene, although you yourself may not show any detrimental effects from it.

4. Explain the difference between dominant and recessive genes.

Dominance and recessiveness are confusing concepts that are commonly misunderstood. Since we have two copies of each of our chromosomes, we have two copies of each of our genes. The problem of dominance occurs when we inherit two different genes. As stated above, the usual case is that one copy will be defective and one will be normal. The confusing aspect of this is that both genes are expressed, that is both make a protein (the job of most genes). Even the defective one will make a protein, but the protein will be defective.

If you have two copies of a defective gene, you can make only defective proteins. If this protein is important, you may exhibit a genetic disorder. But with one defective and one normal gene, you may or may not exhibit that disorder. If you do, then we say that the defective gene is dominant (and that the normal gene is recessive). For example, Huntington's disease (a fatal genetic disorder whose symptoms include progressive dementia) is a genetic disorder caused by a dominant defective gene. If you don't show symptoms of the disease, then we say that the defective gene is recessive (and the normal gene is dominant).

5. *People obsess over particular physical characteristics in selecting an egg or sperm donor (i.e., height, weight, hair color, physique). Can you describe the variety of ways these characteristics are determined for one's offspring?*

Height, weight, and general physique are complicated properties of organisms that are controlled by many, many different proteins (and therefore many, many different genes). In addition, our physiques are dependent on our environment, the foods we eat, and the exercise we do. The only sure thing that can be said about these traits is that their inheritance is complex and that there are many non-inherited components to their expression. Thus you can have a tall, large-boned daughter even if you and your spouse are short and small-boned.

6. *Many recipients do not want to let anybody know they used an egg donor. What are your thoughts about the ability to keep this information secret in the "age of the human genome?"*

You can certainly keep it secret from laypeople. But the tools of genetic diagnosis can reveal maternity and paternity very easily.

7. *What can be said about the way various physical characteristics are determined?*

Eye and hair color are relatively simple traits that are controlled by a few genes. Other physical characteristics, like foot size, tooth structure, length of leg, and breast size are much more complex, and their inheritance is much less understood. In other words, for these traits it isn't certain that having two parents with large feet, for example, will produce offspring with large feet. It just isn't that simple.

8. *What can be said about the way abilities such as musical ability or athletic ability are determined?*

Most of these traits are very complex. The scientific community has little or no idea how many genes are involved and how much of their expression is due to genetics and how much is due to the environment. Take one example: verbal ability. It is all but certain that if a person who has inherited very high verbal ability was put into a deprived environment, that verbal ability wouldn't be expressed. In this case, environment is probably much more important than genetics. If verbal ability or athletic ability were solely genetic, the children of writers would be famous writers and the children of extraordinary athletes would be extraordinary athletes.

EMBRYOLOGY

Answers are provided by Gregory Ryan, Ph.D.

Biographical Notes: Gregory Ryan holds a Ph.D. in molecular biology. He has conducted research at the Albert Einstein Medical College and served as an embryologist at lVF New Jersey.

1. *How are eggs graded?*

Embryologists examine the appearance of the eggs immediately after retrieval usually using a dissecting microscope. Very immature or dying eggs are discarded and the remaining eggs are assigned a grade to help the embryology team determine the timing and methods that will be used to fertilize the eggs. Different laboratories use different grading schemes, so it is sometimes difficult to compare one practice with another. Eggs are usually graded into broad categories depending on the appearance of the egg cytoplasm and the surrounding cumulus and corona cells. Those eggs with the best potential appear light and even in color and have an evenly radiating cumulus cell complex. Dark or dense surrounding cell masses may indicate a less mature egg. Degraded eggs, which appear smaller and have a very dark cytoplasm with tightly clustered, darker-colored surrounding cells, are usually discarded.

2. *How do I know they won't mix up my eggs and sperm with someone else's?*

Great caution is taken in the laboratory to avoid this type of mistake. Each laboratory may use different combinations of procedures, but usually fresh semen specimens to be used for insemination are processed separately from routine sperm-analysis specimens. Each tube for the whole sperm-washing and separation procedure is pre-labeled clearly and prominently color-coded. Pre- and post-insemination sperm are kept in different places so that used sperm preparations cannot be mistaken for the unused ones. Embryologists are required to check and initial the case notes at the appropriate points and to "say the name aloud" as they read the tube label before sperm is used for insemination. Eggs and embryos are kept in clearly and brightly labeled dishes separated from the dishes of other patients, preferably on their own shelf in the incubators. Embryos are removed from the incubators only one case at a time. When the embryologist talks to you before your transfer, he or she will address you by name, and when embryos are finally being prepared for your transfer, the RN who has prepared you for the procedure will be asked to check the dish to ensure it is the correct one.

3. *How do you know when the eggs are fertilized?*

Following successful fertilization of the egg, both the maternal and the paternal nuclear material are briefly visible within the egg under a high-powered microscope. The presence of these so-called pronuclei and the extrusion of an additional polar body are indicators of successful fertilization. Occasionally two sperm may enter an egg, resulting in the visualization of three or more pronuclei. These polyspermic eggs cannot be used and are discarded. Likewise, aberrant processing of genetic material and the presence of more than two pronuclei are sometimes seen in ICSI-inseminated eggs. These multinuclear eggs are likewise discarded to prevent the possibility of their being mixed with the normally fertilized embryos. Any mature eggs that fail to fertilize are also not used.

4. *Is there any way to know which embryos will freeze well?*

Pre-embryos at the stage just after fertilization before the male and female nuclear material combine have the greatest chance of surviving the freezing procedure. As the embryos become more complex in their development, the survival rate after freezing is decreased. About one-half to two-thirds of embryos at the Day 3 stage will survive the process of freezing and thawing. While there has not been a long history to evaluate the success of freezing at the blastocyst stage, the emerging data suggests that only blastocysts with excellent morphology have a good probability of surviving the cryopreservation procedure.

The decision about which embryos to freeze usually rests with the embryologists. Many advanced embryology programs hold up freezing until Day 6 to allow your remaining blastocysts (the ones that were not used for the Day 5 transfer) an additional day to develop into fully expanded blastocysts. Interestingly, during this time some of the blastocysts may hatch from their shell or protective coating, called the zona pellucida. Hatched blastocysts can be frozen, but they are more fragile and some embryologists feel that there is an increased possibility of damaging the embryo during subsequent transfer.

MEDICAL QUESTIONS

Answers are provided by Annette Lee, M.D., Reproductive Medicine Associates, Morristown, New Jersey.

Biographical Notes: Annette Lee, M.D., is a Phi Beta Kappa graduate of Cornell University, where she studied genetics and biology. Dr. Lee graduated with honors from Hahnemann University School of Medicine in Philadelphia, Pennsylvania. She completed her residency in obstetrics and gynecology at Winthrop University Hospital in Mineola, New York. There her interest in infertility and assisted reproductive techniques led her to a fellowship in reproductive endocrinology at Oregon Health Sciences University in Portland, Oregon. Dr. Lee has worked at the Center for Reproductive Endocrinology at Morristown Memorial Hospital. She then joined Drs. Darder and Treiser at IVF New Jersey. In July 2000 she joined

Reproductive Medicine Associates in Morristown, New Jersey. Dr. Lee moderates INCIID's Donor Gametes and General Infertility forums.

1. *Can I "kill" my wife if I give her an injection in the wrong location?*

No. However, it is possible to hit a blood vessel, which could cause bruising or decreased absorption of the medication, or to hit a nerve, which would be painful. For this reason, intramuscular injections should be given in the upper outer quadrant of the buttock and the person performing the injection needs to "pull back" on the plunger. If you see blood flowing into the syringe, simply remove the syringe and choose another spot. You are very unlikely to injure your wife seriously by giving an injection improperly.

2. *How important is it to take my injections at the same time every night?*

Most of the medications can be given at *about* the same time each day. A few hours later or earlier will not make a difference.

3. *What happens if I cannot find anybody to give me an injection and I cannot give it to myself? What should I do?*

You can find an urgent-care center or "drop-in clinic," or you can call your doctor and ask if you can delay your shot. Or you can attempt to give it to yourself. Intramuscular injections can be given in the buttock, the front of the thigh, or the fleshy part of the upper arm.

4. *How soon after a failed cycle can I re-cycle?*

Depending on whether there are any residual follicles left on the ovary, you may be able to start immediately. Some clinics prefer to have you take one cycle "off," depending on your stimulation protocol.

5. *Why is a cycle canceled? Is there anything I can do to decrease the chance that my cycle will be canceled?*

Sometimes the cycle is canceled because the response to the medication is not what the doctor expected, i.e., more—or fewer—eggs than expected, or hormone levels rising too fast or slow. At a certain point, your doctor may decide that the best option is to stop everything and start again from scratch with a different protocol.

6. *If my cycle was canceled last time, does that mean that I have a higher likelihood of having my next cycle canceled?*

It depends on the reason why it was stopped. If it was due to an inadequate response (too few eggs), then there is an increased chance of a poor response again despite changing the protocol.

7. *I'm forty-one years old. I have a normal Day 3 FSH. What are my chances of getting pregnant using my own eggs?*

Even with a normal FSH level the age-related decline in egg quality must be taken into consideration. In general, in the normal population, about 60 to 70 percent of women will be fertile at age forty-one. In a population of women complaining of infertility, of course this number will be much lower.

8. *I'm forty-one years old and have a normal Day 3 FSH. How do I decide whether I am better off doing an IVF procedure or an IUI procedure?*

In general, in patients over age forty most reproductive endocrinologists will tend to become more aggressive earlier. That is, since time is of the essence, they will try at most six cycles of IUI before moving on to IVF. Whether to go directly to IVF depends on many other factors, such as the status of the fallopian tubes, insurance coverage, sperm count, etc. You should sit down with your reproductive endocrinologist (RE) for a consultation to discuss the pros and cons of each option.

9. *How do I know when it is time to leave my OB-GYN?*

In general, once you have had the "basic workup," including an HSG, semen analysis, Day 3 hormone levels, postcoital test, and/or endometrial biopsy, you should consider seeing a reproductive endocrinologist. Also see an RE if your workup reveals any abnormalities that either you or your doctor feels need the attention of a specialist. Finally, if you feel that it is time to "become more aggressive" or feel frustrated with the care you are receiving, it may be a good idea to see an RE.

10. *What's the best tactic for me to try to persuade my clinic to treat me uniquely rather than putting me through a "cookie-cutter" approach?*

Your clinic should take into account all of the various aspects of your case: your age, your level of urgency, your insurance coverage. I would be very wary of any clinic that follows the same workup or treatment for everyone. During your initial consultation, you should feel that your doctor has considered the circumstances of your case and has outlined a treatment plan you are comfortable with. If this is not the case, you should seek a second opinion elsewhere. On the other hand, if you visit several REs and they all give you the same recommendation, it may be that the options are clear-cut even if you do not like what you are hearing.

11. *What's the optimum number of embryos to transfer?*

It depends on the "quality" and the "age" of the embryos. In general, the more developed the embryos (Day 5 versus Day 3) and the better quality, the higher the implantation rate. Therefore, it would make sense to transfer fewer higher-quality ones. Most transfers will be two to six Day 3 embryos or one to three Day 5 embryos (or blastocysts).

12. *What lifestyle restrictions are there after I have my embryos transferred?*

It is recommended that you avoid any strenuous activity for forty-eight hours. Of course, avoid caffeine, tobacco, and alcohol until after the pregnancy test.

13. *Can I fly while I am taking the medication prior to retrieval?*

Yes. If you cross time zones, try to stick to the same schedule as your "home" time.

14. *Can I fly after the embryos are transferred but before I have had my pregnancy test?*

Yes.

15. *Can I fly after a positive pregnancy test but before the end of fourteen weeks?*

Yes, as long as everything is going well, but we recommend that you avoid any unnecessary travel until the second trimester.

16. *Can I use hair dye while I am taking the medication prior to retrieval? Can I use hair dye after the embryos are transferred but before I have had my*

pregnancy test? Can I use hair dye after a positive pregnancy test but before the end of fourteen weeks?

Hair dye has not been definitively tested, so we recommend avoiding it if you can stand it until the second trimester.

17. *Can I exercise while I am taking the medication prior to retrieval?*

Yes, but as the ovaries enlarge or if you become bloated, we recommend avoiding any high-impact or intense exercise.

18. *Can I exercise after the embryos are transferred but before I have had my pregnancy test? Can I exercise after a positive pregnancy test but before the end of fourteen weeks?*

Swimming and walking are okay. We suggest avoiding high-impact exercises or getting your heart rate above 120.

19. *In the time between the transfer and my pregnancy test, what signs indicate that I am likely to be pregnant (e.g., tender breasts, abdominal cramping, vaginal discharge)? What signs are likely indicators that I am not pregnant?*

Because you will most likely be taking progesterone, which causes the *same* symptoms as pregnancy, you will not be able to tell whether you are pregnant by how you feel.

20. *I am worried about taking fertility medications. Am I at increased risk for getting ovarian cancer?*

The theoretical concern that fertility drugs could increase the chance of ovarian cancer has caused a great deal of concern in the medical community. Many studies have been done and *none* have shown that fertility drugs cause a statistically significant increased risk. One problem with conducting these studies is that infertile women are at increased risk of ovarian cancer *even if they never take any fertility medications.* Also, women who never give birth are at increased risk. We suggest you discuss this issue with your doctor and decide for yourself if the small, undefinable chance of an increased risk is worth the potential benefit. Only you can make this decision for yourself.

21. *Are there any family history conditions that would make me more susceptible than other women to have adverse reactions because I am taking fertility medications?*

For women who have a history of ovarian or breast cancer in their families, the theoretical concern about taking fertility medications may be of more concern. This should be discussed with your physician. In some cases, your doctor may ask you to be tested for BRCA1, a gene that has been shown to increase the risk of developing breast or ovarian cancer.

22. *Can I begin a cycle of Clomid when I have a residual cyst? Can I begin a cycle of injectable medication when I have a residual cyst?*

It depends. If the cyst is not too large and if it is not producing any hormones such as estrogen or progesterone, your doctor may decide to begin Clomid or injectables.

23. *What do you think about combining a natural cycle with acupuncture or the use of herbal remedies?*

There is some evidence to suggest that acupuncture may have a beneficial effect; however, there are no well-controlled studies. On the other hand, herbal remedies such as St. John's wort and echinacea have been shown to impede sperm function in the laboratory.

24. *For what purposes and when should baby aspirin be used during a cycle?*

Baby aspirin is thought to "thin the blood" a little bit, thus perhaps increasing the blood supply to the pelvic organs and preventing the formation of very small clots. This in theory is supposed to improve the response to medication and decrease the chance of miscarriage. Again, this has not been definitively proven, but many clinics use a baby aspirin (80 mg.) per day on an empiric or "can't hurt" basis.

25. *I am taking melatonin to help me sleep. Can this have any adverse reactions on my cycle?*

Melatonin, in a "natural" cycle, may interfere with the release of LH and FSH, thus interfering with ovulation. Discuss it with your doctor, but in general it is prudent to avoid any unnecessary medications.

26. *Can I have dental procedures while I am doing an IVF cycle?*

Yes, as long as you let the dentist know you are trying to conceive. In general, the use of Novocaine is okay but nitrous oxide should be avoided and lead shields should be used to block X-rays to the pelvic area.

27. *What gauge needles work best to minimize pain for subcutaneous injections and for intramuscular injections?*

Use a ½-inch 27-gauge or higher needle for subcutaneous (higher number equals smaller needle) and 1½-inch 22-gauge for intramuscular. If you run out of small needles, you can take subcutaneous medications intramuscularly; it will just be more uncomfortable.

28. *I have endometriosis and am planning to have it removed. Is there a "window of opportunity" after removing the endometriosis during which I have a higher likelihood of getting pregnant? What is that window? How aggressive should my treatment be during this time?*

In general, once endometriosis has been removed at the time of surgery, there is thought to be a "honeymoon period" of six to twelve months during which the endometriosis has not really grown back. Your doctor may want to be aggressive and give you fertility medications or do IVF during this time period.

29. *Please explain the relationship between endometrial thickness, endometrial structure (e.g., number of layers) and cycle outcome success. What is the range of acceptable endometrial parameters for cycle success?*

Studies in which the lining of the uterus has been examined prior to transferring embryos in IVF cycles have shown that implantation is more likely to occur when the lining is at least six millimeters thick and when it has a "triple layer" or "trilaminar" appearance. (It literally looks like three layers, somewhat like a layer cake.) Nevertheless, pregnancy can and does occur with linings that are "too thin" or that lack the "trilaminar" appearance.

30. *What is the relationship between cervical mucus quality and cycle outcome? Is there anything that can be done to increase the quality of my cervical mucus?*

Cervical mucus acts as a reservoir for the sperm. Around the time of ovulation, it should be thin, clear, and stretchy. If it is not, there may be a decreased window of opportunity for the sperm to survive inside the woman's body. One way to get around this is to have artificial insemination timed to coincide with ovulation. Some people also will use supplemental estrogen or Robitussin cough syrup in an attempt to improve the mucus quality; however, this has never been proven to work.

31. *Please explain what it means to be board certified or board eligible. How will my doctor's status with respect to board certification or board eligibility affect: (1) his competence, (2) his insurance coverage, (3) his hospital privileges?*

The American Board of Obstetrics and Gynecology issues "board certification" in both general obstetrics and gynecology, and in the subspecialty of reproductive endocrinology. If your doctor is board certified in one or both of these, it means he or she has passed an arduous written and oral examination and been found to be competent by his or her peers. If your doctor is board eligible, then he or she is eligible to take the exam but has not yet passed it. The most likely reason for this status is that the board requires a certain number of years of practice before one can take the exam. Also, since the exam costs several thousand dollars and is given only once per year, your doctor may not have had the opportunity to sit for it yet. Board certification does not guarantee that your doctor will be "good" or compassionate; however, it does indicate that your doctor was examined and tested by experts in his or her field and found to be competent. By the same token, lack of certification does not mean your doctor is less competent; it merely indicates that he or she has not been examined in this way. Many hospitals and insurance companies may require a doctor to be board certified within a certain number of years of becoming board eligible in order to qualify for privileges or in order to become a member of their panel.

32. *What is considered the normal range of fluctuation in FSH level from month to month?*

FSH levels can fluctuate from month to month; however, evidence has shown that as women reach the end of their functional reproductive years (i.e., when there are only a few hundred eggs left in the ovary), the month-to-month variation increases. Evidence in large populations of women has shown that once the Day 3 FSH is abnormally high even one time, the chance of successful pregnancy is very low (less than 5 percent), even if the FSH is normal during other months. For this reason, many REs will recommend that once one elevated Day 3 FSH has been found, the patient may want to consider the use of donor eggs.

33. *I know that FSH levels can be too high. Can they also be too low?*
  In certain conditions, such as hyperprolactinemia (increased levels of prolactin in the blood, which causes discharges of milky fluid from the breast and irregular or absent ovulation) or anovulation (very infrequent or rare ovulation) due to weight loss, the brain will shut down production of either FSH or the hormone that stimulates FSH release (called GnRH). In these cases the FSH will be low or on the low side of normal. A lack of FSH production is usually treated with injectable fertility medications containing FSH.

34. *How long can a sperm sample survive between being produced and being processed? What's the best way to transport a sample from home to the lab?*
  Sperm will generally stay alive and well for sixty to ninety minutes after ejaculation, however they need to be kept as near to body temperature as possible. We recommend obtaining a sterile container from your clinic, then putting the specimen inside the shirt or bra and taking it immediately to the lab for analysis.

AFTERWORD:
PARENTING AFTER INFERTILITY

We wrote our new edition of *Getting Pregnant* to help you *get* pregnant. When you do succeed in realizing your dream, we know that you'll probably be asking a different set of questions, questions having to do with what it is like to be a child conceived through "heroic" means and what it is like to raise such a child. Indeed, one of the fastest-growing areas on the INCIID Web site is the forum devoted to parenting issues. For us, rarely a day goes by that we don't have a phone call or an e-mail posing a question about parenting a child born through infertility treatment.

Although we don't offer the same level of expertise in parenting as we do in dealing with infertility, we can share with you our more than seven years of fielding media questions, as well as the real-life situations of our life with our now seven-year-old egg-donor twins, Nathaniel and Allegra.

What's it like raising these children? Not much different from parenting any set of active, high-energy twins. Exciting. Thrilling. Challenging. Expensive. Better than we ever could have imagined. Raising twins is difficult, but much of the day-to-day routine is no different than if they had been conceived naturally.

Psychologically, however, there are pitfalls to avoid. Infertility has its attributional traps. When you can't get pregnant, you attribute your difficulties to "the abortion I should never have had" or to "my greedy desire to have so much." When you follow our Pointers you dispute these irrational beliefs. But a new set of equally irrational beliefs will crop up *after* you succeed in having a child. Wait until the first time your child says, "I hate you, Mommy!" And if your child is like most seven-year-olds who are not allowed to stay up until midnight, wear that outrageous outfit, or get yet another *Star Wars* character or Barbie doll, you can be sure they *will* say that. The trap to avoid is telling yourself, If they had been conceived the regular way, if I had used my own eggs, my own sperm, if I had carried them instead of that surrogate [you can fill in the other blanks], they would never be saying such things to me. Well, they *would*—because they are typical seven-year-olds!

Also, because these children are so wanted, you may be more likely to spoil them or worry about their well-being. Ellen Glazer, writing about parenting after infertility,[1] says, "Fears of loss seem to arise more readily for parents after infertility than for other parents. Part of this seems to be their fear of retribution—that they will be punished if they forget to be grateful for even a moment." Quite possibly the urge to spoil may follow on the heels of these fears.

Like many other parents of egg-donor babies, we are older parents—often twenty years or more older than the parents of our children's playmates. Helane always says Nathaniel picks the boy with the youngest parents to be his best friend merely as a way to point out to us that we need to stay young. Although we may have less energy than these thirty-year-olds, we have much more patience.

Many of you will not be twenty years older than other parents, but, if your infertility quest does take time, you will be somewhat older than other parents. The age difference, as well as your view of getting pregnant finally, might make you feel slightly different from those other parents, the ones who got pregnant even before they wanted to. Every time we hear someone say they can't wait to find a sitter so they can go out on Saturday night, we realize how different we feel. We've been out on Saturday nights, many of them, both before we were married and while we tried to get pregnant. We can think of nothing more wonderful than to be in on Saturday night and to spend time with our children.

Personally, now the age issue is more pressing than the egg-donor one. Both Nathaniel and Allegra have figured out that their parents are older than most and also that we might die sooner. We tell them that no one knows when he or she will die. We tell them that we hope to live a long time because the joy they bring us is so great that we want to prolong it as much as we can. We assure them that we take care of ourselves. We hope that we are encouraging each of them to become strong and independent, as well as to look to each other as they grow so that they can thrive when we are gone.

Our kids have known since they were old enough to talk that they were conceived through ovum donation. We explained that they were in Mommy's tummy, but we needed the help of the doctors at IVF New Jersey (Auntie Susan and Uncle Michael) and a nice lady who gave us some eggs. Allegra is easier with it. She often talks about all the good things she got from the donor: her "yellow" hair, her athletic ability, her wonderful constitution. She also is able to verbalize about all the good things she got from Mommy: her zest for life, her sense of style, and her ability to talk about almost anything with anybody.

Helane needs to be tough because, in helping Allegra figure out what's good about herself, Allegra often makes negative physical or ability comparisons. "I am a good singer and you're not. The donor must have been a good singer." In fact, we don't know whether the donor sings well or not, but we do know that Daddy is a great singer. We help Allegra through her laundry list of goods and bads and help her see that all people are combinations of daddies and mommies but are ultimately unique.

Nathaniel is less easy with it. He is so bonded with his Mommy and Daddy that he feels like he is being "untrue" if he acknowledges anyone other than his parents being his parents. With him, we don't know the right answers. We reassure him and love him and answer his questions. They are hard ones, but ones we need to grapple with. Nathaniel is much more complex than Allegra, yet developmentally he is less advanced. We know that when he finally gets to dealing with his conception, he will ruminate about it for months and months. All we can say is we will be ready. He is the focus, not us.

We offer this information to reassure you. We want you to know that the decision to try to get pregnant when you think you cannot is a reasonable one and the outcome can be wonderful. We certainly are not experts. We love our children and want them to feel safe. In the evening when they tell us they worry we will die because we are "so old," we let them cuddle with us until they fall asleep assured. Is this the appropriate solution? Maybe yes and maybe no. Outsiders tell us that the kids have our number. They do. But we have theirs as well and are doing our best to raise our children to be strong and happy individuals.

Assisted reproductive technology, particularly the use of some of the more advanced procedures, is relatively new and data are not yet available to inform you of what happens as parents try to raise children conceived this way. New information is available each week. It is impossible to update books often enough to keep up with these developments. For that reason we are committed to maintaining our Web site at www.gettingpregnantbook.com and updating it with the latest information. We urge you to visit it from time to time. Please send us e-mail with your questions, comments, and, most especially, your success stories. Take advantage of the opportunity to talk with a child conceived through ovum donation by clicking on Ask Allegra and sending her e-mail. She will answer honestly! (Although it may take her a while to read and write answers to your queries.) Send us pictures of your new baby. Participate in discussion groups with other readers. Let's all work together to help one another and enable all of us to say, "I got pregnant when I thought I couldn't."

CLINIC RESOURCES

Here is a state-by-state listing of clinics that perform assisted reproductive technology (ART) procedures. Most of these clinics submit reports to the Centers for Disease Control (CDC) so that their success-rate claims can be audited. Clinics choosing not to submit reports to the CDC are noted here as "Non-CDC."

ALABAMA

ART Program of Alabama
(Dr. Kathryn L. Honea, Director)
Women's Medical Plaza, Suite 508
2006 Brookwood Medical Center
   Drive
Birmingham, AL 35209
Phone: (205) 870-9784
Fax: (205) 870-0698
www.artprogram.com
art_program@msn.com

University of Alabama at
   Birmingham
(Dr. Michael P. Steinkampf,
   Director)
IVF Program
Department of OB/GYN
2006 Avenue South
Birmingham, AL 35233
Phone: (205) 934-1030
Fax: (205) 975-5732
www.uabmc.edu

University of South Alabama
(Dr. Peter Rizk, Director)
IVF Program
307 University Boulevard,
   CCCB 326
Mobile, AL 36688
Phone: (334) 460-7173
Fax: (334) 460-7251
http://southmed.usouthal.edu/com/
   obgyn/index.html

Center for Reproductive Medicine
(Dr. George Koulianos)
3 Mobile Infirmary Circle, Suite 312
Mobile, AL 36607
Phone: (334) 438-4200
Fax: (334) 438-4211
http://www.infertilityalabama.com/

ARIZONA

Fertility Treatment Center
(Dr. H. Randall Craig)
3200 North Dobson, Suite F-7
Chandler, AZ 85224
Phone: (480) 831-2445
Fax: (480) 897-1283
www.inciid.org/advisory/johnson.html
MDJFTC@aol.com

Arizona Reproductive Medicine
(Dr. Robert Tamis, Director)
2850 North 24th Street, Suite 503
Phoenix, AZ 85008
Phone: (602) 468-3840
Fax: (602) 468-2449
www.conceive.com/

IVF Phoenix
(Dr. John Couvaras, Director)
4626 East Shea Boulevard,
   Suite C-230

Phoenix, AZ 85028
Phone: (602) 996-2411
Fax: (602) 996-5254
www.ihr.com/ivfphonix
ivfphx@primenet.com

Arizona Reproductive Medicine
   Specialists
(Dr. John H. Mattox, Director)
1300 North 12th Street, Suite 520
Phoenix, AZ 85006
Phone: (602) 343-2767
Fax: (602) 343-2766
www.arizonarms.com

Southwest Fertility Center
(Dr. Sujatha Gunnala, Director)
3125 North 32nd Street, Suite 200
Phoenix, AZ 85018
Phone: (602) 956-7481
Fax: (602) 956-7591
http://www.primenet.com/swfertil/

Arizona Center for Fertility
   Studies
(Dr. Jay S. Nemiro, Director)
8997 East Desert Cove Avenue,
   2nd Floor
Scottsdale, AZ 85260
Phone: (602) 860-4792
Fax: (602) 860-6819
www.acfs2000.com/html/about.html

ARKANSAS

Intravaginal Culture Fertilization
   Program
(Dr. Francisco Batras, Director)
500 South University, Suite 103
Little Rock, AR 72205
Phone: (501) 663-5858
Fax: (501) 663-9007

University of Arkansas for Medical
   Sciences
IVF Program
(Dr. Michael M. Miller, Director)
4301 West Markham, Slot 518
Little Rock, AR 72205-7199
Phone: (501) 296-1705
Fax: (501) 296-1710
www.uams.edu/obgyn
millermichael@exchange.uams.edu

CALIFORNIA

Alta Bates Medical Center
   IVF Program
(Dr. Ryszard Chetkowski, Director)
2999 Regent Street, Suite 101-A
Berkeley, CA 94705
Phone: (510) 649-0440
Fax: (510) 649-8700
www.abivf.com
abivf@pacbell.net

Reproductive Medicine and Surgery
   Associates
450 North Roxbury Drive
Beverly Hills, CA 90210
Phone: 310-777-2393
Fax: 310-274-5112

West Coast Infertility Medical
   Clinic Inc.
(Dr. Michael Kamrava, Director)
250 North Robertson Boulevard,
   Suite 403
Beverly Hills, CA 90211
Phone: (310) 285-0333
Fax: (310) 285-0334
www.westcoastinfertility.com
michael@westcoastinfertility.com

Central California IVF
   Program
(Dr. Carlos Sueldo, Director)
6215 North Fresno,
   Suite 108
Fresno, CA 93710
Phone: (559) 439-1913
Fax: (559) 439-3936

West Coast Fertility Centers
11160 Warner Avenue
   Suite 411
Fountain Valley, CA 92807
Phone: (714) 513-1399
Fax: (714) 513-1393
www.ivfbaby.com
mp545@aol.com

Werlin-Zarutskie Fertility Centers
(Dr. Lawrence Werlin, Director)
4900 Baranca Parkway
Irvine, CA 92604
Phone: (949) 726-0600
Fax: (949) 726-0601
www.wzfertctr.com

Reproductive Science Center of
   San Diego
(Dr. Sam Wood, Director)
4150 Regents Park Row, Suite 280
La Jolla, CA 92037
Phone: (858) 625-0125
Fax: (858) 625-0131

Scripps Clinic Fertility Center
(Dr. Jeffrey S. Rakoff, Director)
10666 North Torrey Pines Road
La Jolla, CA 92037
Phone: (858) 554-8680
Fax: (858) 554-8727
www.scrippsclinic.com/centers/fertil/

Loma Linda University Center for
    Fertility & IVF
(Dr. William Patton, Director)
11370 Anderson Street, Suite 3950
Loma Linda, CA 29354
Phone: (909) 796-4851
Fax: (909) 478-6450
www.llu.edu/llumc/fertility/

Century City Hospital
Center for Reproductive Medicine
(Dr. David Hill, Director)
2070 Century Park East
Los Angeles, CA 90067
Phone: (310) 201-6619
Fax: (310) 201-6657
www.centurycityhospital.com/

Tyler Medical Clinic
(Dr. Jaroslav Marik, Director)
921 Westwood Boulevard
    Suite 300
Los Angeles, CA 90024
Phone: (310) 208-6765
Fax: (310) 208-3648
www.tylermedicalclinic.com
jjmarik@aol.com

University of California–
    Los Angeles
Fertility Clinic
(Dr. Joseph Gambone, Director)
OB/GYN, Room 22-177 CHS
10833 Le Conte Avenue
Los Angeles, CA 90095
Phone: (310) 825-9500
Fax: (310) 206-9731

New Directions in Fertility
    (Non-CDC)
(Bassett Brown, M.D.)

4727 Wilshire Boulevard,
    Suite 310
Los Angeles, CA 90010
Phone: (877) 428-3222
www.1877havebaby.com/

University of Southern
    California
Reproductive Endocrinology and
    Infertility
(Dr. Richard Paulson, Director)
1245 Wilshire Boulevard,
    Suite 403
Los Angeles, CA 90017
Phone: (213) 975-9990
Fax: (213) 975-9997
http://www.uscivf.org

Reproductive Specialty Medical
    Center
(Dr. Beth Ary, Director)
1441 Avocado Avenue, Suite 203
Newport Beach, CA 92660
Phone: (949) 640-7200
Fax: (949) 720-0203
drary@deltanet.com

Southern California Center for
    Reproductive Medicine
(Dr. Robert Anderson, Director)
361 Hospital Road, Suite 333
Newport Beach, CA 92663
Phone: (949) 642-8727
Fax: (949) 642-5413

Northridge Center for
    Reproductive Medicine
(Jirair Konialian, M.D.)
18546 Roscoe Boulevard,
    Suite 240
Northridge, CA 91324
Phone: (818) 701-8181

www.northridgeivf.com/
ivfnridge@aol.com

NOVA In Vitro Fertilization
(Dr. Francis Polansky, Director)
1681 El Camino Real
Palo Alto, CA 94306
Phone: (650) 322-0500
Fax: (650) 322-5404
http://www.novaivf.com

Huntington Reproductive
   Center
(Dr. Joel Batzofin, Director)
301 South Fair Oaks Avenue,
   Suite 402
Pasadena, CA 91105
Phone: (626) 440-9161
Fax: (626) 440-0138
http://www.havingbabies.com/

Reproductive Partners Medical
   Group Inc.
(Dr. Bill Yee, Director)
510 North Prospect Avenue,
   Suite 202
Redondo Beach, CA 90277
Phone: (310) 318-3010
Fax: (310) 798-7304
www.2reproduce.com

Northern California Fertility
   Center
406 Sunrise Avenue,
   Suite 310
Roseville, California 95661
(916) 773-2229
www.ncfmc.com/
doctorg@ncfmc.com (Dr. John
   Gililland)
jandrey@ncfmc.com (Dr. Janice
   Andreyko)

csoto@ncfmc.com (Dr. Carlos Soto-
   Albors)

University of California–Davis
ART Program
Department of OB/GYN
(Dr. Lloyd Smith, Director)
4860 Y, Suite 2500
Sacramento, CA 95817
Phone: (916) 734-6930
Fax: (916) 734-6666
http://medicalgroup.ucdavis.edu/
   offices/

IGO Medical Group of San Diego
(Dr. Benito Villanueva, Director)
9339 Benésee Avenue, Suite 220
San Diego, CA 92121
Phone: (858) 455-7520
Fax: (858) 554-1312
www.igomed.com

Reproductive Endocrine
   Associates
6719 Alvarado Road, Suite 108
San Diego, CA 92120
Phone: (619) 265-1800
Fax: (619) 265-4055
sbronymd@cts.com

Astarte Fertility Medical Center
(Dr. Alex Steinleitner, Director)
450 Sutter Street, Suite 2215
San Francisco, CA 94108
Phone: (415) 773-3413
Fax: (415) 837-1155
http://www.astarte.com

Pacific Fertility Medical Center
(Dr. Vicken Sahakian, Director)
55 Francisco Street, Suite 500
San Francisco, CA 94133

Phone: (415) 834-3000
Fax: (415) 834-3099
www.pfmc.com

San Francisco Center for
Reproductive Medicine
(Dr. Carol Herbert, Director)
390 Laurel Street, Suite 205
San Francisco, CA 94118
Phone: (415) 771-1483
Fax: (415) 771-8421
www.sffertility.com/

University of California–
San Francisco
(Dr. Eldon Schriock, Director)
350 Parnassus Avenue, 300
San Francisco, CA 94117
Phone: (415) 476-5405
Fax: (415) 502-4944
www.ihr.com/ucsfivf

Zouves Fertility Center
(Non-CDC)
(Christo Zouves, M.D.)
901 Campus Drive, Suite 214
Daly City, California 94015
Phone: (800) 800-1160
http://www.goivf.com/index.html

Fertility Physicians of Northern
California
(Dr. David Adamson, Director)
2516 Samaritan Drive, Suite A
San Jose, CA 95125
Phone: (408) 358-2500
Fax: (408) 356-8954
www.fpnc.com

Forest Fertility Center (Non-CDC)
(Dr. Vincent Nola, Director)
2110 Forest Avenue, Suite A

San Jose, CA 95128
Phone: (408) 288-9933
Fax: (408) 286-7730

Reproductive Science Center of
Bay Area
(Dr. Louis Weckstein, Director)
3160 Crow Canyon Road,
Suite 150
San Ramon, CA 94583
Phone: (925) 867-1800
Fax: (925) 275-0933
www.ihr.com/bafertil/medicalt.html
bafertil@ccnet.com

Center for Assisted Reproductive
Medicine
1250 16th Street, Suite 2129
Santa Monica, CA 90404
Phone: (310) 319-4482
Fax: (310) 319-4123

Center for Reproductive Health &
Gynecology (Non-CDC)
(Melvin Thornton, M.D.)
2121 Wilshire Boulevard
Santa Monica, CA 90403
Phone: (310) 264-0699
www.reproductive.org/

North Bay Fertility Center Inc.
(Dr. Steven Dodge, Director)
1111 Sonoma Avenue, Suite 212
Santa Rose, CA 95405
Phone: (707) 575-1729
Fax: (707) 575-4379
www.cnbfma.com/

Stanford University Medical
Center
IVF Program
(Dr. Amin Milki, Director)

GYNOB HH333
300 Pasteur Drive
Stanford, CA 94305-5387
Phone: (650) 725-5983
Fax: (650) 498-5024
www.stanford.edu/dept/GYNOB/rei/

Center for Fertility and
    Gynecology
(Dr. Michael Vermesh, Director)
18370 Burbank Boulevard,
    Suite 301
Tarzana, CA 91356
Phone: (818) 881-9800
Fax: (818) 881-1857
www.centerforhumanreprod.com/
    low_speed/CHRlowspeed/
    gyncormap/chrca/chrca.htm

The Fertility Institutes
18370 Burbank Boulevard,
    Suite 414
Tarzana, CA 91356
Phone: (818) 776-8700
Fax: (818) 776-8754
www.fertility-docs.com

San Antonio Fertility Center
(Non-CDC)
510 North 13th Avenue, Suite 201
Upland, CA 91786
Phone: (909) 920-4858
Fax: (909) 985-7137
http://pages.ivillage.com/lefmg/
    infertinfo.html

COLORADO

Colorado Springs Center for
    Reproductive Health
(Drs. Robert Hahn and
    Eric Silverstein)

1625 Medical Center Point,
    Suite 290
Colorado Springs, CO 80907
Phone: (719) 636-0080
Fax: (719) 636-3030
www.fertilitynetwork.com

Colorado IVF at Rose
(Dr. Sam Alexander, Director)
4600 East Hale Parkway, Suite 350
Denver, CO 80220
Phone: (303) 321-7115
Fax: (303) 321-9519
www.fertilitycolorado.cnchost.com/
crecares@concentric.net

Reproductive Genetics In Vitro
(Dr. George Henry, Director)
455 South Hudson Street, Level 3
Denver, CO 80246
Phone: (303) 399-1464
Fax: (303) 399-1465
www.reprogen.com

Center for Reproductive Medicine
(Dr. William Schlaff, Director)
4701 East Ninth Avenue,
    University Pavillion 254 South
Denver, CO 80220
Phone: (303) 372-1483
Fax: (303) 372-1499
www.uchsc.edu/sm/smobsgyn/rei.htm

Colorado Center for Reproductive
    Medicine
(Dr. John Yumans, Director)
799 East Hampden Avenue,
    Suite 300
Eaglewood, CO 80110
Phone: (303) 788-8300
Fax: (303) 788-8310
www.colocrm.com

Rocky Mountain Center for
Reproductive Medicine
(Dr. Bachus)
1080 East Elizabeth
Fort Collins, CO 80524
Phone: (970) 493-6366
Toll Free: (800) 624-9035
www.drbachus.com/
rmcrm@aol.com

Conceptions: Reproductive
Associates
Women's Health and Fertility
Specialists
(Dr. Betty John, Director)
7720 South Broadway, Suite 580
Littleton, CO 80122
Phone: (303) 794-0045
Fax: (303) 794-2054
www.conceptionsrepro.com

CONNECTICUT

University of Connecticut Health
Center
Department of OB/GYN
263 Farmington Avenue
Farmington, CT 06032
Phone: (860) 679-4580
Fax: (860) 679-1436
www.fertilitycenter-uconn.org

Hartford Fertility & Reproductive
Endocrinology (Non-CDC)
100 Retreat Avenue, Suite 900
Hartford, CT 06106
Phone: (860) 525-8283
Fax: (860) 525-1930
www.harthosp.org/womens/
phys_directory

New Britain General Hospital
(Non-CDC)
(Dr. Anthony A. Luciano, Director)
100 Grand Street
New Britain, CT 06050
Phone: (860) 224-5467
www.nbgh.org/fertile.htm

Yale University IVF Program
Reproductive Center
333 Cedar Street
New Haven, CT 06510
Phone: (203) 785-4708
Fax: (203) 785-3560
http://info.med.yale.edu/yfp/
referral/obst/rep.html

Michael P. Doyle, M.D.
148 East Avenue
Norwalk, CT 06851
Phone: (203) 855-1200
Fax: (203) 866-3668

New England Fertility Institute
(Dr. Gad Lavy, Director)
1275 Summer Street
Stamford, CT 06905
Phone: (203) 325-3200
Fax: (203) 323-3130

DELAWARE

Delaware Institute for Reproduc-
tive Medicine
(Dr. Jeffrey Russell, Director)
4745 Stanton-Ogletown Road,
Suite 111
Newark, DE 19713
Phone: (302) 738-4600
Fax: (302) 738-3508

DISTRICT OF COLUMBIA

Columbia Hospital for Women
ART Program
(Dr. Richard Falk, Director)
2440 M. Street NW, Suite 401
Washington, D.C. 20037
Phone: (202) 293-6567
Fax: (202) 778-6190
fertdocs@erols.com

The George Washington University
    Medical Center
IVF Program
(Dr. Paul Gindoff, Director)
2150 Pennsylvania Avenue, NW
Washington, DC 20037
Phone: (202) 994-4614
Fax: (202) 994-0817
www.gwumc.edu/mfa/refi/index.htm

Reproductive Science Center
    Walter Reed Army Medical
    Center
Reproductive Endocrinology
6900 Georgia Avenue, NW
Washington, DC 20307
Phone: (202) 782-5090
Fax: (202) 782-4833

FLORIDA

Boca Fertility
(Dr. Moshe Peress)
875 Meadows Road, Suite 334
Boca Raton, FL 33428
Phone: (561) 368-5500
Fax: (561) 368-4793
www.bocafertility.com
frontdest@bocafertility.com

CHR-Florida
(Dr. Edward Zbella, Director)
2454 McMullen Booth Road,
    Suite 601
Clearwater, FL 33759
Phone: (727) 796-7705
Fax: (727) 796-8764

Specialists in Reproductive
    Medicine & Surgery, P.A.
(Dr. Craig Sweet, Director)
12611 World Plaza Lane,
    Building 53
Fort Myers, FL 33907
Phone: (941) 275-8118
Fax: (941) 275-5914
www.dreamababy.com

University of Florida/Park Avenue
    Women's Center
807 Northwest 57th Street
Gainesville, FL 32605
Phone: (352) 392-6200
Fax: (352) 392-6204
www.med.ufl.edu/obgyn/endo/
    main.html
williams@obgyn.med.ufl.edu

Fertility Institute of Northwest
    Florida
(Dr. Robert Pile, Director)
1110 Gulf Breeze Parkway
Gulf Breeze, FL 32561
Phone: (850) 934-3900
Fax: (850) 932-3753

Florida Institute for Reproductive
    Medicine
(Dr. Kevin Winslow, Director)
836 Prudential Drive, Suite 902
Jacksonville, FL 32207

Phone: (904) 399-5620
Fax: (904) 399-5645
www.firmjax.com/

North Florida Gynecologic
    Specialists (Non-CDC)
Dr. Michael Fox
1820 Barrs Street, Suite 350
Jacksonville, FL
Phone: (904) 388-4695
www.fertilitynetwork.com/Open/
    Jacksonville.htm

Florida Institute for Reproductive
    Science and Technology
    (F.I.R.S.T.)
9900 Stirling Road, Suite 300
Cooper City, FL 33024
Phone: (954) 436-2700
Fax: (954) 436-6663

IVF Florida/Northwest Center for
    Infertility and Reproductive
    Endocrinology
(Dr. Wayne Maxson, Director)
2825 North SR 7, Suite 302
Margate, FL 33063
Phone: (954) 247-6200
Fax: (954) 247-6262
www.ivfflorida.com

Fertility & IVF Center of Miami
(Dr. Michael Jacobs, Director)
8950 North Kendall Drive,
    Suite 103
Miami, FL 33176
Phone: (305) 596-4013
Fax: (305) 596-4557
fivf@msn.com

South Florida Institute for
    Reproductive Medicine
6250 Sunset Drivve, Suite 202

South Miami, FL 33143
Phone: (305) 662-7901
Fax: (305) 662-7910
www.ivfmd.com/

Arnold Palmer Hospital Fertility
    Center
(Dr. Mark Trolice, Director)
22 Underwood Street
Orlando, FL 32806
Phone: (407) 649-6995
Fax: (407) 841-3367
jconway@orhs.org

Center for Infertility &
    Reproductive Medicine
(Dr. Gary W. DeVane, Director)
3435 Pinehurst Avenue
Orlando, FL 32804
Phone: (407) 740-0909
Fax: (407) 740-7262
www.ivforlando.com/
cirm@aol.com

Reproductive Medicine & Fertility
    Center
(Dr. Mark Jutras, Director)
615 East Princeton Street,
    Suite 225
Orlando, FL 32803
Phone: (407) 896-7575
Fax: (407) 894-2692
mark.jutras@obgyn.net

Fertility Center of Sarasota
(Julio E. Pabon, M.D.)
5664 Bee Ridge Road, Suite 103
Sarasota, FL 34233
Phone: (941) 342-1568
Fax: (941) 342-8296

Palm Beach Fertility Center
    (Non-CDC)

(Mark S. Denker, M.D.)
22023 State Road 7, Suite 104
Boca Raton, FL 33428
(561) 477-7728
http://members.icanect.net/
~pbfertil/

Center for Advanced Reproductive
Endocrinology
(Dr. Mick Abaé, Director)
6738 West Sunrise Boulevard,
Suite 106
Plantation, FL 33313
Phone: (954) 584-2273
Fax: (954) 587-9630
www.care-life.com
carelife@bellsouth.net

Fertility Institute of Fort
Lauderdale
4100 South Hospital Drive,
Suite 209
Plantation, FL 33317
Phone: (954) 791-1442
Fax: (954) 791-1887

The Reproductive Medicine
Group
(Dr. Marc Bernhisel, Director)
2919 Swann Avenue, Suite 305
Tampa, FL 33609
Phone: (813) 870-3553
Fax: (813) 872-8727
www.floridafertility.com/

Genetics and IVF of Florida
5500 Village Boulevard,
Suite 103
West Palm Beach, FL 33407
Phone: (561) 697-4200
Fax: (561) 686-8525

GEORGIA

Emory Center for Reproductive
Medicine and Fertility
(Dr. Aida Schanti, Director)
20 Linden Avenue NE,
Suite 4701
Atlanta, GA 30308
Phone: (404) 686-3229
Fax: (404) 686-4297
www.emory.edu/WHSC/MED/
GYN-OB/divisions/
endocrinology.htm

Medical College of Georgia
Department of OB/GYN
(Dr. Lawrence Layman, Section
Director)
1120 15th Street, Room BB-7514
Augusta, GA 30912-3360
Phone: (706) 721-3832
Fax: (706) 721-6830
www.oiri.mcg.edu/pfl/Queries/
Med/OBGYN/OBGYN05.asp

Reproductive Biology Associates
5505 Peachtree Dunwoody Road,
Suite 400
Atlanta, GA 30342
Phone: (404) 843-3064
Fax: (404) 256-1528
www.rba-online.com

ILLINOIS

Advanced Institute of Fertility
1700 West Central Road, Suite 40
Arlington Heights, IL 60005
Phone: (847) 394-5437
Fax: (847) 394-5478
www.advancedfertility.com
info@aiof.com

Center for Human Reproduction
(Dr. Norbert Gleicher, Director)
750 North Orleans Street
Chicago, IL 60610
Phone: (312) 397-8000
Fax: (847) 486-7541
www.centerforhumanreprod.com/
    gyncormap/chril/chril.htm

IVF Illinois
(Dr. Aaron Lifchez)
836 West Wellington
Chicago, IL 60657
Phone: (773) 296-7096
Fax: (773) 296-7478

UIC Medical Center
Center for Women's Health (Non-
    CDC) IVF Laboratory
Fertility Center
1801 West Taylor Street,
    Suite 4A
Chicago, IL 60612
Phone: (312) 413-7500
www.obgyn.uic.edu/rendo/rendo.htm

Rush Center for Advanced Repro-
    ductive Care
1725 West Harrison,
    Suite 408 East
Chicago, IL 60612
Phone: (312) 997-2229
Fax: (312) 997-2354
www.rushcopley.com/doctors/
    radwanskae.html

Midwest Fertility Center
(Dr. Amos Madanes, Director)
4333 Main Street
Downers Grove, IL 60515
Phone: (630) 810-0212

Fax: (630) 810-1027
www.midwestfertilitycenter.com
midwfert@aol.com

Fertility Centers of Illinois
(Dr. Aaron Lifchez, Director)
3703 West Lake Avenue, Suite 106
Glenview, IL 60025
Phone: (847) 998-8200
Fax: (847) 998-6880

Advanced Fertility Center of
    Chicago
6440 Grand Avenue, Suite 102
Gurnee, IL 60031
Phone: (847) 855-1818
www.advancedfertility.com
doctor@advancedfertility.com

Highland Park Hospital
(Dr. Scott Hansfield, Chairman)
Department of OB/GYN
718 Glenview Avenue
Highland Park, IL 60035
Phone: (847) 480-3950
Fax: (847) 480-2608
www.hphosp.org/fertility/index.html

Hinsdale Center for Reproduction
(Dr. Jay Levin, Director)
121 North Elm Street
Hinsdale, IL 60521
Phone: (630) 856-3535
Fax: (630) 856-3545
www.hinsdalereprod.com/

Oak Brook Fertility Center
(Dr. W. Paul Dmowski, Director)
2425 West 22nd Street,
    Suite 102
Oak Brook, IL 60523

Phone: (630) 954-0054
Fax: (630) 954-0064
www.oakbrookfertility.com

Reena Jabamoni, M.D.
(Director, Anil Dubey)
120 Oak Brook Center,
    Suite 308
Oak Brook, IL 60521
Phone: (630) 574-3633
Fax: (630) 574-3660
ivfrj@aol.com

Fertility and Reproductive
    Medicine Center of Central
    Illinois (Non-CDC)
(Romaine B. Bayless, M.D.)
Physicians' Medical Plaza
214 N.E. Glen Oak Avenue,
    Suite 606
Peoria, IL 61603-4309
Phone: (309) 672-4752
www.fertilitynetwork.com/DrHTML/
    Peoria.htm

Advanced Reproductive
    Center, Ltd.
(Director, John P. Holden)
435 North Mulford,
    Suite 9
Rockford, IL 61107
Phone: (815) 229-1700
Fax: (815) 229-1831
arcltd@bossnt.com

Reproductive Health and Fertility
    Center
(Dr. Ronald Burmeister, Director)
2350 North Rockton Avenue,
    Suite 408
Rockford, IL 61103

Phone: (815) 971-7234
Fax: (815) 971-7425
www.reprohealth-fertility.org

Reproductive Endocrinology
    Associates, S.C.
IVF Program
(Dr. Maryann McRay, Director)
340 West Miller Street
Springfield, IL 62702
Phone: (217) 523-4700
Fax: (217) 523-9025

Division of Reproductive
    Endocrinology and Infertility
Department of OB/GYN
Southern Illinois University School
    of Medicine
751 North Rutledge Street,
    Suite 2100
Springfield, IL 62794
Phone: (217) 782-5117
Fax: (217) 788-5561
www.siumed.edu/ob

INDIANA

Associated Fertility-
    Gynecology P.C.
(Dr. Shelby Cooper, Director)
7910 West Jefferson,
    Suite 301
Fort Wayne, IN 46804
Phone: (219) 432-6250
Fax: (219) 436-7220

Advanced Fertility Group
(Dr. William Gentry, Director)
201 North Pennsylvania Parkway,
    Suite 205

Indianapolis, IN 46280
Phone: (317) 817-1300
Fax: (317) 817-1306

Indiana University
Department of OB/GYN
(Dr. Frederick Stehman, Chairman)
550 North University Boulevard,
    Room 2440
Indianapolis, IN 46202-5274
Phone: (317) 274-4875
Fax: (317) 278-3787
www.medlib.iupui.edu/obgyn/
fstehman@iupui.edu

Midwest Reproductive Medicine
(Dr. Leo Bonaventura, Director)
8081 Township Line Road
Indianapolis, IN 46260
Phone: (800) 333-1415
Fax: (317) 872-5063
www.fertilitymrm.com/

Advanced Reproductive Health
    Centers, Ltd.
(Joel G. Brasch, M.D.)
2428 Lake Avenue
Ft. Wayne, IN 46805
Phone: (219) 423-4368
www.infertilityarc.com/

Reproductive Endocrinology
    Associates
(Dr. Donald Cline, Director)
2020 West 86th Street,
    Suite 310
Indianapolis, IN 46260
Phone: (317) 872-1515
Fax: (317) 879-2784
www.womenshospital.org/
    physdirectory/dcline.html

Center for Assisted Reproduction
(Dr. Jan Reineke, Director)
615 North Michigan Street,
    Suite 115
South Bend, IN 46601
Phone: (219) 284-3633
Fax: (219) 284-6927
www.qualityoflife.org/infertility/
    infertil.htm
assistrep@memorialsb.org

IOWA

McFarland Clinic, P.C.
(Dr. Dale Anderson, Director)
1215 Duff Avenue
Ames, IA 50010
Phone: (515) 239-4414
Fax: (515) 239-4786
www.mcfarlandclinic.com/
    MedicalSpecialties/Spec/
    InfertilityReproductive-
    Medicine.htm

Center for Advanced Reproductive
Care
University of Iowa Hospitals
    & Clinics
Department of OB/GYN
200 Hawkins Drive
Iowa City, IA 52242
Phone: (319) 356-8483
Fax: (319) 356-6659
www.uihc.uiowa.edu/arc/

Mid Iowa Fertility, P.C.
(Dr. Donald Young, Director)
3408 Woodland Avenue,
    Suite 302
West Des Moines, IA 50266
Phone: (515) 222-3060

Fax: (515) 222-9563
www.midiowasfertility.com

KANSAS

University of Kansas Medical
  Center
Women's Reproductive Center
(Dr. Valerie Montgomery Rice,
  Director)
3901 Rainbow Boulevard
Kansas City, KS 66160-7316
Phone: (913) 588-6272
Fax: (913) 588-3242
www.kumc.edu/wichita/dept/wri/
  crm.html

Reproductive Resource Center of
  Greater Kansas City
(Dr. Rodney Lyles, Director)
12200 West 106th Street,
  Suite 120
Overland Park, KS 66215
Phone: (913) 894-2323
Fax: (913) 894-0841
www.rrc-gkc.com/

The Center for Reproductive
  Medicine
(Dr. David Grainger, Director)
2903 East Central
Wichita, KS 67124
Phone: (316) 687-2112
Fax: (316) 687-1260
www.kumc.edu/wichita/dept/wri/
  wri.html#center

KENTUCKY

Fertility and Endocrine Associates
(Dr. Robert Homm, Director)

1780 Nicholasville Road,
  Suite 402
Lexington, KY 40503
Phone: (606) 278-9151
Fax: (606) 278-8946
www.fertilitynetwork.com/DrHTLM/
  Lexington.htm

University of Kentucky Chandler
  Medical Center
Department of OB/GYN
Reproductive Center
(Dr. Berry Campbell, Director)
800 Rose Street
Lexington, KY 40536
Phone: (606) 260-1515
Fax: (606) 260-1425
www.kyinfertility.com/contact.htm
louivf@aol.com

University OB/GYN Associates
  Fertilily Center
315 East Broadway
P.O. Box 35070
Louisville, KY 40202-5070
Phone: (502) 629-3830
Fax: (502) 629-3713

University OB/GYN Associates
  (Non-CDC)
(Marvin A. Yussman, M.D.)
University OB/GYN Associates
601 South Floyd Street, Suite 300
Louisville, KY 40202
Phone: (502) 629-8154
www.kyinfertility.com/

LOUISIANA

Fertility and Laser Center
IVF Program
(Dr. Heber Dunaway, Director)

4720 I-10 Service Road,
Suite 100
Metairie, LA 70001
Phone: (504) 454-2165
Fax: (504) 888-2250
www.fertilityandlasercenter.com

Women's Center for Fertility
Woman's Hospital (Non-CDC)
Airline Highway at Goodwood
Blvd.
9050 Airline Highway
Baton Rouge, LA 70815
Phone: (225) 927-1300
www.womans.com/fert/fert.htm

The Center for Fertility and
Advanced Reproduction
(Dr. William Roniger, Director)
2820 Napoleon Avenue,
Suite 920
New Orleans, LA 70115
Phone: (504) 891-1181
Fax: (504) 887-7055

Fertility Institute of New Orleans
(Dr. Richard Dickey, Director)
6020 Bullard Avenue
New Orleans, LA 70128
Phone: (504) 246-8971
Fax: (504) 246-9778
www.fertilityinstitute.com/

Center for Fertility and
Reproductive Health
(Dr. David Vandermolen,
Director)
2401 Greenwood Road
Shreveport, LA 71103
Phone: (318) 632-8270
Fax: (318) 632-8275
http://obg.lsumc.edu/art/

MARYLAND

Center for Advanced Reproductive
Technology
University of Maryland
(Dr. Howard McClamrock,
Director)
405 West Redwood Street,
3rd Floor
Baltimore, MD 21201
Phone: (410) 328-2304
Fax: (410) 328-8389
hmcclamr@umm001.ummc.
umaryland.edu

GBMC Fertility Center
(Dr. Eugene Katz, Director)
6569 North Charles Street
Physicians Pavilion West,
Suite 406
Baltimore, MD 21204
Phone: (410) 828-2484
Fax: (410) 828-3067
www.gbmc.org/fertilitycenter
fertility@gbmc.org

Helix Center for Assisted
Reproductive Technology
Union Memorial Hospital—
OB/GYN
(Dr. Sanford Markham, Director)
201 East University Parkway
Baltimore, MD 21218-2895
Phone: (410) 554-2271
Fax: (410) 554-2900
www.unionmemorial.org

Division of Reproductive
Endocrinology
(Dr. Jairo Garcia, Director)
The Johns Hopkins Medical
Institute

Houck Building, Room 249
600 North Wolfe Street
Baltimore, MD 21287
Phone: (410) 955-7570
Fax: (410) 614-9684
jgarica@jhmi.edu

CHR-Mid Atlantic
(Drs. Frank Chang & Rafat Abbasi)
10215 Fernwood Road,
   Suite 303-304
Bethesda, MD 20817
Phone: (301) 897-8850
Fax: (301) 530-8105
www.midatlanticfertility.com

Shady Grove Fertility Centers
(Dr. Robert J. Stillman, Director)
15001 Shady Grove Road,
   Suite 400
Rockville, MD 20850
Phone: (301) 340-1188
Fax: (301) 340-1612
www.shadygrovefertility.com

Fertility Center of Maryland
(Dr. Santiago L. Padilla, Director)
110 West Road, Suite 102
Towson, MD 21204
Phone: (410) 296-6400
Fax: (410) 296-6405
www.erols.com/fcmivf

MASSACHUSETTS

Brigham and Women's Hospital
(Dr. Robert Barbieri, Director)
Department of OB/GYN
75 Francis Street, ASB1-3

Boston, MA 02115
Phone: (617) 732-4222
Fax: (617) 975-0825
rbarbieri@partners.org

Massachusetts General Hospital
Vincent IVF Unit
(Dr. Thomas Toth, Director)
210 Vincent Building
55 Fruit Street
Boston, MA 02114
Phone: (617) 724-3500
Fax: (617) 724-8882
www.mgh.harvard.edu/ivf/

Boston IVF
(Dr. Michael Alper, Director)
40 Second Avenue, Suite 200
Waltham, MA 02451
Phone: (781) 434-6400
Fax: (781) 890-5016
www.bostonivf.com
michaelalper@bostonivf.com

New England Fertility &
   Endocrinology Associates
(Dr. Gary L. Gross, Director)
One Brookline Place,
   Suite 421
Brookline, MA 02445
Phone: (617) 277-1778
Fax: (617) 734-9951

Fertility Center of New England
20 Pond Meadow Drive,
   Suite 101
Reading, MA 01867
Phone: (781) 942-7000
   ext. 229
www.fertilitycenter.com

Reproductive Science Center of
  Boston
(Dr. Patricia McShane, Director)
Deaconess Waltham Hospital
20 Hope Avenue
Waltham, MA 02254
Phone: (781) 647-6263
Fax: (781) 647-6323
www.cris.com/~rscbostn/

New England Medical Center
(David L. Keefe, M.D., Medical
  Director)
750 Washington Street,
  NEMC #036
Boston, MA 02111
Phone: (617) 636-0053
www.nemc.org/home/departments/
  adult/reprodu.htm

MICHIGAN

University of Michigan Medical
  Center
Suite 1442
(Dr. John Randolph, Director)
1500 East Medical Center Drive
1324 Taubman, Box 0384
Ann Arbor, MI 48109-0384
Phone: (734) 763-4323
Fax: (734) 763-7682
www.med.umich.edu/obgyn/
  repro-endo/reproend.html

Center for Reproductive
  Medicine
(Dr. David Magyar, Director)
Oakwood Hospital
18181 Oakwood Boulevard,
  Suite 109
Dearborn, MI 48124

Phone: (313) 593-5880
Fax: (313) 593-8837
www.oakwood.org

Michigan Reproductive & IVF
  Center
(Dr. William Dodds, Director)
221 Michigan, Suite 406
Grand Rapids, MI 49503
Phone: (616) 391-2558
Fax: (616) 391-2552
www.michiganivf.com

Grand Valley Gynecology
(Dr. Curtis Struyk)
1900 Wealthy Street SE,
  Suite 330
Grand Rapids, MI 49506
Phone: (616) 774-0700
Fax: (616) 774-0651

West Michigan Reproductive
  Institute, P.C.
(Dr. R. Donald Eward, Director)
885 Forest Hill Avenue SE
Grand Rapids, MI 49546
Phone: (616) 942-5180
Fax: (616) 942-2450

Infertility and Gynecology Center
  of Lansing, P.C.
(Drs. Fereshteh Fahimi and
  Mohammad Mohsenian)
1200 East Michigan Avenue,
  Suite 305
Lansing, MI 48912
Phone: (517) 484-4900
Fax: (517) 364-5785

Michigan State University
Reproductive Endocrinology
Department of OB/GYN

200 East Michigan Avenue,
Suite 700
East Lansing, MI 48912
Phone: (517) 364-5888
Fax: (517) 364-5889
harold.sauer@ht.msu.edu

Beaumont Center for Fertility
and Reproductive Medicine
(Dr. William Keye, Director)
3535 West Thirteen Mile Road,
Suite 344
Royal Oak, MI 48073
Phone: (810) 551-0515
Fax: (810) 551-3616
www.beaumont.edu/women/
fertil_index.html

F.I.R.S.T. IVF
(Drs. Michael Fakih and
Inderbir Gill)
5400 Mackinaw, Suite 2400
Saginaw, MI 48604
Phone: (517) 792-8771
Fax: (517) 792-3377
www.first-ivf.com/home.htm

Henry Ford Reproductive
Medicine
(Dr. Ronald Strickler, Director)
1500 West Big Beaver, Suite 105
Troy, MI 48084
Phone: (248) 637-4050
Fax: (248) 637-4025
www.henryford.com

Ann Arbor Reproductive Medicine
IVF Program
(Drs. Peterson, Ayers, & Shamma)
4990 Clark Road, Suite 100
Ypsilanti, MI 48197
Phone: (737) 434-4871
Fax: (734) 434-8848

University Center for Reproductive
Medicine (Non-CDC)
8800 Ryan Road, Suite 320
Warren, Michigan 48092
Phone: (810) 558-1100
http://obg.med.wayne.edu/
fertility.htm

MINNESOTA

Center for Reproductive Medicine
(Dr. Paul Kuneck, Director)
Abbott Northwestern Hospital
2800 Chicago Avenue, 3rd Floor
Minneapolis, MN 55407
Phone: (612) 863-5390
Fax: (612) 863-2697
www.abbottnorthwestern.com/ahs/
anw.nsf/page/rm_home

The Midwest Center for
Reproductive Health, P.A.
(Dr. Randle Corfman, Director)
Oakdale Medical Building,
Suite 550
3366 Oakdale Avenue North
Minneapolis, MN 55422
Phone: (612) 520-2600
Fax: (612) 520-2606
www.mcrh.com

Mayo Clinic
200 First St. S.W.
Rochester, MN 55905
Phone: (507) 284-4520
www.mayo.edu/repro/remain.htm

MISSISSIPPI

University of Mississippi Medical
Center
IVF Program

(Dr. Brian Cowan, Director)
Department of OB/GYN
2500 North State Street
Jackson, MS 39216-4505
Phone: (601) 984-5330
Fax: (601) 984-5965
www2.umsmed.edu/dept/obgyn/
  ivf.html

MISSOURI

Saint Luke's Hospital
Advanced Reproductive Specialists
(Dr. Jorge Pineda, Director)
226 South Woods Mill Road,
  Suite 64W
Chesterfield, MO 63017
Phone: (314) 542-9422
Fax: (314) 205-6800
www.chesterfield.mo.us/html/
  healthcare.html

University of Missouri–Columbia
(Dr. Leonard Wayne Heff,
  Director)
Department of OB/GYN
N610 HSC
Columbia, MO 65212
Phone: (573) 882-4141
Fax: (573) 882-5952
www.muhealth.org/~outreach/
  rependo.shtml
heffL@heff.missouri.edu

Infertility & IVF Center
(Dr. Ronald Wilbois, Director)
3009 North Ballas Road,
  Suite 359C
Saint Louis, MO 63131
Phone: (314) 225-5483
Fax: (314) 872-9040

www.ivfctrstl.org
drwilbois@ivfctrstl.org

The Infertility Center of St. Louis
(Sherman Silber, M.D.)
St. Luke's Hospital
224 S. Woods Mill Rd., Suite 730
St. Louis, MO 63017
Phone: (314) 576-1400
www.infertile.com/

NEBRASKA

Methodist Hospital Reproductive
Endocrinology/Infertility
(Dr. C. Maud Doherpy, Director)
8111 Dodge Street, Suite 237
Omaha, NE 68114
Phone: (402) 354-5210
Fax: (402) 354-5221
www.bestcare.org/methhosp.html

University of Nebraska Medical
  Center
Olson Center for Women's Health
983255 Nebraska Medical Center
Omaha, NE 68198-3255
Fax: (402) 559-4520
Toll Free: (800) 981-5858
www.unmc.edu/Olson/reinf.htm

NEVADA

Fertility Center of Las Vegas
(Dr. Bruce Shapiro, Director)
8851 West Sahara, Suite 100
Las Vegas, NV 89117
Phone: (702) 254-1777
Fax: (702) 254-1213
www.fertilitycenterlv.com

Northern Nevada Fertility Center
(Non-CDC)
(Dr. Scott Jacobs, Director)
75 Pringle Way, Suite 803
Reno, NV 89502
Phone: (775) 688-5600
Fax: (775) 322-3603
www.nevadanet.com/HealthSource/
Services/165.html

NEW HAMPSHIRE

Dartmouth-Hitchcock Medical
Center
(Dr. Misty Blanchette-Porter,
Director)
One Medical Center Drive
Lebanon, NH 03756
Phone: (603) 650-8162
Fax: (603) 650-2079
www.hitchcock.org
Misty.B.Porter@Hitchcock.org

NEW JERSEY

Center for Reproductive
Endocrinology (Non-CDC)
(Alexander Dlugi, M.D., and
Walid Saleh, M.D.)
One Robertson Drive, Suite 24
Bedminster, NJ 07921
Phone: (317) 621-2280
Fax: (317) 621-2283
www.ivfcenter.net

Reproductive Gynecologists, P.C.
(Dr. Wesley Chodos)
Kennedy Health System
2201 Chapel Avenue West,
Suite 206

Cherry Hill, NJ 08002
Phone: (609) 662-6662
Fax: (609) 661-0661

North Jersey Center for
Reproductive Endocrinology
and Fertility
(Dr. Mark Ransom, Director)
10-35 Route 46 East
Clifton, NJ 07013
Phone: (973) 470-0303
Fax: (973) 916-0488

Center for Reproductive Medicine
(Dr. Gerson Weiss, Director)
214 Terrace Avenue, 2nd Floor
Hasbrouck Heights, NJ 07604
Phone: (888) 777-8922
Fax: (201) 393-7410
www.arcfertility.com/membership/
newjersey.html

Princeton Center for Infertility and
Reproductive Medicine
(Dr. Althea O'Shaughnessy,
Director)
3131 Princeton Pike, Building 4,
Suite 204
Lawrenceville, NJ 08648
Phone: (609) 895-1114
Fax: (609) 895-1196
www.fertilitext.org/oshaugh.html

East Coast Infertility
and IVF, P.C.
(Dr. Miguel Damien, Director)
200 White Road, Suite 214
Little Silver, NJ 07739
Phone: (732) 758-6511
Fax: (732) 758-1048
www.eastcoastivf.com

The Institute for Reproductive
Medicine and Science
Saint Barnabas Medical Center
94 Old Short Hills Road
East Wing, Suite 403
Livingston, NJ 07039
Phone: (973) 322-8286
Fax: (973) 322-8890
www.sbhcs.com/hospitals/obgyn/
about/endo.htm

Cooper Center for IVF, P.C.
(Dr. Jermone Check, Director)
8002 Greentree Commons
Marlton, NJ 08053
Phone: (609) 751-5575
Fax: (609) 751-7289
www.cooperhealth.org/referral/
reproductive.html

Delaware Valley Institute of
Fertility and Genetics
(Dr. George Taliadouros,
Director)
2001 Greentree Exec Campus,
Suite F
Route 73 & Lincoln Drive West
Marlton, NJ 08053
Phone: (609) 988-0072
Fax: (609) 988-0056
www.startfertility.com

South Jersey Fertility Center, P.A.
(Dr. Robert Skaf, Director)
512 Lippincott Drive
Marlton, NJ 08053
Phone: (609) 596-2233
Fax: (609) 596-2411
www.sjfert.com
sjfert@erols.com

Diamond Institute for Infertility
and Menopause

(Dr. Matan Yemini, Director)
89 Millburn Avenue
Millburn, NJ 07041
Phone: (973) 761-5600
Fax: (973) 761-5100
www.diamondinstitute.com

Robert Wood Johnson Medical
School IVF Program
303 George Street, Suite 250
New Brunswick, NJ 08901
Phone: (732) 235-7300
Fax: (732) 235-7318
www.fertilityucref.com

IVF New Jersey
(Drs. Susan Treiser & Michael
Darder)
1527 Highway 27, Suite 2100
Somerset, NJ 08873
Phone: (732) 220-9060
Fax: (732) 220-1122
www.ivfnj.com

CHR–New Jersey
(Dr. Daniel Navot, Director)
400 Old Hook Road
Westwood, NJ 07675
Phone: (201) 666-4200
Fax: (201) 666-2262

Advanced Fertility Institute
(Dr. Chong S. Lee, Director)
158 Linwood Plaza, 318
Fort Lee, NJ 07024
Phone: (201) 363-1810
Fax: (201) 363-1115

NEW MEXICO

Southwest Fertility Services
4705 Montgomery Boulevard
Northeast, Suite 101

Albuquerque, NM 87109
Phone: (505) 837-1510
Fax: (505) 888-4486
www.southwestfertility.com

NEW YORK

Women's Health Center of Albany
  Medical Center
Division for Reproductive
  Endocrinology and Infertility
(Dr. Gordon Kuttner, Director)
58 Hackett Boulevard
Albany, NY 12209
Phone: (518) 462-0084
Fax: (518) 462-0174
www.amc.edu/Patient/womens_Health
  /womens_health_center.htm

Leading Institute for Fertility
  Enhancement (L.I.F.E.)
130 Everett Road
Albany, NY 12205
Phone: (518) 482-1008
Fax: (518) 489-6210

The Fertility Institute at the
  Brooklyn Hospital
(Dr. George D. Kofinas, Director)
161 Ashland Place
Brooklyn, NY 11201
Phone: (718) 237-4593
Fax: (718) 250-8756

Hartsdale Fertility and Fetal
  Medicine Institute
(Dr. David Barad, Director)
141 South Central Avenue
Hartsdale, NY 10530
Phone: (914) 997-1060
Fax: (914) 997-1099
www.montefiore.org/prof/clinical/

obsgyn/progserv/hartsdale/
index.html

Garden City Center for Advanced
  Reproductive Technologies
394 Old Country Road
Garden City, NY 11530
Phone: (516) 248-8307
Fax: (516) 248-5007
www.matherhospital.com/patient.
  html

Center for Human Reproduction
(Dr. David Rosenfeld, Director)
North Shore University Hospital
300 Community Drive
Ambulatory Building, Lower Level
Manhasset, NY 11030
Phone: (516) 562-2229
Fax: (516) 562-1710
www.northshorelij.com

Advanced Fertility Services, P.C.
(Dr. Hugh D. Melnick, Director)
1625 Third Avenue
New York, NY 10128
Phone: (212) 369-8700
Fax: (212) 562-5587
www.infertilityny.com

Brooklyn/Central Park West
  Fertility Center
(Dr. Dov Goldstein, Director)
55 Central Park West,
  Suite 1C
New York, NY 10023
Phone: (212) 721-4545
Fax: (212) 721-4598

Columbia Presbyterian Medical
  Center
Division of Assisted Reproduction

(Dr. Mark V. Sauer, Director)
622 West 168th Street, PH-1630
New York, NY 10032
Phone: (212) 305-4665
Fax: (212) 305-3695
mvs9@columbia.edu

Cornell University Medical Center
The Center for Reproductive
   Medicine and Infertility
(Dr. Zev Rosenwaks, Director)
505 East 70th Street
New York, NY 10021
Phone: (212) 746-1762
Fax: (212) 746-8860
www.ivf.org

Lillian D. Nash, M.D.
315 West 57th Street
New York, NY 10019
Phone: (212) 247-3111
Fax: (212) 247-3255

Mount Sinai (Non-CDC)
Department of Reproductive
   Endocrinology
1212 Fifth Avenue
New York, NY 10029
Phone: (212) 241-5927
www.mssm.edu/ivf/

New York Fertility Institute
1016 Fifth Avenue
New York, NY 10028
Phone: (212) 734-5555
Fax: (212) 734-6059

NYU Medical Center Program for
   In Vitro Fertilization
600 First Avenue at 38th Street,
   5th Floor
New York, NY 10016

Phone: (212) 263-8990
Fax: (212) 263-7853
www.nyudh.med.nyu.edu/
   obgyn.htm

Offices for Fertility and
   Reproductive Medicine
88 University Place, 9th Floor
New York, NY 10003
Phone: (212) 243-5550
Fax: (212) 243-0009
ofrm@aol.com

Brandeis Center (Non-CDC)
(Dr. Vincent Brandeis, Director)
606 Columbus Avenue,
   2nd Floor
New York, NY 10024
Phone: (212) 362-4848
Fax: (212) 724-1315

New York Medical Services for
   Reproductive Medicine
(Dr. Niels Lauerson, Director)
784 Park Avenue
New York, NY 10021
Phone: (212) 744-4222
Fax: (212) 288-3608

Montefiore's Fertility and
   Hormone Center (Non-CDC)
(914) 693-8820
www.aecom.yu.edu/obgyn/divdep/
   endocrin.html
dbarad@montefiore.org

Long Island IVF Associates
(Dr. David Kreiner, Director)
625 Belle Terre Road, Suite 200
Port Jefferson, NY 11777
Phone: (516) 331-7575
Fax: (516) 331-1332
www.longislandivf.com

Institute for Reproductive Health
and Infertility
(Drs. Muechler & Hayes)
1561 Long Pond Road, Suite 410
Rochester, NY 14626
Phone: (716) 723-7468
Fax: (716) 723-7043

Strong Infertility & IVF Center
(Dr. Vivian Lewis, Director)
601 Elmwood Avenue,
Ambulatory Center—5th Floor,
Box 685
Rochester, NY 14642
Phone: (716) 275-1930
Fax: (716) 756-4146
www.urmc.rochester.edu/
stronghealth/ivf/

Reproductive Endocrinology
(Dr. Richard Bronson, Director)
SUNY at Stony Brook
Stony Brook, NY 11794-7555
Phone: (516) 444-2737
Fax: (516) 444-6121
http://www.obgyn.sunysb.edu/
obgyn/ReprodEndo.html

Westchester Fertility and
Reproductive Endocrinology
(Dr. Michael Blotner, Director)
136 South Broadway,
Suite 100
White Plains, NY 10605
Phone: (914) 949-6677
Fax: (914) 949-5758

Reproductive Medicine
and IVF
(Dr. John Wieckowski, Director)
1321 Millersport Highway,
Suite 102

Buffalo, NY 14221
Phone: (716) 634-4351
www.repmedivf.com

NORTH CAROLINA

North Carolina Center for
Reproductive Medicine
(Dr. Sameh Toma, Director)
400-200 Asheville Avenue
Cary, NC 27511
Phone: (919) 233-1680
Fax: (919) 233-1685
www.nccrm.com/nccrm/index.
shtml

University of North Carolina ART
Clinic
(Dr. Marc A. Fritz, Director)
OB/GYN: CB 7570
Chapel Hill, NC 27599-7570
Phone: (919) 966-1150
Fax: (919) 966-1259
http://www.med.unc.edu/obgyn/
re.htm

Institute for Assisted Reproduction
1918 Randolf Road, 5th Floor
Charlotte, NC 28207
Phone: (704) 343-3400
Fax: (704) 343-3428
www.ivfsuccess.com

Women's Institute
Carolinas Medical Center
(Dr. Ronald Wade, Director)
1000 Blythe Boulevard
Charlotte, NC 28232-2861
Phone: (704) 355-3153
Fax: (704) 355-3141

Chapel Hill Fertility Center
    (Non-CDC)
(Dr. Gary Berger, Director)
109 Conner Drive, Suite 2200
Chapel Hill, NC 27514
Phone: (919) 968-4656
Fax: (919) 967-8637
www.chapelhillfertility.com

Duke University Division of
    Reproductive Endocrinology
    and Infertility (Non-CDC)
Box 3143
Durham, NC 27710
Phone: (919) 684-5327
www2.mc.duke.edu/ivf/index.htm

Wake Forest University School of
    Medicine
Department of OB/GYN
Reproductive Endocrinology
(Dr. Eberhard Mueller-Heubach,
    Director)
Medical Center Boulevard
Winston-Salem, NC 27157-1066
Phone: (336) 716-2368
Fax: (336) 716-0194
www.wfubnc.edu

NORTH DAKOTA

MeritCare Medical Group Fertility
    Center
(Dr. Steffen Christiensen, Director)
737 Broadway
Fargo, ND 58123
Phone: (701) 234-2700
Fax: (701) 234-2783

Med Center One (Non-CDC)
(They don't have reproductive
    endocrinology anymore—only a
    monthly doctor.)

Department of OB/GYN
(Dr. Shari Orser, Director)
414 North 7th Street
Bismark, ND 58506
Phone: (701) 323-6880
Fax: (701) 323-6508

OHIO

Bethesda Center for Reproductive
    Health and Fertility
(Dr. Glen Hofmann, Director)
619 Oak Street, 3 South
Cincinnati, OH 45206
Phone: (513) 569-6433
Fax: (513) 569-6386
www.bethesdafertility.com

University Fertility Institute
Camelot Women's Health Center
4775 Knightsbridge Boulevard,
    Suite 103
Columbus, OH 43214
Phone: (614) 442-5761
Fax: (614) 442-1080

Greater Cincinnati Institute for
    Reproductive Health at the
    Christ Hospital
(Dr. Sherif Awadalla, Director)
MOB 2, 2123 Auburn Avenue,
    Suite 044
Cincinnati, OH 45219
Phone: (513) 585-4400
Fax: (513) 585-4457
www.cincinnatifertility.com

Department GYN/OB
(Dr. Jerome Belinson,
    Director)
Cleveland Clinic Foundation
9500 Euclid Avenue

Cleveland, OH 44195
Phone: (216) 444-8374
Fax: (216) 444-8551
www.ccf.org/obgyn/infertilitymain.
htm

University Hospitals of
Cleveland
MacDonald Women's Hospital
(Dr. James Goldfarb, Director)
111000 Euclid Avenue
IVF Department, Room 1204
Cleveland, OH 44106
Phone: (216) 844-1741
Fax: (216) 844-5809

Ohio Reproductive Medicine
(Dr. Steve Williams, Director)
4830 Knightsbridge Boulevard,
Suite E
Columbus, OH 43214
Phone: (614) 451-2280
Fax: (614) 451-4352
www.ohiorepromed.com
cg@ohiorepromed.com

Genetics and IVF Institute
of Ohio
(Dr. C. Roger Moriz, Director)
369 West First Street, Suite 120
Dayton, OH 45402
Phone: (937) 228-4483
Fax: (937) 496-1404
givf@erinet.com

Fertility Center of Northwest Ohio
(Dr. Joseph Karnitif, Director)
2142 North Cove Boulevard
Toledo, OH 43606
Phone: (419) 479-8830
Fax: (419) 479-6005

OKLAHOMA

Presbyterian Hospital Laboratory for
Assisted Reproductive Technologies
1000 North Lincoln Boulevard,
Suite 300
Oklahoma City, OK 73104
Phone: (405) 271-9200
Fax: (405) 271-9222

The University of Oklahoma Health
Sciences Center (Non-CDC)
Department of OB/GYN
2410 WP 920 Stanton L. Young Blvd.
Oklahoma City, OK 73104
Phone: (405) 271-5277
http://w3.ouhsc.edu/endo/

Henry G. Bennett, Jr., Fertility
Institute
IVF Program
3433 Northwest 56th Street,
Suite 200B
Oklahoma City, OK 73112
Phone: (405) 949-6060
Fax: (405) 949-6872
www.integres-health.com

Tulsa Center for Fertility and
Women's Health
(Dr. Stanly Prough, Director)
1145 South Utica, Suite 1209
Tulsa, OK 74104
Phone: (918) 584-2870
Fax: (918) 587-3602
www.tulsafertility.com

OREGON

Women's Care (Non-CDC)
590 Country Club Parkway,
Suite A

Eugene, OR 97401
Phone: (541) 683-1559
http://womenscare.com/
    infertilitymds.html

Northwest Fertility Center
(Dr. Eugene Stoelk, Director)
1750 SW Harbor Way, Suite 200
Portland, OR 97201
Phone: (503) 227-7799
Fax: (503) 227-5452

University Fertility Consultants
(Dr. Kenneth Burry, Director)
Oregon Health Sciences University
1750 SW Harbor Way, Suite 100
Portland, OR 97201-5133
Phone: (503) 418-3700
Fax: (503) 418-3708
www.ihr.com/oregon

PENNSYLVANIA

Abington Reproductive Medicine
    (Non-CDC)
1245 Highland Avenue,
    Suite 404
Abington, PA 19001
Phone: (215) 887-2010
www.abington-repromed.com/

Infertility Solutions, P.C.
(Dr. Bruce Rose, Director)
2200 Hamilton Street, Suite 105
Allentown, PA 18104-6329
Phone: (610) 776-1217
Fax: (610) 776-4149
www.infertilitysolutions.com

Reprotech, Inc.
440 South 15th Street

Allentown, PA 18102
Phone: (610) 437-7000
Fax: (610) 437-6381
www.babiesforyou.com

Family Fertility Center
(Dr. H. Christina Lee, Director)
95 Highland Avenue, Suite 100
Bethlehem, PA 18017
Phone: (610) 868-8600
Fax: (610) 868-8700
familyfertility@enter.net

Geisinger Medical Center Fertility
    Program
(Dr. Latif Awad, Director)
100 North Academy Avenue
Danville, PA 17822-0116
Phone: (570) 271-5620
Fax: (570) 271-5629

Reproductive Sciences In Vitro
    Fertilization
(Dr. Steven Somkuti, Director)
1200 Old York Road
Abington, PA 19001
Phone: (215) 481-2349
Fax: (215) 481-7550

The Milton S. Hershey Medical
    Center
P.O. Box 850
Hershey, PA 17033
Phone: (717) 531-6731
Fax: (717) 531-6286
www.hmc.psu.edu/obgyn/
    repend.htm

Jefferson Center for Women's
    Medical Specialties
(Dr. Thomas Klein, Director)
834 Chestnut Street, Room 300

Philadelphia, PA 19107
Phone: (215) 955-4108
Fax: (215) 923-1089

Pennsylvania Reproductive
  Associates
(Dr. Steven Corson, Director)
819 Locust Street
Philadelphia, PA 19107
Phone: (215) 922-3173
Fax: (215) 627-7554
www.womensinstitute.org

Allegheny General Hospital
  IVF Program
(Dr. Anthony N. G. Wakim,
  Director)
One Allegheny Square, Suite 280
Pittsburgh, PA 15212
Phone: (412) 359-1900
Fax: (412) 359-1915
www.allhealth.edu

The Fertility Center at Saint Clair
  Hospital
(Dr. Miguel Marrero, Director)
Professional Office Building,
  Suite 304
1050 Bower Hill Road
Pittsburgh, PA 15243
Phone: (412) 572-6565
Fax: (412) 572-6591

The University of Pittsburgh
  Physicians
Reproductive Endocrinology
(Dr. Carolyn Kubik, Director)
300 Halket Street
Pittsburgh, PA 15213
Phone: (412) 641-4726
Fax: (412) 641-1133

Reproductive Endocrinology and
  Fertility Center
(Dr. Albert El-Roeiy, Director)
Crozer Chester Medicine Center
1 Medical Center Boulevard
Upland, PA 19013-3995
Phone: (610) 447-2727
Fax: (610) 447-6549
aelroeiy@crozer.org

Reproductive Science Institute of
  Suburban Philadelphia
(Dr. Abraham Munabi, Director)
950 West Valley Road,
  Suite 2401
Wayne, PA 19087
Phone: (610) 964-9663
Fax: (610) 964-0536
www.ihr.com/rsi

RHODE ISLAND

Reproductive Medicine &
  Infertility
(Dr. David Keefe, Director)
Women & Infants Hospital
101 Dudley Street
Providence, RI 02905
Phone: (401) 453-7500
Fax: (401) 453-7598

SOUTH CAROLINA

Southeastern Fertility Center
(Dr. Grant Patton)
1375 Hospital Drive
Mount Pleasant, SC 29464
Phone: (843) 881-3900
Fax: (843) 881-4729

SOUTH DAKOTA

University Physicians Fertility
  Specialists
(Dr. LuAnn Eidsness, Director)
1310 West 22nd Street
Sioux Falls, SD 57105
Phone: (605) 782-2284
Fax: (605) 782-2270

TENNESSEE

Reproductive Medicine and
  Fertility
(Dr. John Lucas)
935 Springcreek Road,
  Suite 205
Chattanooga, TN 37412
Phone: (423) 899-0500
Fax: (423) 499-5521

Appalachian Fertility &
  Endocrinology
(Dr. Pickens Gantt, Director)
2204 Pavilion Drive, Suite 307
Kingsport, TN 37660
Phone: (423) 392-6330
Fax: (423) 392-6400

University of Tennessee Fertility
  Center
(Dr. Gayla Harris, Director)
200 Blount Street
Suite 301
Knoxville, TN 37920
Phone: (423) 544-6756
Fax: (423) 544-6757

University Fertility Associates
909 Ridgeway Loop Road
Memphis, TN 38120
Phone: (901) 767-6868

Fax: (901) 682-2231
www.universityfertility.org
wkutteh@utmem.edu

Nashville Fertility Center
2400 Patterson Street, Suite 319
Nashville, TN 37203-1546
Phone: (615) 321-4740
Fax: (615) 320-0240

The Center for Reproductive
  Health
(Dr. Jaime Vasquez, Director)
326 21st Avenue North
Nashville, TN 37203
Phone: (615) 321-8899
Fax: (615) 321-8877
www.reproductivehealthctr.com

Vanderbilt University Center for
  Reproductive Medicine
(Dr. Steven Entman, Director)
C-1100 MCN
Nashville, TN 37232-2515
Phone: (615) 322-6576
Fax: (615) 343-8881

TEXAS

Texas Fertility Center
(Drs. Vaughn, Silverberg, &
  Hansard)
3705 Medical Parkway, Suite 420
Austin, TX 78705
Phone: (512) 451-0149
Fax: (512) 451-0977
www.txfertility.com

Center for Assisted Reproduction
(Dr. Kevin Doody, Director)

1701 Park Place Avenue
Bedford, TX 76022
Phone: (817) 540-1157
Fax: (817) 267-0522
www.embryo.net

Trinity IVF Program
4325 North Josey Lane, Suite 308
Carrollton, TX 75010
Phone: (972) 394-3699
Fax: (972) 394-6517
wfhoward@juno.com

Baylor Center for Reproductive
  Health
(Dr. Samuel Marynick, Director)
3707 Gaston Avenue, Suite 310
Dallas, TX 75246
Phone: (214) 821-2274
Fax: (214) 821-2373

Dallas In Vitro Associates
Presbyterian Hospital Dallas
(Dr. James Madden)
8160 Walnut Hill Lane, 6th Floor
  Perot
Dallas, TX 75231
Phone: (214) 345-2624
Fax: (214) 345-8317

National Fertility Center of Texas,
  P.A.
(Dr. Brian Cohen, Director)
Building C-638
7777 Forest Lane
Dallas, TX 75230-2517
Phone: (972) 566-6686
Fax: (972) 566-6670

University of Texas Southwestern
  Fertility Associates

(Dr. Debora Smith, Director)
Department of OB/GYN
5323 Harry Hines Boulevard
Dallas, TX 75235
Phone: (214) 648-8846
Fax: (214) 648-2813

University of Texas Houston
  Medical School (Non-CDC):
OB/GYN & Reproductive Sciences
(Dr. Allen Katz, Director)
6431 Fannin, MSB R3-060
Houston, TX 77030
Phone: (713) 500-6400
Fax: (713) 500-0797
www.obg.med.uth.tmc.edu

Baylor Assisted Reproductive
  Technology
(Dr. John Buster, Director)
Department of OB/GYN
6550 Fannin, Suite 821
Houston, TX 77030
Phone: (713) 798-8232
Fax: (713) 798-8231
www.bcm.tmc.edu/obgyn/
  obgyn-ce/rei.html

Center for Reproduction at
  Gramercy
(Dr. Robert McWilliams, Director)
2727 Gramercy, Suite 200
Houston, TX 77025
Phone: (713) 661-3111
Fax: (713) 661-2218

North Houston Center for
  Reproductive Medicine
(Dr. Dorothy J. Roach, Director)
530 Wells Fargo Drive,
  Suite 116

Houston, TX 77090-4042
Phone: (281) 444-4784
Fax: (281) 444-0429
www.ihr.com/nhcrm

OB & GYN Associates ART
    Program
(Dr. George Grunert, Director)
7550 Fannin Street
Houston, TX 77054
Phone: (713) 512-7914
Fax: (713) 512-7853
grunert@ivfhouston.com

Houston Infertility Clinic
    (Non-CDC)
(Dr. Sonja Kristiansen)
1631 North Loop West,
    Suite 410
Houston, TX 77008
Phone: (713) 862-6181
http://www.infertilityivf.com/

Wilford USF Medical Center
(Dr. William Barth, Director)
59th MDW/MNO
2200 Bergquist Drive,
    Suite 1
Lackland Air Force Base,
    TX 78236-5300
Phone: (210) 292-7547
Fax: (210) 292-7547

The Center for Reproductive
    Medicine
(Dr. Janelle Dorsett, Director)
3506 21st Street, Suite 605
Lubbock, TX 79410
Phone: (806) 788-1212
Fax: (806) 788-1253

Texas Tech University Health
    Science Center
IVF Program
(Dr. Kathy Porter, Director)
3601 4th Street
Lubbock, TX 79430
Phone: (806) 743-1200
Fax: (806) 743-3200

Scott & White Memorial Hospital
    (Non-CDC)
Phone: (254) 724-2111
Toll Free: (800) 792-3710
www.sw.org/depts/obgyn/
    obgyn.htm

Institute for Women's Health
    Science
7940 Floyd Curl Drive
San Antonio, TX 78229
Phone: (210) 616-0680
Fax: (210) 616-0684

Center for Reproductive Medicine
(Dr. Vicki Schnell, Director)
450 Medical Center Boulevard,
    Suite 202
Webster, TX 77598
Phone: (281) 332-0073
Fax: (281) 332-1860
www.home1.gte.net

UTAH

Utah Center for Reproductive
    Medicine
(Dr. Herry Hatafaka, Director)
50 North Medical Drive,
    Suite 2355

Salt Lake City, UT 84132
Phone: (801) 581-4838
Fax: (801) 585-2231
http://medstat.med.utah.edu/kw/
utah_center/

VERMONT

University of Vermont College of
    Medicine
IVF Program
1 South Prospect Street
Burlington, VT 05401
Phone: (802) 847-0986
Fax: (802) 847-8433
phil.mead@vtmednet.org

VIRGINIA

The Fertility and Reproductive
    Health Center
(Dr. Pierre Asmar, Director)
4316 Evergreen Lane
Annandale, VA 22003
Phone: (703) 658-3100
Fax: (703) 658-3103
www.erols.com/frhc

Dominion Fertility &
    Endocrinology
(Drs. Michael Dimattina & John
    Gordon, Directors)
46 South Glebe Road, Suite 301
Arlington, VA 22204
Phone: (703) 920-3890
Fax: (703) 892-6037
www.dominionfertility.com
info@dominionfertility.com

Genetics & IVF Institute
    (Non-CDC)

(Dr. David Bick, Director)
3020 Javier Road
Fairfax, VA 22031
Phone: (703) 698-7355
Fax: (703) 698-0418
www.givf.com

Jones Institute for Reproductive
    Medicine
(Dr. Suheil Muasher, Director)
Department of OB/GYN
601 Colley Avenue
Norfolk, VA 23507
Phone: (757) 446-7116
Fax: (757) 446-8998
www.jonesinstitute.org

Fertility Institute of Virginia
(Drs. Michael Edelstein & Kenneth
    Steingold)
10710 Midlothian Turnpike,
    Suite 33
Richmond, VA 23235-4766
Phone: (804) 379-9000
Fax: (804) 379-9031

Richmond Center for Fertility &
    Endocrinology
(Dr. Stanford Rosenberg, Director)
7603 Forest Avenue, Suite 301
Richmond, VA 23229
Phone: (804) 285-9700
Fax: (804) 285-9745
www.eggdoc.com

LifeSource Fertility Center
(Dr. Joseph Gianfortoni, Director)
7603 Forest Avenue, Suite 204
Richmond, VA 23229
Phone: (804) 673-2273
Fax: (804) 285-3109

Medical College of Virginia
IVF/Assisted Reproduction
   Program
(Dr. John Seeds, Director)
Box 980034, MCV Station
Richmond, VA 23298
Phone: (804) 828-9636
Fax: (804) 828-0573

The Beach Center for Infertility,
   Endocrinology and
   IVF (Non-CDC)
Virginia Beach, VA 23451
Phone: (757) 428-0002
www.beachcenter.com

WASHINGTON

Washington Center for
   Reproductive Medicine
(Dr. James Kustin, Director)
1370 116th Avenue NE,
   Suite 202
Bellevue, WA 98004
Phone: (425) 462-9292
Fax: (425) 635-0742

Olympia Women's Health
(Dr. James Moruzzi, Director)
403 Black Hills Lane, SW
Olympia, WA 98502
Phone: (360) 786-1515
Fax: (360) 754-7476

Pacific Gynecology Specialists
(Dr. Jane Uhlir, Director)
1101 Madison Street,
   Suite 1500
Seattle, WA 98104
Phone: (206) 215-3200
Fax: (206) 215-6590

University of Washington
Fertility and Endocrine
   Center
(Dr. Michael Soules, Director)
4225 Roosevelt Way NE,
   Suite 101
Seattle, WA 98101
Phone: (206) 548-4225
Fax: (206) 548-6081
http://depts.washington.edu/reidiv/

Virginia Mason Center for Fertility
   and Reproductive Endocrinology
(Dr. Lori Marshall, Director)
1100 9th Avenue, X11-FC
Seattle, WA 98101
Phone: (206) 223-6190
Fax: (206) 341-0596
www.vmc.org/fertility

GYFT Clinic, P.L.L.C.
(Dr. Jacque Wilson, Director)
P.O. Box 8550
Tacoma, WA 98418-6715
Phone: (253) 475-5433
Fax: (253) 473-6715

WEST VIRGINIA

Center for Reproductive Medicine
(Dr. Reed Heywood, Director)
West Virginia University Health
   Sciences Center
830 Pennsylvania Avenue,
   Suite 304
Charleston, WV 25302
Phone: (304) 344-1515
Fax: (304) 344-1570

WISCONSIN

Family Fertility Program
Appleton Medical Center

(Dr. Michael West, Director)
1818 North Meade Street
Appleton, WI 54911
Phone: (920) 738-6242
Fax: (920) 831-5149

Gundersen/Lutheran Medical
  Center
Department of OB/GYN
(Dr. Charles Schauberger,
  Chairman of Department)
1836 South Avenue
LaCrosse, WI 54601
Phone: (608) 782-7300
Fax: (608) 791-6611

University of Wisconsin Hospitals
  & Clinics
Women's Endocrine Clinic
(Dr. Sander Shapiro, Director)
600 Highland Avenue
Madison, WI 53792
Phone: (608) 263-1217
Fax: (608) 263-0191

Advanced Institute of Fertility
Saint Luke's Medicine Center
(Dr. K. Paul Katayama, Director)
Professional Office Building,
  Suite 535
2801 West KK River Parkway
Milwaukee, WI 53215
Phone: (414) 645-5437

Fax: (414) 645-5401
aiof@aiof.com

Reproductive Specialty Center
(Drs. Charles Koh and Grace
  Janik)
2315 North Lake Drive,
  Suite 501
Milwaukee, WI 53211
Phone: (414) 289-9668
Fax: (414) 289-0974
www.reproductivecenter.com/

WomenCare, S.C.
(Dr. Pat Thomas, Director)
20611 Watertown Road
Waukesha, WI 53186
Phone: (414) 798-1910
Fax: (414) 798-8660

Women's Health Care, S.C.
(Dr. Mathew Meyer)
721 American Avenue, Suite 304
Waukesha, WI 53188
Phone: (414) 549-2229
Fax: (414) 549-1657

Clinic of OB/GYN
(Drs. Lee, Lamping, & Sprotiello)
8800 West Lincoln Avenue
West Allis, WI 53227
Phone: (414) 545-8808
Fax: (414) 545-4920

GLOSSARY

---

abortion: The loss of a pregnancy before a fetus can survive on its own.

ACA: See Anticardiolipin Antibodies.

acrosin: An enzyme in the head of a sperm that dissolves the coating around the egg in order to allow the sperm to penetrate the egg.

acrosome reaction: The chemical changes that enable the sperm to penetrate the egg.

adhesions: Bands of scar tissue attached to the surface of organs such as the ovary, the bowels, or the fallopian tubes.

adrenaline: A hormone secreted by the adrenal medulla during strong emotion. This hormone causes bodily changes such as increased blood pressure.

agglutination of sperm: When sperm cells clump or stick together.

AI: See Artificial Insemination, Donor Insemination, Intrauterine Insemination (IUI).

AID: artificial insemination donor. See Artificial Insemination, Donor Insemination, Intrauterine Insemination (IUI).

AIH (artificial insemination by husband): A procedure in which a wife is inseminated with her husband's sperm, in contrast to being inseminated by the sperm of a donor.

alloimmune factors: Natural killer cells, leukocyte antigen cross match. Alloimmune factors can lead to pregnancy loss in two different ways. First, the body fails to recognize a pregnancy, and, second, there is an abnormal immunological response to the pregnancy. A patient may be tested for leukocyte antibodies, natural killer cells, and embryo toxic factor. Possible treatments are intravenous immunoglobulin (IVIg) or paternal white-blood-cell immunization.

amenorrhea: Absence of menstrual cycles.

The American Society for Reproductive Medicine (ASRM): An organization of more than 10,000 health-care specialists interested in reproductive medicine. This organization was previously known as the American Fertility Society (AFS).

ampulla: The outer end of the fallopian tube that is the widest part of the tube.

ANA: See Antinuclear Antibodies.

andrologist: A doctor specializing in male reproductive problems.

anesthesia (general): An agent that produces unconsciousness and complete loss of sensation throughout the body.

anesthesia (local): The use of medication to induce a loss of sensation in a specific part of the body without loss of consciousness.

anovulatory: A term describing a woman who rarely or never ovulates.

antagon: A GnRH (gonadotropin releasing hormone) antagonist that can prevent a premature LH surge. A GnRH antagonist needs to be injected less often than Lupron, which is a GnRH agonist. GnRH antagonists need to be injected during the time period when an LH surge is likely to occur.

antibodies: Chemicals made by the body to fight or attack foreign substances entering the body. Normally they prevent infection; however, when they attack the sperm or fetus, they cause infertility. Sperm antibodies may be made by either the man or the woman.

anticardiolipin antibodies: Proteins produced by the mother's body that are directed against the fat cells of the fetus. These antibodies are associated with repeated miscarriages.

antigen: A substance that causes antibodies to form.

antinuclear antibodies (ANA): Antinuclear antibodies react against normal components of the cell nucleus. They may be present in a number of immunologic diseases such as systemic lupus erythematosus, rheumatoid arthritis, and certain collagen diseases, and in about 1 percent of normal individuals. If you have systemic lupus erythematosus, it can be transmitted through the placenta to the baby, resulting in heart problems.

antiovarian antibodies (AOA, AVA): Antibodies against ovarian targets. Such antibodies would bind to important functional sites in the ovary and granulosa cells and impair the normal response.

antiphospholipid antibodies (APA): Antibodies that attack phospholipids. The presence of antiphospholipid antibodies may indicate that there is an underlying process that results in recurrent pregnancy loss. Phospholipids work to hold dividing cells together and are necessary for growth of the placenta into the wall of the uterus. They also filter nourishment from the mother's blood to the baby, and filter the baby's waste back through the placenta. There are seven antiphospholipid antibodies: anticardiolipin (ACA), phosphoethanolamine, phosphoinositol, phosphatidic acid, phosphoglycerol, phosphoserine, and hosphocholine.

antisperm antibodies: Protective agents produced by the body's immune system that attach to the sperm and prevent them from moving and fertilizing the egg.

AOA: See Antiovarian Antibodies.

APA: See Antiphospolipid Antibodies.

ART: Assisted reproductive technology. ART encompasses various techniques to stimulate the production of multiple eggs and enhance their likelihood of being fertilized. The list of techniques include IVF, GIFT, ZIFT, TET, and PROST.

artificial insemination: The introduction of sperm into a woman's vagina or cervix using a special instrument rather than their introduction through intercourse.

Asherman's syndrome: A condition where adhesions form inside the cavity of the uterus.

aspiration: The application of light suction to the ovarian follicle to remove the eggs.

ASRM: See The American Society for Reproductive Medicine.

assertiveness training: A behavior-therapy technique for helping individuals become more self-assertive in their interpersonal relationships.

assisted hatching (AH, AZH): Thinning out the zona pellucida prior to transferring the embryo into the uterus.

assisted reproductive technology (ART): Several procedures employed to bring about conception without sexual intercourse, including IUI, IVF, GIFT, and ZIFT.

asymptomatic: Having no symptoms.

automatic thoughts: Thoughts that occur in your stream of consciousness that are rarely questioned. They include "should"s and "must"s and are difficult to tune out.

AVA: See Antiovarian Antibodies.

azoospermia: The absence of sperm in the ejaculate.

baby aspirin: Low-dose aspirin (80 to 100 milligrams) used in infertility treatment to increase blood flow to the uterus. Often used in conjunction with heparin in patients with immune problems.

bacteria: Microscopic single-celled organisms that can cause infections.

balanced translocation (BT): When a person has the correct number of chromosomes but the pieces are joined up incorrectly. The problem can be inherited from one parent and then balanced out by the other. If both partners have similar problems, recurrent miscarriage may occur.

basal body temperature (BBT): The body temperature at rest. Some female infertility patients are asked to complete a BBT chart showing their temperature, taken orally, on consecutive days for one or more months.

BBT: See Basal Body Temperature.

behavioral medicine: An interdisciplinary field concerned with the relation between physical health and psychological aspects of individuals who have, or are at risk for, physical disease.

behavior modification: Techniques used to change specific behaviors.

beta HCG: A pregnancy test that determines the presence of hCG in the woman's bloodstream.

bicornuate uterus: A congenital malformation of the uterus where there are two small horn-shaped bodies, each having one fallopian tube.

biochemical pregnancy: When a patient's pregnancy test is positive but no pregnancy is visible on ultrasound.

biofeedback: Treatment techniques in which data regarding an individual's biological activity are collected, processed, and conveyed back so that one can modify that activity.

biphasic: Having two phases. Used to describe BBT charts that show a clear shift from the follicular phase (before ovulation) to the luteal phase (after ovulation).

blastocyst: The stage of development when the embryo consists of many cells packed inside a tough outer membrane.

blastocyst transfer: Allowing in vitro fertilized embryos to reach blastocyst stage, usually taking five days, before transferring the embryos into the uterus.

blastomere: A cell produced during cleavage of a fertilized egg.

blighted ovum: A pregnancy that stops developing very early on. The amniotic sac may only contain fluid and no fetal tissue when the miscarriage occurs.

bromocriptine (Parlodel): A drug used to suppress the production of prolactin.

BT: See Balanced Translocation.

Buserelin: A long-acting GnRH available in Europe as a nasal spray and used to create the pseudomenopause desirable for reducing the size and number of endometriotic lesions. It can also be used to treat fibroid tumors, PMS, hirsutism, and ovulation induction, and for in vitro fertilization.

capacitation: The alteration of sperm during their passage through the female reproductive tract that gives them the capacity to penetrate and fertilize the egg.

catheter: A flexible tube used for aspirating or injecting fluids.

CCT/CCCT: See Clomiphene Citrate Challenge Test.

centrifuge: A machine that separates materials with different densities by spinning them at high speed. Used in sperm washing.

cerclage: A surgical stitch (suture) used to try to keep cervix tightly closed. Used for women with incompetent cervix.

cervical mucus: A secretion produced by the lining of the cervical canal.

cervical smear: A sample of the cervical mucus examined microscopically to assess the presence of estrogen and white blood cells, indicating possible infection.

cervical stenosis: A blockage of the cervical canal from a congenital defect or from complications of surgical procedures. See also Cervix.

cervicitis: An inflammation of the cervix.

cervix: The lower section of the uterus, which protrudes into the vagina and dilates during labor to allow the passage of the infant.

cetrorelix: A GnRH antagonist that can prevent a premature LH surge. A GnRH antagonist needs to be injected less often than Lupron, which is a GnRH agonist. GnRH antagonists need to be injected during the time period when an LH surge is likely to occur.

chemical pregnancy: A pregnancy where hCG levels are detected but the pregnancy is lost before a heartbeat is seen on an ultrasound. This is a very early miscarriage—often before the woman misses a period.

chlamydia: A type of bacteria that is transmitted often between sexual partners.

chocolate cyst: A cyst on the ovary that is filled with old blood.

chorionic vallae sampling (CVS): An alternative to amniocentesis that can be done earlier in the pregnancy. It is a biopsy of the placenta that is used to check for genetic abnormalities in the fetus. Some OB-GYNs claim that, compared to amniocentesis, CVS could cause limb damage in the developing fetus.

chromosome: Strands of DNA in a cell's nucleus that transmit hereditary information.

cilia: Microscopic hair-like projections from the surface of a cell capable of beating in a coordinated fashion.

cleavage: The division of a fertilized egg. The egg size remains unchanged; the cleavage cells become smaller with each division.

clinical pregnancy: A pregnancy confirmed by an increasing level of hCG and the presence of a gestational sac detected by ultrasound.

clinical psychology: A field of psychology concerned with understanding, assessing, treating, and preventing maladaptive behavior.

Clomid: The brand name for clomiphene citrate.

clomiphene citrate challenge test (CCCT, CCT): This test entails the oral administration of 100 milligrams of clomiphene citrate on menstrual cycle Days 5 to 9. Blood levels of FSH are measured on cycle Day 3 and again on cycle Day 10. Elevated blood levels of FSH on cycle Day 3 or cycle Day 10 are associated with very low probability of pregnancy. (Also called Clomid challenge test.)

cognitive activation: Setting into motion mental processes including perception, memory, and reasoning by which a person acquires knowledge, solves problems, and makes plans.

cognitive psychotherapy: Treatment approach to psychological problems where a patient identifies his "warped thinking" and learns more realistic ways to formulate his experiences.

COH: Controlled ovarian hyperstimulation.

colposcopy: Use of a scope to examine the cervix for abnormal cells.

conception: The fertilization of a woman's egg by a man's sperm resulting in a new life.

cone biopsy: A surgical procedure used to remove precancerous cells from the cervix. The procedure may damage the cervix and thus disrupt normal mucus production or cause an incompetent cervix, which may open prematurely during pregnancy.

congenital defect: A birth defect acquired during pregnancy but not necessarily hereditary.

controlled ovarian hyperstimulation (COH): Using fertility medications to stimulate the growth of multiple follicles for ovulation. Also called superovulation.

corpus luteum: The "yellow body" formed in the ovary following ovulation that produces the supply of progesterone needed to sustain a pregnancy.

CPT codes: Medical codes used to refer to a standard list of medical procedures. Insurance companies refer to these codes to determine the reasonable cost for a medical procedure.

creative visualization: See Guided Fantasy.

cryopreservation: Freezing at a very low temperature, such as in liquid nitrogen ($-196°C$), to keep embryos, eggs, or sperm viable.

cycle day: The day of a woman's menstrual cycle. The first day (Day 1) is when full flow starts before mid-afternoon.

cycle synchronization: A procedure for ensuring that an egg donor and an egg recipient reach the middle of their menstrual cycle at the same time.

cyst: A fluid-filled sac.

cytoplasmic transfer: An extension of in vitro fertilization that takes the genetic material from a mother's egg and combines it with the cytoplasm of a donor egg. Two methods of cytoplasm transfer were developed, one transferring a small amount of cytoplasm by tiny needle from the donor to the recipient egg, the other transferring a larger amount of cytoplasm, which is then fused to the recipient cytoplasm with electricity.

Danazol (danocrine): A drug used to treat endometriosis.

D&C: See Dilation and Curettage.

Day 1: The first day of a woman's cycle with menses in full flow (not just spotting). Flow should begin before mid-afternoon or the next day would be considered Day 1.

days post-ovulation (DPO): The number of days a woman is past ovulation. Counting begins the day after ovulation, so if ovulation is on Wednesday, Saturday would be 3 DPO.

days post-transfer (DPT): The number of days a woman is past embryo transfer. Counting begins the day after transfer, so if the transfer takes place on Monday, Friday would be 4 DPT.

Day 3 FSH: A woman's follicle-stimulative hormone (FSH) level taken on Day 3 of her cycle. This reading is an indication of the woman's ovarian reserve. A high level indicates a possible fertility problem.

DES (diethylstilbestrol): A synthetic form of estrogen that was prescribed in the 1950s and 1960s to prevent miscarriages. Tragically, this drug caused malformation of the reproductive system of women born to mothers who took this drug. DES was banned for pregnant women by the Food and Drug Administration in 1971.

dilation and curettage (D&C): A procedure performed after a miscarriage. It involves opening the cervix, stretching (or dilating) it, and scraping (curetting) the lining of the uterus.

direct intraperitoneal insemination (DIPI, IPI): Injection of sperm into the peritoneal cavity. A form of artificial insemination that may be used with low sperm counts and motility.

direct oocyte-sperm transfer (DOST): Involves transvaginal retrieval of eggs from the stimulated ovary, just as in standard IVF. However, following retrieval, instead of inseminating the eggs with sperm and placing them into the incubator, the eggs are inseminated and transferred directly into the uterus nonsurgically two hours later. This allows the eggs to fertilize within the uterus, making it acceptable for women with damaged, nonfunctional, or absent fallopian tubes, just as in IVF.

dominant follicle: The largest follicle among developing follicles in the ovary.

donor egg: Eggs donated by one woman to another.

donor insemination: Artificial insemination with donor sperm. See Artificial Insemination, Intrauterine Insemination.

downregulation: The use of the drug Lupron to inhibit the woman's body from producing its own follicle-stimulating hormone (FSH) and luteinizing hormone (LH). Downregulation enables the doctor to have complete control over the woman's menstrual cycle.

doxycycline: An antibiotic used to prevent infection during an ART procedure.

dysmenorrhea: Painful menstruation.

dyspareunia: Difficult or painful coitus.

ectopic pregnancy: A pregnancy in the fallopian tube or elsewhere outside the lining of the uterus. Also called a tubal pregnancy.

egg donation: Surgical removal of an egg from one woman for transfer into the fallopian tube or uterus of another woman.

egg harvest: The procedure where eggs are obtained by inserting a needle into the ovarian follicle and removing the fluid and the egg by suction. Also called ova aspiration.

egg retrieval: The procedure for obtaining eggs by using a needle to puncture each ovarian follicle and suck out the fluid containing the egg.

ejaculate: The seminal fluid and sperm released from the penis during orgasm.

embryo: A fertilized egg that has begun cell division, often called a pre-embryo (for "pre-implantation embryo"). An embryo is now defined as a later stage, i.e., at the completion of the pre-embryonic stage, which is considered to end at about Day 14. The term *embryo* is used to describe the early stages of fetal growth, from conception to the eighth week of pregnancy.

embryologist: A scientist who specializes in embryo development.

embryo transfer: Placement of the pre-embryos into the uterus or, in the case of ZIFT and TET, into the fallopian tube.

endocrine system: System of glands including the thymus, pituitary, thyroid, adrenals, testicles, or ovaries.

endometrial biopsy: removal of a portion of the uterine lining in order to study the tissue under a microscope.

endometriosis: A disease where normal endometrial tissue (the lining of the uterus) grows outside the uterus. It may be associated with infertility.

endometrium: The mucous membrane lining the uterus.

epididymis: An elongated organ in the male lying above and behind the testicles. It contains a highly convoluted canal four to six meters in length, where, after production, sperm are stored, nourished, and ripened for a period of several months.

estimated due date (EDD): An approximate date for when a baby is due to be born. It is generally calculated based on LMP (last menstrual period), when LMP is two weeks before ovulation. To figure the due date, take your LMP and add nine months plus one week. To figure EDD based on ovulation, add nine months and subtract one week. When using ARTs, one would consider the day of insemination to be ovulation and the day of egg retrieval to be ovulation.

estradiol (E2): A hormone released by follicles in the ovary. Plasma estradiol levels are used to help determine progressive growth of the follicle during ovulation induction.

estrogen: The female hormone largely responsible for thickening the uterine lining during the first half of the menstrual cycle.

fallopian tubes: A pair of tubes attached to the uterus, one on each side, where sperm and egg meet in normal conception.

falloposcopy: The visual examination of the inside of the fallopian tube. A tiny flexible catheter is inserted through the cervical canal and uterine cavity into the fallopian tube. A small flexible fiberoptic endoscope is threaded through the catheter into the fallopian tube. A camera at the end of the falloscope transfers images of the inside of the tube to a monitor so the surgeon can thoroughly visualize and examine the inside of the tube. If problems are found, surgical repairs can be made at the same time.

fertility specialist: A physician specializing in the practice of fertility. The American Board of Obstetrics and Gynecology certifies a subspecialty for OB-GYNs who receive extra training in endocrinology (the study of hormones) and infertility. Those who acquire certification are reproductive endocrinologists (REs).

fertility treatment: Any method or procedure used to enhance fertility or increase the likelihood of pregnancy, such as ovulation-induction treatment, varicocele repair, and microsurgery to repair damaged fallopian tubes. The goal of fertility treatment is to help couples have a child.

Fertilization: The penetration of the egg by the sperm and fusion of genetic material to result in the development of an embryo.

Fertinex: FSH injectable fertility medication.

FET (frozen embryo transfer): Embryos not transferred during an IVF procedure can be frozen. During a subsequent cycle these frozen embryos are thawed and are replaced in the uterus in a procedure called FET (frozen embryo transfer).

fetus: The stage of development of a pregnancy from the third month until delivery.

fibroid (myoma or leiomyoma): A benign (noncancerous) tumor found in the wall of the uterus.

fimbria: The fringed and finger-like outer ends of the fallopian tubes.

fimbrioplasty: Plastic or reconstructive surgery to repair the fimbria that may be damaged or causing a blockage within the fallopian tubes.

follicle: A fluid-filled, cyst-like structure or sac just beneath the ovary's surface in which the egg grows to maturity.

follicle-stimulating hormone (FSH): The pituitary hormone responsible for the stimulation of the follicle cells around the egg.

follicular phase: The first portion of the menstrual cycle, occurring from the time of menstruation to just prior to ovulation. During this phase the egg follicle develops and the egg matures.

follicular fluid: The fluid inside the follicle that cushions and nourishes the ovum. When released during ovulation, the fluid stimulates the fimbria to grasp the ovary and coax the egg into the fallopian tube.

follicular phase: The first half of the menstrual cycle (beginning on Day 1 of bleeding) during which the dominant follicle secretes large amounts of estrogen.

Follistim: Recombinant FSH injectable fertility medication used for superovulation.

frozen embryo transfer (FET): The transfer to the uterus of an embryo that has been frozen (cryopreserved) and then thawed out.

fructose test: A test to determine whether fructose sugar is present in the semen. The test helps to determine whether an obstruction is preventing sperm from getting into the ejaculate.

FSH: See Follicle-Stimulating Hormone.

gamete: The male or female reproductive cells—the sperm or the ovum (egg).

gamete intrafallopian transfer (GIFT): A method of assisted reproduction that involves surgically removing an egg from the woman's ovary, combining it with sperm, and immediately placing the egg and sperm into the fallopian tube. Fertilization takes place inside the tube.

gene: A structure within the nucleus of a cell that contains hereditary characteristics. Genes consist of DNA and are found at specific locations on chromosomes.

genetic abnormality: A disorder resulting from a chromosomal error or a mistake in the structure of a gene.

genetic counseling: The advice offered by experts in genetics on the detection, consequences, and risk of recurrence of chromosomal and genetic disorders.

germ cell: In the male testicular cell that divides to produce the immature sperm cells; in the woman the ovarian cell that divides to form the egg (ovum). The male germ cell remains intact throughout the man's reproductive life; the woman uses up her germ cells at the rate of about one thousand per menstrual cycle, although usually only one egg matures each cycle.

Gestalt psychotherapy: A type of psychotherapy that emphasizes the wholeness of the person and the integration of thought, feeling, and action.

gestational sac: A fluid-filled structure that develops within the uterine cavity early in pregnancy.

GIFT: See Gamete Intrafallopian Transfer.

gland: An organ that produces a hormone.

GnRH: See Gonadotropin Releasing Hormone.

GnRH analogues: Synthetic hormones similar to the naturally occurring gonadotropin releasing hormone (GnRH). Examples are Lupron and Synarel.

gonadotropin: A hormone capable of stimulating the testicles or the ovaries to produce sperm or an egg, respectively.

gonadotropin releasing hormone (GnRH): Hormone secreted by the hypothalamus, a control center in the brain, that prompts the pituitary gland to release follicle-stimulating hormone (FSH) and luteinizing hormone (LH) into the bloodstream.

Gonal-F: Recombinant FSH injectable fertility medication used for superovulation.

gonorrhea: A venereal disease characterized by inflammation of the mucous membrane of the genitourinary tract.

GPST (Getting Pregnant Self-Talk): Words a person says to him- or herself in the mind's ear to motivate the person to act. These self-statements combat the negative automatic thoughts that prevent the person from taking necessary actions.

guided fantasy: Using mental images to help you relax, get motivated, and develop an upbeat attitude.

gynecologist: A physician who specializes in treating female disorders.

hamster penetration test: A test to determine the penetrating ability of a man's sperm. The test uses a hamster egg rather than a human egg to assess the sperm's penetrating ability.

hCG/HCG: See Human Chorionic Gonadotropin.

heparin: A blood thinner given as an injection to prevent blood clots from forming.

heparin therapy: The use of heparin to thin blood in women with recurrent pregnancy loss or presence of an autoimmune problem, such as antiphospholipid antibodies.

herpes: A sexually transmitted virus infection.

hirsutism: The overabundance of body hair, such as a mustache or pubic hair growing upward toward the navel, found in women with excess androgens.

hMG: Human menopausal gonadotropin, which is another name for drugs such as Pergonal.

home pregnancy test (HPT): A test a woman can use at home to test urine for the presence of hCG.

hormone: A chemical, produced by an endocrine gland, that circulates in the blood and has widespread action throughout the body.

hostile mucus: Cervical mucus that impedes the natural progress of sperm through the cervical canal.

host uterus: Also called a "surrogate gestational mother." A couple's embryo is transferred to another woman, who carries the pregnancy to term and returns the baby to the genetic parents immediately after birth.

HSG: See Hysterosalpingogram.

Huhner test: A postcoital test (PCT) to determine whether sperm are surviving in the cervical mucus after intercourse.

human chorionic gonadotropin (hCG): A hormone produced by the placenta during pregnancy; its detection is the basis for most pregnancy tests. HCG is often used with clomiphene or hMG for the treatment of ovulation problems. HCG is also used during ovulation induction to trigger ovulation.

human menopausal gonadotropin (hMG): An ovulation drug, containing follicle-stimulating hormone and luteinizing hormone, derived from the urine of postmenopausal women. Pergonal is a brand name.

Humegon (hMG): Similar to Pergonal: the luteinizing and follicle-stimulating hormones recovered from the urine of postmenopausal women. Used to stimulate multiple ovulation in some fertility treatments.

hydrosalpinx: A fluid-filled, club-shaped fallopian tube that is closed at its end near the ovary. This condition is a contributor to infertility.

hyperprolactenemia: Increased levels of prolactin in the blood that causes discharges of milky fluid from the breast and irregular or absent ovulation.

hyperstimulation syndrome: A possible side effect of treatment with human menopausal gonadotropin in which the ovaries become painful and swollen and fluid may accumulate in the abdomen and chest.

hypothalamus: A thumb-sized area in the base of the brain that controls many body functions and regulates the pituitary gland.

hysterosalpingogram (HSG): A test to determine whether the fallopian tubes are open (patent). The test involves injecting dye and taking an X-ray of the tubes and uterus.

hysteroscope: Examination of the inner part of the uterus by means of a telescopic instrument inserted through the vagina and the cervical canal.

ICSI: See Intracytoplasmic Sperm Injection.

idiopathic (unexplained) infertility: When no cause for infertility can be found after substantial testing.

IF: See Infertility (bulletin board abbreviation).

IM: See Intramuscular.

immature oocyte retrieval (IOR): A procedure where immature eggs are aspirated from the ovaries and treated in the laboratory with fertility drugs to bring them to maturity. At maturity they are mixed with sperm and any resulting embryos are transferred into the uterus.

immature sperm (germinal cell): A sperm that has not matured and gained the ability to swim. In the presence of illness or infection such sperm may appear in the semen in large numbers.

immune system: The body's means of defending itself against injury or invasion by foreign substances.

immunobead test: A test to check for the presence of antibodies on the sperm.

immunologist: One who studies the functioning of the immune system.

immunoglobulins: Antibodies.

immunosuppressive drug: A drug that interferes with the normal immune response.

immunotherapy: A medical treatment for an immune-system disorder that involves transfusing donor white blood cells into a woman who has recurrent miscarriages.

implantation: The embedding of the fertilized egg in the endometrium of the uterus.

implantation spotting: Bleeding associated with an embryo implanting into the endometrium around five to ten days after ovulation. It is not uncommon, but it is not the norm.

impotence: The inability of the man to achieve or maintain an erection and to ejaculate due to physical or emotional problems, or a combination thereof. This is not the same thing as being sterile.

incompetent cervix: A weakened cervix that opens prematurely during pregnancy and can cause the loss of the fetus. A cervical cerclage is a procedure in which a stitch or two is put around the cervix to prevent its opening until removed when the pregnancy is at term.

incomplete abortion: A miscarriage where some tissue has passed but some remains in the uterus.

infertility: The inability of a couple to achieve a pregnancy after one year of regular unprotected sexual relations, or the inability of the woman to carry a pregnancy to live birth.

inflammation: Swelling, redness, heat, and pain caused by injury, such as infection.

inhibin: A male feedback hormone made in the testicles to regulate FSH production by the pituitary gland.

inhibin-B: Inhibin-B is secreted by the granulosa cells while estradiol is secreted by several other cell types in the ovary. Women with low levels of the hormone were found to have more impaired ovulation in the course of the IVF cycle, lower pregnancy rates, and higher cancellation rates and miscarriage rates. Often tested in conjunction with antiovarian antibodies to determine ovarian reserve.

inhibin-F (folliculostatin): A female feedback hormone made in the ovary to regulate FSH production by the pituitary gland.

injectables/injectable fertility medications: Medications given by injection. On INCIID and other infertility forums, the word "injectables" is commonly used to refer to ovulation induction medications such as hMG (brands Pergonal, Humegon, and Repronex), urofollitropins (brands Fertinex and Metrodin), and recombinant FSH follitropins alpha and beta (brands Follistim and Gonal-F).

insemination: The installation of semen into a woman's vagina for the purpose of conception.

insomnia: The inability to sleep.

intracervical insemination: Artificial insemination of sperm into the cervical canal.

intracytoplasmic sperm injection (ICSI): A micromanipulation procedure where a single sperm is injected into the egg to enable fertilization with very low sperm counts or with nonmotile sperm.

intramuscular (IM): An IM medication is given by needle into the muscle. This is as opposed to a medication that is given by a needle, for example, into the skin (intradermal) or just below the skin (subcutaneous) or into a vein (intravenous).

intrauterine insemination: Artificial insemination of sperm into the uterine cavity, bypassing the cervix.

intravenous immunoglobulin (IVIg): Intravenous transfer of immunoglobulin (antibodies), used for some immune problems.

in vitro fertilization (IVF): A method of assisted reproduction that involves surgically removing an egg from the woman's ovary and combining it with sperm in a laboratory dish. If the egg is fertilized, resulting in a pre-embryo, the pre-embryo is transferred to the woman's uterus.

IOR: See Immature Oocyte Retrieval.

Isthmus: The narrow portion of the fallopian tube, which is attached to the uterus.

IVIg: See Intravenous Immunoglobulin.

karyotype: The chromosomal characteristics of a cell.

karyotyping: A chromosome analysis where cells are studied to look for abnormalities. Testing a fetus may show if there is a chromosomal reason for the pregnancy loss, which causes about 50 percent of miscarriages. Testing the parents can help determine if there is an underlying chromosomal problem that increases the chances of repeated losses, which occurs in about 3 percent of couples with recurrent pregnancy loss.

Klinefelter's syndrome: A genetic abnormality characterized by having one Y (male) and two X (female) chromosomes or a mosaic (a combination of 46XY and 47XX). Klinefelter's often causes a fertility problem, though some men will produce sperm. ART and donor insemination are possible (using donor sperm). The condition can be passed on (if ART is done using the husband's sperm).

laparoscope: A small telescopic instrument used to perform a laparoscopy.

laparoscopy: The direct visualization of the ovaries and the exterior of the fallopian tubes and uterus by means of inserting a surgical instrument through a small incision below the navel.

laparotomy: Major abdominal surgery where reproductive-organ abnormalities can be corrected and fertility restored, such as tubal repairs and the removal of adhesions.

last menstrual period (LMP): The calendar date for the first day of full menstrual flow (cycle Day 1).

legitimation: The feeling that your partner considers your concerns to be legitimate and valid.

Leveling: Sharing one's inner world with one's partner during communication.

LH: See Luteinizing Hormone.

LH surge: See Luteinizing Hormone Surge.

Listening: Actively trying to understand one's partner's inner world of experience.

Lisuride: A drug having properties similar to those of Parlodel.

LMP: See Last Menstrual Period.

low responder: A woman who does not produce many follicles with injectable fertility medications.

LPD: See Luteal Phase Defect.

LUF syndrome: See Luteinized Unruptured Follicle Syndrome.

Lupron: The trade name for leuprolide acetate, a GnRH analog. This medicine is injected daily during superovulation to prevent premature ovulation and to allow the doctors to control the follicular phase of the menstrual cycle.

luteal phase: The phase of the menstrual cycle occurring after ovulation.

luteal phase defect (LPD): Inadequate functioning of the corpus luteum that can hamper the fertilized egg's ability to implant in the endometrium.

luteinized unruptured follicle (LUF) syndrome: A condition where the follicle develops and changes into the corpus luteum without releasing the egg. This sometimes goes hand-in-hand with PCO. The use of non-steroidal anti-inflammatory drugs such as Advil, Motrin, and Aleve near ovulation may also contribute to LUFS.

luteinizing hormone (LH): A hormone secreted by the anterior lobe of the pituitary throughout the menstrual cycle. Secretion of LH increases in the middle of the cycle to induce release of the egg.

luteinizing hormone surge (LH surge): The spiking release of luteinizing hormone (LH) that causes release of a mature egg from the follicle. Ovulation test kits detect the sudden increase of LH, signaling that ovulation is about to occur (usually within twenty-four and thirty-six hours).

meditation: A practice of uncritically attempting to focus attention on one thing at a time. The technique is used to reduce stress.

meiosis: When gametes lose half their chromosomes before fertilization.

menses: A woman's menstrual flow or period.

menstrual cycle: A cycle involving the development of an egg and its ovulation, terminating in the shedding of the lining of the uterus.

menstruation: The regular shedding of the lining of the uterus, usually occurring each month.

mental imagery: The ability to reproduce internally a variety of sensations when the object that stimulated them is no longer physically present.

mental rehearsal: Constructing a "movie in your mind" of a future event and rehearsing your behavior in that situation.

methotrexate: A toxic anti-cancer drug that is an analogue of folic acid and an anti-metabolite. Used as an anti-neoplastic agent (to attack abnormal tissue growth). Sometimes used to treat ectopic and molar pregnancies.

Metrodin: A fertility drug consisting of pure follicle-stimulating hormone (FSH). This drug is no longer being manufactured.

microsurgical epididymal sperm aspiration (MESA): Using microsurgery to remove sperm from the epididymis for use in in vitro fertilization, often with ICSI.

miscarriage: Spontaneous abortion.

mitosis: When cells divide in half as the embryo grows.

mittelschmerz: The discomfort felt on one or both sides of the lower abdomen at the time of ovulation.

molar pregnancy (trophoblastic disease): The fertilization of an egg without a nucleus. A baby (usually anomalous) may or may not be present, and the placenta develops into a non-malignant tumor called a hydatidiform mole. The layer of cells that line the gestational sac and normally give rise to the chorionic villi convert into a mass of clear, tapioca-like vesicles instead of into a healthy placenta. The fertilized egg then deteriorates. Probably caused by a chromosomal abnormality in the fertilized egg. A continuous or intermittent brownish discharge is the prime symptom. Treated by a D&C and sometimes methotrexate.

morphology: The shape of sperm as studied in a semen analysis.

morula: The stage of cell division prior to blastocyst. It is a solid mass of blastomeres formed by cleavage of a fertilized egg.

motility of sperm: The ability of the sperm to move about.

mucus: Secretions from a gland that can be watery, gel-like, stretchy, sticky, or dry. Fertile mucus resembles raw egg whites (watery and stretchy).

mycoplasma: An agent causing a sexually transmitted infection.

Negative Self-Talk: Inner negative self-defeating statements a person thinks about.

neuromuscular activation: A process where neural activity stimulates the contraction of skeletal muscles.

neuromuscular relaxation: A process where an individual can perform a series of exercises to reduce neural activity and contractile tension in skeletal muscles.

neuropeptides: Peptide hormones produced by the immune system that influence immune activity.

OB-GYN: See Obstetrician-Gynecologist.

obstetrician-gynecologist (OB-GYN): A doctor who specializes in the diseases and the routine physical care of the reproductive system of women, including treating women through pregnancy and childbirth.

OHSS: See Ovarian Hyperstimulation Syndrome.

olfactory: Involving the sense of smell.

oligospermia: An abnormally low number of sperm in the ejaculate of the male.

oocyte: The egg.

oocyte retrieval: A surgical procedure, usually under IV sedation, to collect the eggs contained within the ovarian follicles. A needle is inserted into the follicle and the fluid and egg are aspirated into the needle, then placed into a culture medium-filled dish.

OPK/OPT: See Ovulation Predictor Kit/Test.

Orgasm: The sexual climax involving male ejaculation and female experience of intense sexual pleasure and excitement.

ovarian cyst: A fluid-filled sac inside the ovary. An ovarian cyst may be found in conjunction with ovulation disorders, tumors of the ovary, and endometriosis. See also Chocolate Cyst.

ovarian failure: The failure of the ovary to respond to FSH stimulation from the pituitary because of damage to or malformation of the ovary. Diagnosed by elevated FSH in the blood.

ovarian hyperstimulation syndrome (OHSS): See Hyperstimulation Syndrome.

ovarian wedge resection: Surgical removal of a pie-shaped wedge of a polycystic ovary in order to help ovulation.

ovary: The sexual gland of the female that produces the hormones estrogen and progesterone, and in which the ova are developed. There are two ovaries, one on each side of the pelvis, and they are connected to the uterus by the fallopian tubes.

ovulation: The release of a mature egg from the surface of the ovary.

ovulation induction: Medical treatment performed to initiate ovulation. See also Clomid, Humegon, Pergonal, Repronex, Follistim, Gonal-F, Fertinex.

ovulation predictor kit/test (OPK/OPT): A test kit a woman can use at home to predict forthcoming ovulation based on a surge of luteinizing hormone.

ovulatory dysfunction: A problem existing in the ovary where either something is abnormal in the process of developing the follicle or the egg is not released from the follicle.

ovum: The egg; the reproductive cell from the ovary; the female gamete; the sex cell that contains the woman's genetic information.

ovum donation: A procedure where eggs are retrieved from a fertile donor and fertilized in a laboratory dish by a husband's sperm, then the resulting embryo is replaced in the recipient woman's uterus.

panic attacks: A situation in which a person experiences intense anxiety and feels immobilized.

Pap smear: A procedure where cells are removed from the surface of the cervix and studied under a microscope.

Parlodel: A drug (also known as bromocriptine) used to suppress prolactin secretion.

partial zona dissection (PZD): A predecessor to ICSI where the zona pellucida, or outer covering, surrounding a woman's egg is opened, using either chemical dissolution or a sharp instrument to file through the outer covering, in order to allow easier access for sperm. Can result in too many sperm entering the egg.

patent: The condition of being open, as with tubes that form part of the reproductive organs. An HSG, for example, is done to see if the fallopian tubes are patent.

pelvic inflammatory disease (PID): An infection of the pelvic organs that causes severe illness, high fever, and extreme pain. PID may lead to tubal blockage and pelvic adhesions.

penis: The male organ of sexual intercourse.

percutaneous epididymal sperm aspiration (PESA): A small needle is passed directly into the head of the epididymis and fluid is aspirated. Any sperm found are used in conjunction with in vitro fertilization with ICSI.

Pergolide: A drug, similar to Parlodel, used to suppress prolactin secretion.

Pergonal: A fertility drug consisting of a combination of FSH and LH.

perinatologist: A doctor specializing in treating the fetus/baby and mother during pregnancy, labor, and delivery, particularly when the mother and/or baby are at a high risk for complications.

PI: See Primary Infertility.

PID (pelvic inflammatory disease): A condition where a female pelvic organ becomes inflamed, usually as a result of a sexually transmitted disease.

pituitary gland: An organ lying at the base of the brain that secretes hormones. This particular gland is known as the "master gland." The pituitary gland controls most of the other endocrine glands in the body.

placenta: A spongy organ attached to the wall of the uterus. The bloodstream passes oxygen through this organ to nourish the developing fetus.

polycystic ovarian syndrome (PCO): Development of multiple cysts in the ovaries due to arrested follicular growth. There is an imbalance in the amount of LH and FSH released during the ovulatory cycle.

polyp: A small growth in the uterus or cervix.

polyspermia: Fertilization of the egg by more than one sperm.

postcoital test (PCT): An examination under the microscope of cervical mucus obtained shortly after intercourse during the time of maximum fertility to determine the number of sperm surviving in the mucus following intercourse.

premature ovarian failure (POF): The cessation of menses associated with high levels of gonadotropins and low levels of estrogen before age forty. The ovary may intermittently produce mature follicles.

primary infertility (PI): Refers to those struggling with infertility without ever having conceived. Popular usage has been extended to include those who have conceived but not had a live birth.

Profasi: The trade name for hCG (human chorionic gonadotropin). See hCG.

progesterone (P4): A hormone secreted by the corpus luteum of the ovary after ovulation has occurred. Also produced by the placenta during pregnancy.

progestin: A synthetic substance that chemically resembles progesterone.

progressive relaxation: A deep muscle relaxation technique where the individual identifies anxiety by noticing muscle tension and reduces anxiety by relaxing the tense muscles.

prolactin: The pituitary hormone that in large amounts stimulates milk production.

PROST (pronuclear stage transfer): A procedure where embryos are transferred at the pronuclear stage. Also referred to as ZIFT.

prostaglandin: Hormone-like substances which can be responsible for cramping if they are not washed away from sperm samples used for intrauterine inseminations.

psychoneuroendocrinology: A branch of medicine based on the interaction of the brain, the endocrine system, and the immune system.

psychotherapy: Treatment of mental disorders by psychological methods.

PZD: See Partial Zona Dissection.

radiologist: A physician who takes X-rays and specializes in their interpretation.

RE: See Reproductive Endocrinologist.

recombinant (human) follicle-stimulating hormone (R-FSH, R-hFSH): Genetically engineered follicle-stimulating hormone, as opposed to FSH extracted from the urine of postmenopausal women. It is synthesized in vitro by cells into which genes encoding for FSH subunits have been inserted. Brand names are Gonal-F and Follistim.

recurrent pregnancy loss (RPL), recurrent miscarriage, recurrent spontaneous abortion (RSA): Repeated miscarriages. Testing can be done to try to determine the cause of such losses. If an underlying condition is found, the woman may need to be treated for the problem before a pregnancy can be carried to term.

reproductive endocrinologist (RE): Obstetrician-gynecologists with advanced education (usually a two-year fellowship), and research in reproductive endocrinology. These highly trained and qualified physicians treat reproductive disorders that affect children, young women, men, and mature women. Some physicians describing themselves as reproductive endocrinologists have not completed certification with the American Board of Obstetrics and Gynecology in the subspecialty of reproductive endocrinology and infertility.

reproductive immunologist (RI): A medical specialty combining obstetrics and gynecology with immunology to treat reproductive disorders that are related to immune problems.

Repronex (hMG): A medication used to replace the pituitary hormones LH and FSH. Similar to Humegon and Pergonal. May be used to induce ovulation in women who do not respond to clomiphene citrate. Most frequently used with women who do not normally produce estrogen because of pituitary gland or hypothalamic malfunction. May also be used with men to stimulate sperm production.

resistant ovary: An ovary that cannot respond to the follicle-stimulating message sent by FSH. Primitive germ cells will be present in the ovary; however, they will not respond to FSH stimulation.

RESOLVE Inc.: The national organization devoted to education and advocacy about infertility.

retrograde ejaculation: A male fertility problem that allows the sperm to travel into the bladder instead of out the opening of the penis due to a failure in the sphincter muscle at the base of the bladder.

retroverted uterus: Uterus that is tilted back toward the rectum.

reversal: Term used in infertility for undoing a sterilization procedure such as a tubal ligation or vasectomy.

Rh factor: Any of one or more genetically determined antigens present in the red blood cells of most persons and capable of inducing intense immunologic reactions. Some women develop a sensitization to Rh during pregnancy. If a woman is Rh-negative and her husband is Rh-positive, she is a candidate for Rh-incompatibility problems. After the first pregnancy, the Rh factor enters the Rh-negative mother's circulatory system during the delivery (or miscarriage) of a child who has inherited the Rh factor from his father. The mother's body then produces antibodies against it. If she becomes pregnant with another Rh-positive baby, the antibodies cross the placenta and attack the baby's red blood cells, causing mild to serious anemia in the baby. The medication Rhogam (called "Anti-D" in Britain and New Zealand) is given to prevent these problems.

Rhogam (Anti-D): An immunization given to Rh-negative women after a miscarriage, stillbirth, or live birth to prevent production of antibodies in any Rh-positive babies they may have in future pregnancies.

RI: See Reproductive Immunologist.

RPL: See Recurrent Pregnancy Loss.

RSA: See Recurrent Spontaneous Abortion.

secondary Infertility: The inability to conceive or carry a pregnancy after having successfully conceived and carried one or more pregnancies.

semen: The sperm and seminal secretions ejaculated during orgasm.

semen analysis: The study of fresh ejaculate under the microscope to count the number of sperm (millions per milliliter or cubic centimeter) to check the shape and size of the sperm, and to note their ability to move (motility).

semen density: How many sperm are present per milliliter of volume.

semen viscosity: How thick or watery the semen sample is.

semen volume: How much liquid is produced in the semen sample. Normal is two to eight milliliters.

seminal vesicles: Two glands in the male that produce the secretion of a fluid containing fructose and store some sperm prior to ejaculation.

septum: A wall in the uterus that should not be there.

Serophene: A commercial name for the drug clomiphene citrate.

sexually transmitted disease (STD): An infectious disease transmitted during sex.

social support: The resources that are provided by other people to help an individual cope with a stressful situation. These resources can be informational (such as how to get insurance claims reimbursed), emotional (such as comforting a woman when her treatment did not succeed), or tangible (such as lending money to pay for a procedure a couple could not otherwise afford).

sonogram (ultrasound): Use of high-frequency sound waves for creating an image of internal body parts. Used to detect and count follicle growth (and disappearance) in many fertility treatments. Also used to detect and monitor pregnancy.

sonohystogram (SonoHSG): An ultrasound/sonogram in which saline is injected into the uterus. It is used to check for abnormalities. It has some similarity to a hysterosalpingogram in purpose, but does not require iodine dye injection or radiation. A safer alternative to hysterography.

sperm: A male reproductive cell.

sperm bank: A place where sperm are kept frozen in liquid nitrogen for later use in artificial insemination.

sperm count: The number of sperm in ejaculate. Also called sperm concentration or sperm density and given as the number of sperm per milliliter.

sperm maturation: A process during which the sperm grow and gain their ability to swim. Sperm take about ninety days to reach maturity.

sperm morphology: The shape of a sperm cell.

sperm precursors: Sperm that are not fully developed and still have twice the number of chromosomes (forty-six rather than twenty-three) they should have when they attempt to fertilize an egg.

sperm washing: A technique that separates the sperm from the seminal fluid.

spontaneous abortion: A miscarriage.

STD: See Sexually Transmitted Disease.

Stein-Leventhal disease: Another name for polycystic ovaries.

sterility: An irreversible condition that prevents conception.

stillbirth: The death of a fetus between the twentieth week of gestation and birth.

stress: A dynamic relationship between a person and the environment in which the person judges that the demands of a situation exceed his or her resources for coping with the situation. Because the demands seem overwhelming, the person's sense of well-being feels endangered.

subzonal insertion (SUZI): A predecessor to ICSI where the zona pellucida is punctured and sperm is inserted into the area between the zona and the egg. Having more than one sperm enter the egg is a potential problem with this procedure.

superovulation: Another name for controlled ovarian hyperstimulation, which is the method of using fertility drugs to stimulate the production of many egg cells.

surrogate gestational: Carrier woman who gestates an embryo that is not genetically related to her and then turns over the child to its genetic parents.

surrogate mother: A woman who is artificially inseminated and carries to term a baby who will be adopted and raised by its genetic father and his partner. The term is usually used for a woman who is the biological mother of the baby she is carrying, while a gestational host carries a fetus that is not genetically hers.

SUZI: See Subzonal Insertion.

swim-up technique: A method of extracting the best sperm from a sperm sample. After a sperm sample has been washed, a small amount of culture media is placed in a test tube, which is placed in an incubator. The most actively motile sperm swim up from the bottom of the tube and the sluggish ones, as well as any debris, remain on the bottom.

Synarel: The commercial name for a GnRH analogue, similar to Lupron.

syphilis: A sexually transmitted disease that can lead to paralysis, insanity, and death within several years.

TDI (therapeutic donor insemination): Artificial insemination by donor.

termination: The ending of a pregnancy by choice by induced labor (resulting in a live birth or stillbirth) or abortion.

TESA: See Testicular Sperm Aspiration.

testes: The male sexual glands, of which there are two. Contained in the scrotum, they produce the male hormone testosterone and produce the male reproductive cells, the sperm.

TESE: See Testicular Sperm Extraction.

testicular biopsy: The removal of a piece of testis by a surgical procedure in order to study it microscopically.

testicular sperm aspiration (TESA): A needle biopsy of the testicle used to obtain small amounts of sperm. A small incision is made in the scrotal skin and a spring-loaded needle is fired through the testicle. Usually does not result in enough sperm to freeze for later use.

testicular sperm extraction (TESE): An open biopsy where a small piece of testicular tissue is removed through a skin incision. The tissue is placed in culture media and separated into tiny pieces. Sperm are released from within the seminiferous tubules, where they are produced, and are then extracted from the surrounding testicular tissue. This procedure can be done using local anesthetic or IV sedation. It is possible to get enough sperm to freeze for future use.

testicular stress pattern: A semen analysis result showing depressed sperm production, poor sperm motility, and poor sperm morphology. The pattern is consistent with secondary testicular failure or illness.

testicular torsion: When a testicle twists on itself, cutting off its own blood supply. Causes extreme pain and requires immediate surgical repair to reduce damage to the testicle.

testosterone: The male hormone responsible for the formation of secondary sex characteristics and for supporting the sex drive. Testosterone is also necessary for spermatogenesis.

TET: See Tubal Embryo Transfer.

therapeutic abortion: A termination of a pregnancy due to severe abnormalities in the fetus or where the mother's health is at risk.

tubal embryo transfer (TET): The placement of an embryo inside the fallopian tube after in vitro fertilization. The process is meant to mimic the natural process of a fertilized embryo traveling down the tube and implanting in the uterus.

tubal ligation: Surgical sterilization of a woman by obstructing or tying the fallopian tubes.

tubal patency: Unobstructed fallopian tubes.

Turner's syndrome: The most common genetic defect contributing to female fertility problems. The ovaries fail to form and appear as slender threads of atrophic ovarian tissue, referred to as streak ovaries. Karyotyping will reveal that this woman has only one female (X) chromosome instead of two or a mosaic (46XX and 45X).

ultrasound: A technique for viewing the follicles in the ovaries and the fetus in the uterus, allowing the estimation of size.

unexplained infertility: The diagnosis given to a couple who have had extensive diagnostic tests that fail to determine a cause for their infertility.

urologist: A physician who specializes in diseases of the urinary tract.

uterus: A hollow muscular structure that is part of the female reproductive tract. The major function of the uterus is to protect and nourish the developing fetus.

vagina: A tubular passageway in the female connecting the external sex organs with the cervix and uterus.

vaginismus: A spasm of the muscles around the opening of the vagina making penetration during sexual intercourse either impossible or very painful. Can be caused by physical or psychological conditions.

vaginitis: An inflammation of the vagina. Yeast, bacterial vaginosis, or trichomonas infections of the vagina. Frequent vaginitis may indicate the presence of pelvic adhesions and tubal blockage from other infections, such as chlamydia. Vaginitis may interfere with sperm penetration of the cervical mucus, and the symptoms may even interfere with the ability and desire to have intercourse.

varicocele: A varicose vein in the testicles, sometimes a cause of male infertility.

varicocelectomy: A surgical procedure to correct a varicocele.

vas deferens: A pair of thick-walled tubes about forty-five centimeters long in the male that lead from the epididymis to the ejaculatory duct in the prostate. During ejaculation, the ducts make wave-like contractions to propel sperm forward.

venereal disease: Any infection that can be sexually transmitted, such as chlamydia, gonorrhea, ureaplasma, and syphilis. Many of these diseases will interfere with fertility and some will cause severe illness. See also PID.

viable: Capable of sustaining life. Often used to describe an early pregnancy in which a heartbeat has been seen.

virus: A microscopic infectious organism that reproduces inside living cells.

viscosity: The thickness of semen.

X chromosome: The congenital, developmental, or genetic information in the cell that transmits the information necessary to make a female. All eggs contain one X chromosome, and half of all sperm carry an X chromosome. When two X chromosomes combine, the baby will be a girl.

Y chromosome: The genetic material that transmits the information necessary to make a male. The Y chromosome can be found in one-half of the man's sperm cells. When an X and a Y chromosome combine, the baby will be a boy.

ZIFT: See Zygote Intrafallopian Transfer.

Zoladex: Like Lupron and Synarel, Zoladex (goserelin acetate) is sometimes used for treatment of endometriosis. It works by suppressing estrogen and reducing estrogen to a postmenopausal level. Its side effects are similar to those reported for Synarel.

zona pellucida: The outer covering of the ovum that the sperm must penetrate before fertilization can occur.

Zygote: An embryo in early development state.

ZIFT (zygote intrafallopian transfer): The transfer of a fertilized egg in an early stage of development (called a zygote) into the fallopian tube so that it can migrate to the uterus and implant. ZIFT is also sometimes referred to as PROST.

ENDNOTES

Chapter 1

1. In the first edition of *Getting Pregnant When You Thought You Couldn't* we used a thirty-six item Getting Pregnant quiz based on nine Pointers. We asked four questions for each pointer. Our subsequent research showed that we get more useful information by asking only one question about each Pointer. We used the nine-item inventory for a survey of a large international sample that we conducted on the Internet. We found that responses to the inventory as a whole as well as to many of the individual items were highly correlated with how depressed people felt. The more closely people followed our Pointers, the less depressed they felt. Also, in the past few years our work has taught us that we need to add a tenth Pointer: Make Decisions. Thus the quiz in this book consists of ten items—one for each of the ten Pointers.

2. Menning, B. 1988. *Infertility: A Guide for the Childless Couple.* New York: Prentice Hall (second edition).

3. Sandelowski, M. 1987. "The Color Gray: Ambiguity and Infertility," *IMAGE: Journal of Nursing Scholarship,* 19, 2, 70–74.

4. Emotional Bulletin Board Archives, International Council on Infertility Information Dissemination, December 1998.

5. Sandelowski, M. 1986. "Women's Experiences of Infertility," *IMAGE: Journal of Nursing Scholarship,* 18, 4, 140–144.

6. Posters on Internet bulletin boards frequently use abbreviations. This helps them write rapidly but also creates the sense of a shared community of "insiders" who have their own secret communication system. If you are a part of this group, you know this inside information. In this posting, "pg" refers to "pregnant." In our chapter on on-line infertility resources we discuss various abbreviations commonly used.

7. Emotional Bulletin Board Archives, International Council on Infertility Information Dissemination, December 1998.

8. Emotional Bulletin Board Archives, International Council on Infertility Information Dissemination, December 1998.

9. Payne, N. 1997. *The Language of Fertility.* New York: Crown Publishers.

10. Domar, A., and H. Dreher 1996. *Healing Mind, Healthy Woman.* New York: Henry Holt & Company, p. 229.

11. Ellis, A., and Harper, R. 1979. *A New Guide to Rational Living.* Englewood Cliffs, NJ: Prentice Hall.

12. Cohen, S., and Syme, S. (eds.). 1985. *Social Support and Health.* New York: Academic Press.

13. Jourard, S. 1964. *The Transparent Self.* Princeton, NJ: Van Nostrand Reinhold.

14. Greil, A. 1991. *Not Yet Pregnant.* New Brunswick: Rutgers University Press, p. 11.

15. Alberti, R., and Emmons, M. 1990. *Your Perfect Right: A Guide to Assertive Living.* San Luis Obispo, CA: Impact Books.

16. Suinn, R. 1983. "Imagery and Sports." In Sheikh, A. (ed.). *Imagery: Current Theory, Research, and Application.* New York: Wiley, p. 507–534.

17. Chekhov, M. 1953. *To the Actor.* New York: Harper and Row.

18. Rosenberg, Helane S. "Visual Artists and Imagery," *Imagination, Cognition, and Personality,* 7, 1, 1987–88, 77–93.

Chapter 2

1. Salzer, L. 1991. *Surviving Infertility.* New York: HarperCollins.

2. Holmes, T., and Rahe, R. 1967. "The Social Readjustment Rating Scale," *Journal of Psychosomatic Research* 11, 213–218.

3. Andrews, F., Abbey, A., and Halman, J. 1992. "Is Fertility Problem Stress Different? The Dynamics of Stress in Fertile and Infertile Couples," *Fertility and Sterility* 57, 1,247–1,253.

4. Abbey, A., Halman, J., and Andrews, F. 1992. "Psychosical, Treatment, and Demographic Predictors of the Stress Associated with Infertility," *Fertility and Sterility* 57, 122–128.

5. Boivin, J., Takefman, J. E., Tulandi, T., and Brender, W. 1995. "Reactions to Infertility Based on Extent of Treatment Failure," *Fertility and Sterility,* 63, 4, 801–807.

6. Lazarus, R. 1966. *Psychological Stress and the Coping Process.* New York: McGraw-Hill.

7. Tunks, E., and Bellissimo, A. 1991. *Behavioral Medicine: Concepts and Procedures.* New York: Pergamon Press, p. 13.

8. Pert, C. 1990. "The Wisdom of the Receptors: Neuropeptides, the Emotions, and Body-Mind," in Ornstein, R., and Swencionis, C. (eds.). *The Healing Brain: A Scientific Reader.* New York: Guilford Press, p. 147–158.

9. Siegel, B. 1986. *Love, Medicine & Miracles.* New York: Harper and Row.

10. Cousins, N. 1989. *Head First: The Biology of Hope and the Healing Power of the Human Spirit.* New York: Penguin Books.

11. Solomon, G. 1990. "Emotions, Stress, and Immunity," in R. Ornstein and C. Swencionis (eds.) *The Healing Brain.* New York: Guilford Press.

12. Pennebaker, J. 1997. *Opening Up: The Healing Power of Expressing Emotions.* New York: Guilford Press.

13. Domar A., Clapp D., Slawsky E., Dusek J., Kessel B., and Freizinger, M. 2000. "Impact of Group Psychological Interventions on Pregnancy Rates in Infertile Women," *Fertility and Sterility,* 73, 4, 805–811.

14. Posted on the emotional issues bulletin board of the International Council on Infertility Information Dissemination (INCIID), December 1998.

15. D'Zurilla, T. 1986. *Problem-Solving Therapy.* New York: Springer.

16. Jacobson, E. *Progressive Relaxation.* Chicago: University of Chicago Press, 1938.

17. Woolfolk, R., and Richardson, F. 1978 *Stress, Sanity, and Survival.* New York: Monarch Books, p. 179.

18. Beck, A. 1976. *Cognitive Therapy and the Emotional Disorders.* New York: New American Library.

19. Meichenbaum, D. 1985. *Stress Inoculation Training.* New York: Pergamon Press.

20. In her book *The Language of Fertility,* Niravi B. Payne encourages readers to create a self-discovery journal as an essential aspect of the Whole Person Fertility Program. In the journal, she suggests readers chart their unexpressed emotions and try other self-exploration activities.

21. Pennebaker, J. 1997. *Opening Up: The Healing Power of Expressing Emotions.* New York: Guilford Press.

22. Greil, A. 1991. *Not Yet Pregnant.* New Brunswick, NJ: Rutgers University Press, p. 63.

23. Ibid., p. 64.

24. Schwan, K. 1988. *The Infertility Maze: Finding Your Way to the Right Help and the Right Answers.* New York: Contemporary Books.

25. Edwards, W. 1961. "Behavioral Decision Theory," *Annual Review of Psychology,* 12, 473–498.

26. Tversky, A., and Kahneman, D. 1981. "The Framing of Decisions and the Psychology of Choice," *Science,* 211, 453–458.

27. Wilson-Barnett, J. "Diagnostic Procedures." In Johnston, M., and Wallace, L. (eds.). 1990. *Stress and Medical Procedures.* New York: Oxford University Press, p. 91.

28. If you have experienced a diagnostic test, you know what to expect. If you would like to share this information with others who could use it to create a script to rehearse, please e-mail that information and we will post it on our Web site. Similarly, you can read descriptions posted by other readers to help you construct a scenario of a procedure you are about to undergo. By sharing this information on our Web site, we can all help one another. And as an added benefit, we will all feel better knowing that we can help one another. Send e-mail to helane@gettingpregnantbook.com or yepstein@rci.rutgers.edu.

29. Zoldbrod, A. 1990. *Getting Around the Boulder in the Road: Using Imagery to Cope with Fertility Problems.* Lexington, MA: Center for Reproductive Problems, p. 23.

Chapter 3

1. Speroff, L., Glass, R., and Kase, N. 1989. *Clinical Gynecologic Endocrinology and Infertility.* Baltimore: Williams and Wilkins, p. 124.

2. The interval between pulses actually varies considerably depending upon the phase of the menstrual cycle. For a discussion of this issue see Speroff, L., Glass, R., and Kase, N. 1989. *Clinical Gynecologic Endocrinology and Infertility.* Baltimore: Williams and Wilkins, p. 58.

3. *On average,* many women ovulate about half the time from the left ovary and half the

time from the right ovary. Some women may alternate sides each month. Other women may have several consecutive ovulations from the right side followed by several consecutive months of ovulation from the left side.

4. Dr. Sherman Silber likens the sperm-production process to an assembly-line procedure. He states, "If one can imagine an automobile assembly line with a slow, steady, unstoppable movement from one stage to progressively more complex stages of production until the final car comes out for inspection, then one will have a pretty good understanding of how sperm are produced and indeed how sloppy the results can often be. In fact, one might speculate that one reason for the extravagant number of sperm produced by the testicles is that only a small percentage will actually have all their nuts and bolts in the right place." See Silber, S. 1991. *How to Get Pregnant with the New Technology*. New York: Warner Books, p. 116.

5. According to Dr. Jonathan Scher, an expert on miscarriage, "Because we know so little about miscarriage and the real number of occurrences, most people ask this question [i.e., how often do miscarriages happen]. The answer, unfortunately, is that no one knows for certain. Every scientific article that comes out, every magazine article, offers a different statistic. What we do know is that every day many more miscarriages happen than we record, because some may appear as just a heavy period." Scher, J., and Dix, C. 1990. *Preventing Miscarriage: The Good News*. New York: HarperPerennial, p. 8.

6. Statistics about the proportion of the population who are unable to conceive because of various problems differ from one study to another. We base our figure on the data provided by the Centers for Disease Control and the Society for Assisted Reproductive Technology. Please bear in mind that these were obtained from patients who were in treatment with doctors and clinics doing so-called high-tech procedures. They may not accurately represent the entire population of infertile people, especially since the majority of them do not engage in high-tech treatments.

Chapter 4

1. One book that discusses these matters is Toni Wechsler's *Taking Charge of Your Fertility: The Definitive Guide to Natural Birth Control and Pregnancy Achievements* (1995, Harper-Collins paperback). You can find additional material in the form of a list of frequently asked questions about "low-tech" ways to become pregnant on the Internet Web site called Fertile Thoughts, which you can find at http://www.fertilityplus.org/faq/lowtechfaq.html.

2. Drs. Speroff, Glass, and Kase believe ovulation occurs between thirty-four and thirty-six hours after the LH surge. See Speroff, L., Glass, R., and Kase, N. 1989. *Clinical Gynecologic Endocrinology and Infertility*. Baltimore: Williams and Wilkins, p. 107.

3. According to Drs. Bill Yee and Gregory Rosen, it is important to identify the first day of the LH surge "because LH can still be detected 24 hours after its onset." See Yee, B., and Rosen, G. 1990. "Monitoring Stimulated Cycles," in Yee, B. *Infertility and Reproductive Medicine: Clinics of North America*. 1, 1, 15–36. Recall that ovulation will occur about thirty-six hours after the beginning of the surge. So if you perform the test just as the surge is beginning, ovulation will take place thirty-six hours later. But if you perform the test twelve hours after the surge began, ovulation will take place about twenty-four hours later.

4. All prices mentioned in this chapter were obtained in the fall of 1999 and may differ from current pricing.

5. Research by Wilson-Barnett has shown that patients find diagnostic testing even more stressful than treatment itself. Surveys have found that the following information about testing can make them feel less anxious: the purpose of the test, what will happen, how long it will take, where it will be performed, who will do the test, what they will feel physically, and what they may feel emotionally. For a discussion of the stress diagnostic testing see Wilson-Barnett, J., in Johnston, M. and Wallace, L., (eds.). 1990. *Stress and Medical Procedures.* New York: Oxford University Press.

6. Be aware that several studies have found that the postcoital test does not correlate with pregnancy. The problem may be the result of poor timing. Reproductive endocrinologist Samuel Thatcher suggests not including this testing in your routine fertility workup.

7. A third but less commonly used assay is Immunolite.

8. Information about semen analysis is taken from Ohl, D., and Menge, A. 1996. "Assessment of Sperm Function and Clinical Aspects of Impaired Sperm Function," *Frontiers of Bioscience,* 1, 96–108.

9. Drs. Speroff, Glass, and Kase discuss a controversy among physicians as to the best time to perform the PCT. On the one hand, testing after two hours may provide maximal information, but the results may also be deceptive because factors in the mucus that can immobilize sperm may not show up until some time later. Therefore, other physicians recommend doing the test sixteen to twenty-four hours after intercourse. See Speroff, K., Glass, R., and Kase, N. 1989. *Clinical Gynecologic Endocrinology and Infertility.* Baltimore: Williams and Wilkins, p. 519.

10. For a discussion of the falloposcopy procedure see Kerin, J., and Surrey, E. 1992. "Clinical Applications of the Falloscope," *Seminars in Reproductive Endocrinology (New Technologies in Reproductive Endocrinology),* 10, 1, 51–57.

11. Trolice, M., et. al. 2000. "Intrauterine Lidocaine Effective during Endometrial Biopsies," *Obstetrics and Gynecology,* 95, 345–347.

12. Scher, J., and Dix, C. 1990. *Preventing Miscarriage: The Good News.* New York: HarperPerennial.

Chapter 5

1. For a complete description of the drugs of infertility, the proper dosage, methods of administration, and side effects see Rivlin, M. 1990. *Handbook of Drug Therapy in Reproductive Endocrinology and Infertility.* Boston: Little Brown.

2. Information about medications discussed in this chapter is based on material in Kearney, B. 1998. *High-Tech Conception.* New York: Bantam Books.

3. In June of 1999. Poet's Pharmacy can be contacted at 1-800-427-7638 for current costs. Information on the cost of fertility medications was obtained from Poet's Pharmacy in Freehold, New Jersey. This particular pharmacy tends to have prices that are somewhat lower than average.

4. Adashi, E. 1990. "Ovulation Initiation: Clomiphene Citrate," in Seibel, M. *Infertility: A Comprehensive Text.* Norwalk, Conn.: Appleton and Lange, p. 308.

5. Gysler, M., March C., Mishell, D., and Bailey, E. 1982. "A Decade's Experience with an Individualized Clomiphene Treatment Regimen Including Its Effect on the Postcoital Test," *Fertility and Sterility,* 37, 161.

6. Taymor, M. 1990. "The Use and Misuse of Ovulation-Inducing Drugs," in Yee, B. *Infertility and Reproductive Medicine: Clinics of North America.* 1, 1, 165–186.

7. Centers for Disease Control and Prevention. December 1998. *1996 Assisted Reproductive Technology Rates: National Summary and Fertility Clinic Reports.* Atlanta, p. 14.

8. Felberbaum, R., and Diedrich, K. 1998. "Ovulation Stimulation in ART: Use of GnRH-Antagonists," in Kempers, R., Cohen, J., Haney, A., and Younger, J. *Fertility and Reproductive Medicine: Proceedings of the XVI World Congress on Fertility and Sterility.* New York: Elsevier, p. 113–125.

9. Taymor, M. 1990. *Infertility: A Clinician's Guide to Diagnosis and Treatment.* New York: Plenum Medical Books, p. 194.

10. Allen, N., Herbert, C., Maxson, W., Rogers, B., Diamond, M., and Wentz, A. 1985, "Intrauterine Insemination: A Critical Review," *Fertility and Sterility.* 44, 5, 569–580.

11. Nuojua-Huttunen, S., Tomas, C., Bloigu, R., Tuomivaara, L., and Martikainen, H. 1999. "Intrauterine Insemination Treatment in Subfertility: An Analysis of Factors Affecting Outcome," *Human Reproduction,* 14, 3, 698–703.

12. Wolmer, D., and Dodson, W. 1990. "Superovulation and Intrauterine Insemination," in Yee, B. *Infertility and Reproductive Medicine: Clinics of North America,* 1, 1, 135–144.

13. Vollenhoven, B., Selub, M., Davidson, O., Lefkow, H., Henault, M., Serpa, N., and Hung, T. 1996. "Treating Infertility: Controlled Ovarian Hyperstimulation Using Human Menopausal Gonadotropin in Combination with Intrauterine Insemination," *Journal of Reproductive Medicine,* 41, 9, 658–664.

14. Silber, S. 1998. *How to Get Pregnant with the New Technology.* New York: Warner Books, p. 372–389.

15. For a discussion of the importance of Day 3 FSH in predicting the success of infertility treatment see the following articles:

Toner, J., Philput, C., Jones, G., and Musaher, S. 1991. "Basal Follicle-Stimulating Hormone Level Is a Better Predictor of In Vitro Fertilization Performance Than Age," *Fertility and Sterility,* 56, 4, 784–791.

Rosenwaks, Z. 1991. "The Use of Gonadotropin and Estradiol Levels in Prediction of Stimulation Response and IVF Results," in the American Fertility Society's *Course II Assisted Reproductive Technologies—An Advanced Course.* Orlando, Florida, October 19–20, 1991.

16. McArdle, C. "Ultrasound in Infertility," in Seibel, M. *Infertility: A Comprehensive Text.* Norwalk, Conn. Appleton & Lange, p. 274.

Chapter 6

1. The ASRM points out that "some physicians listing their practice description as Reproductive Endocrinology and Infertility have not completed certification with the American Board of Obstetrics and Gynecology in the Subspecialty of Reproductive Endocrinology and Infertility." If board certification is important to you, you should find out this information. Please see the Society for Reproductive Endocrinology and Infertility (SREI) for a list of board-certified subspecialists and more information on this subject. The SREI maintains a list of 570 accredited members.

2. For information about obtaining a copy of the *Membership Directory* of the American Society for Reproductive Medicine (ASRM) contact this organization at 2140 Eleventh Avenue South, Suite 200, Birmingham, Alabama 35205-2800. Tel: (205) 933-8494.

3. This activity is based upon an exercise described by Virginia Satir. See Satir, V. 1988. *The New Peoplemaking.* Mountain View, CA: Science and Behavior Books, p. 71–72. It also draws upon ideas about productive dialogue and empathic communication discussed by Cohen and Epstein. See Cohen, B., and Epstein, Y. 1981. "Empathic Communication in Process Groups," *Psychotherapy: Theory, Research, and Practice,* 18, 4, 493–500.

4. The presumption is made that Amanda and Al do *not* have a problem that would *never* allow them to get pregnant. The formula for computing their odds of getting pregnant after X attempts is:

$1 - (1 - y)^x$ where y = probability of success on any given month and ^{x} represents the number of attempts. In Amanda and Al's example, they were using the Duke University procedure that had a 14% /month success statistic for six months. Therefore, the odds for their success is $1 - (1 - .14)^6$ or $1-(.86)^6$, which equals $1 - (.404) = .595$ or 60%.

5. For a discussion of Gestalt psychotherapy and the concept of human polarities, see Polster, E., and Polster, M. 1973. *Gestalt Therapy Integrated: Contours of Theory and Practice.* New York: Brunner/Mazel.

6. Ibid., p. 62.

Chapter 7

1. Louise Brown's sister, also conceived through IVF, has delivered a baby, the first baby born to a "test tube" baby.

2. Devroey, P., Silber, S., Nagy, Z., Liu, J., Tournaye, H., Joris, H. et al. 1995. "Ongoing Pregnancies and Birth After Intracytoplasmic Sperm Injection with Frozen-Thawed Epididymal Spermatoxzoa," *Human Reproduction,* 10, 903–906.

Holden, C., Fuscaldo, G., Jackson, P., Cato, A., Southwick, G., Hauser, R., Temple-Smith, P., and McLachlan, R. 1997. "Frozen-Thawed Epididymal Spermatozoa for Intra-cytoplasmic Sperm Injection," *Fertility and Sterility,* 1, 81–87.

(*Note:* This study cautions that frozen extracted sperm whose vitality is less than 20 percent will have a poor outcome when used with ICSI. If the vitality is greater than 20 percent, the pregnancy rate is just as good as it is with freshly collected sperm.)

3. Cha, K., Oum, K., and Kim, H. 1997. "Approaches for Obtaining Sperm in Patients with Male Factor Infertility," *Fertility and Sterility,* 67, 6, 985–995.

4. Bonduelle, M. Wilkens, A., Buyesse, A., Van Assche, E., Wisanto, A., Devroey, P., Van Steirteghem, A., Liebaers, I. 1996. "Prospective Follow-up Study of 877 Children Born After Intracytoplasmic Sperm Injection (ICSI) with Ejaculated Epididymal and Testicular Spermatozoa and After Replacement of Cryopreserved Embryos Obtained After ICSI," *Human Reproduction,* 11 (supplement 4), 131–159.

5. Ibid., p. 131.

6. Cummins, J. 1997. "Controversies in Science: ICSI May Foster Birth Defects," *Journal of the National Institutes of Health Research,* 8, 38–42.

7. Palermo, G., Colombero, L., Schattman, G., and Rosenwaks, Z. 1996. "Evolution of Pregnancies and Initial Follow-up of Newborns Delivered After Intracytoplasmic Sperm Injection," *Journal of the American Medical Association,* 276, 1893–1897.

8. Ibid., p. 1893.

9. Tripp, B., Kolon, T., Bishop, C., Lipshulz, L., Lamb, D. 1997. "Intracytoplasmic Sperm Injection and Potential Transmission of Genetic Disease," *JAMA,* 277, 963–964.

10. Bonduelle, M., Joris, H., Liebaers, I., Van Steirteghem, A. 1998. "Mental Development of 201 ICSI Children at 2 Years of Age," *The Lancet,* 351, 1553–1554.

11. Sutcliffe, A., Taylor, B., Li, J., Thornton, S., Grudzinskas, J., Lieberman, B. 1999. "Children Born After Intracytoplasmic Sperm Injection: Population Control Study," *British Medical Journal,* 318, 704–705.

12. Roh, S. 1998. "Biochemical Assisted Hatching," Kempers, R., Cohen, J., Haney, A., Younger, J. (eds). *Fertility and Reproductive Medicine.* New York: Elsevier, pp. 637–648.

13. Nakayama, T., Fujiwara, H., Shigetoshi, Y., Tastumi, K., Honda, T., Fuji, S. 1999. "Clinical Application of a New Assisted Hatching Method Using a Piezo-Micromanipulator for Morphologically Low-Quality Embryos in Poor-Prognosis Infertile Patients," *Fertility and Sterility,* 71, 1,014–1,018.

14. Kearney, B. 1998. *High-Tech Conception.* New York: Bantam p. 293.

15. Kovacs, G., Downing, B., Krins, A., and Freeman, L. 1991. "Triplets or Sequential Siblings?: A Case Report of Three Children Born after One Episode of In Vitro Fertilization," *Fertility and Sterility,* 56, 5, 987–988.

16. Wennerholm, Albertsson-Wikland, K., Bergh, C., Hamberger, L., Niklasson, A., Nilsson, L., Thiringer, K., Wennergren, M., Wikland, M., Borres, M. 1998. "Postnatal Growth and Health in Children Born after Cryopreservation as Embryos," *The Lancet,* 351, 1,085–1,090.

17. Berkowitz, R., Lynch, L., Stone, J., Alvarez, M. 1996. "The Current Status of Multifetal Pregnancy Reduction," *American Journal of Obstetrics and Gynecology,* 174, 4, 1,265–1,272.

Chapter 8

1. We use "Pergonal" to denote any injectable follicle-stimulating hormone medication.

2. Social psychologist Kurt Lewin pioneered the use of *field theory* to apply psychological concepts to the process of changing attitudes and behavior. Discussing Lewin's concepts, social psychologists Morton Deutsch and Robert Krauss note that "Lewin's analysis of the *status quo* as a quasi-stationary equilibrium . . . points out that change from the *status quo* can be produced either by adding forces in the desired direction or by diminishing opposing forces." Deutsch and Krauss point out that of the two approaches, removing impediments to change is the more desirable strategy. For a discussion of field theory and the way its concepts are applied to the process of change, see Deutsch, M., and Krauss, R. 1965. *Theories in Social Psychology.* New York: Basic Books, p. 37–76.

3. Seligman writes about learned optimism as an antidote to learned helplessness. He discusses the health benefits that result from maintaining an optimistic attitude. Seligman indicates that social support and attempts to exert control over the difficult situation can promote an optimistic attitude. Our Pointers are designed to increase the likelihood of getting support and of exerting control. For a discussion of Seligman's important ideas we urge you to read Seligman, M. 1990. *Learned Optimism: How to Change Your Mind and Your Life.* New York: Pocket Books.

4. Damewood, M. 1991. "In Vitro Fertilization: Insurance and Financial Considerations," *Assisted Reproduction Reviews,* 1, 1, 38–49.

5. Johnson, J. "Insurance and the Cost of Infertility," *New York Times,* March 5, 1989.

6. The formula for calculating the odds is: $1 - (1 - y)^x$ where y = probability of success on any given attempt and x represents the number of attempts. So in this example the doctor was advising that you have a 30 percent chance of any given attempt (the national average IVF success rate according to the latest available CDC statistics) and you will be trying IVF three times. The calculation is: $1 - (1 - .3)^3 = (.7)^3 = .657 = 66$ percent.

Chapter 9

1. Greil, A. L. 1991. *Not Yet Pregnant.* New Brunswick: Rutgers University Press, p. 153.

2. Vatican, 1987. *Congregation for the Doctrine of the Faith: Instruction on the Respect for Human Life in Its Origin and on the Dignity of Procreation.* Vatican City: Vatican Press.

3. Lyrics of "Soliloquy" by Richard Rodgers and Oscar Hammerstein II. Copyright © 1945 Williamson Music. Copyright renewed, international copyright secured. Reprinted by permission. All rights reserved.

Chapter 10

1. These statistics are based on the success rate at IVF New Jersey for 1999 as of the date we were writing this chapter.

2. Epstein, Y. 1998. *Depression in Non-Donor College Women and in Their College Donor Counterparts.* Unpublished manuscript. Rutgers University, New Brunswick, NJ.

Chapter 11

1. In an article tracing the history of artificial insemination, it is stated that "in 1884, William Pancoast of Jefferson Medical College, Philadelphia, used AID (artificial insemination by donor) to treat a case of postgonococcal azoospermia. The insemination apparently came about as a result of jokes made by medical students, one of whom, the 'best looking member of the class,' was the semen donor. An intrauterine insemination was performed without the knowledge of the couple. When a pregnancy resulted, the husband was informed. Fortunately, he was pleased, although he asked that his wife not be told. The insemination was not reported until twenty-five years later by one of the medical students involved." See Arny, M., and Quagliarello, J. 1987. "History of Artificial Insemination: A Tribute to Sophia Kleegman, M.D.," *Seminars in Reproductive Endocrinology,* 5, 1, 1–3.

2. Sehnert, B., and Chetkowski, R. 1998. "Secondary Donation of Frozen Embryos Is More Common after Pregnancy Initiation with Donated Eggs than after In Vitro Fertilization–Embryo Transfer and Gamete Intrafallopian Transfer," *Fertility and Sterility,* 69, 2, 350–352.

3. Cooper, S., and Glazer, E. 1998. *Choosing Assisted Reproduction.* Indianapolis, IN: p. 328.

Chapter 12

1. Our definition is essentially the same as that of the World Health Organization's scientific group. They define secondary infertility as "Couple has previously conceived, but is subsequently unable to conceive despite cohabitation and exposure to pregnancy for a period of two years."

2. Mosher, W., and Pratt, W. 1990. "Fecundity and Infertility in the United States, 1965–88," *Advanced Data from the Vital and Health Statistics of the National Center for Health Statistics,* 192, December 4, 1990.

3. One of the few books that focuses almost exclusively on secondary infertility is Harriet Fishman Simons' *Wanting Another Child: Coping with Secondary Infertility,* published by Lexington Books in 1995.

4. Krech, D., and Crutchfield, R. 1948. *Theory and Problems of Social Psychology.* New York: McGraw-Hill, p. 488.

5. Mosher, W., and Pratt, W. 1990. "Fecundity and Infertility in the United States, 1965–88," *Advance Data from the Vital and Health Statistics of the National Center for Health Statistics,* 192, December 4, 1990.

6. For additional help in developing good negotiation skills, we suggest that you read Harvard law professor Roger Fisher's excellent book, which teaches these skills. See Fisher, R., and Ury, W. 1981. *Getting to Yes.* New York: Penguin Books.

Chapter 13

1. When a woman has several miscarriages, the phenomenon is known as recurrent pregnancy loss. Statistics about this problem and a definition are provided in Wheeler, J. 1991. "Epidemiologic Aspects of Recurrent Pregnancy Loss," in Freedman, A. (ed.), *Infertility and Reproductive Medicine: Clinics of North America,* 2, 1, 1–18.

2. Ibid., p. 2.

3. Rein, M. 1991. "Luteal Phase Defect and Recurrent Pregnancy Loss," *Infertility and Reproductive Medicine Clinics of North America,* 2, 1, p. 123.

4. Lauersen, N., and Bouchez, C. 1991. *Getting Pregnant: What You Need to Know Right Now.* New York: Rawson Associates, p. 217.

5. Ibid., p. 218.

6. A critical review of the literature does not support the claims that infections cause miscarriage or that antibiotics can prevent miscarriage. After examining numerous studies on the contribution of mycoplasma to miscarriage, Drs. Laura E. Riley and Ruth Tuomala conclude that "the existing data do not substantiate that Mycoplasma colonization causes recurrent pregnancy loss or that eradication of colonization improves outcome." See Riley, L., and Tuomala, R. 1991. "Infectious Diseases and Recurrent Pregnancy Loss," *Infertility and Reproductive Medicine Clinics of North America,* 2, 1, p. 168.

7. Herbst, A., Senekjian, E., and Frey, K. 1989. "Abortion and Pregnancy Loss among Diethylstilbestrol-Exposed Women," *Seminars in Reproductive Endocrinology,* 7:124.

8. Opponents of the approach dispute these contentions. They claim that the treatment is not needed since there is no evidence that such genetic similarity is problematical. In his review of the causes of recurrent pregnancy loss, Dr. Wheeler points out that "Human Leukocyte Antigen (HLA) overcompatibility was once thought to be an extremely attractive theory of recurrent pregnancy loss. Unfortunately, further research

failed to demonstrate causation." Wheeler, J. 1991. "Epidemiologic Aspects of Recurrent Pregnancy Loss," in Freedman, A. (ed.), *Infertility and Reproductive Medicine: Clinics of North America,* 2, 1, p. 8.

9. From Warburton, D., Kline, J., Stein, Z., and Strobino, B. 1986. "Cytogenic Abnormalities in Spontaneous Abortions of Recognized Conceptions," in Porter, I., and Wiley, A. (eds.), *Perinatal Genetics: Diagnosis and Treatment.* New York: Academic Press, p. 133.

10. Scher, J., and Dix, C. 1990. *Preventing Miscarriage: The Good News.* New York: HarperPerennial, p. 11.

11. Schweibert, P., and Kirk, P. 1985. *When Hello Means Goodbye: A Guide for Parents Whose Child Dies Before Birth, at Birth, or Shortly After Birth.* Available from Perinatal Loss, 2116 N.E. 18th Avenue, Portland, OR 97212. (503) 284-7426.

Chapter 14

1. Liszt's Usenet Newsgroups Directory, July 24, 2000.

Afterword

1. Glazer, E. 1998. *Experiencing Infertility.* San Francisco: Jossey-Bass Publishers, p. 253.

INDEX

ABOUT THE AUTHORS

HELANE ROSENBERG and YAKOV EPSTEIN are a married couple who have eight-year-old twins conceived through an egg donor procedure. Helane is associate professor of education at Rutgers University and egg donor coordinator at IVF New Jersey. She is a member of the advisory board of the International Council for Infertility Information Dissemination (INCIID) and has served as the ovum donor contact person for RESOLVE, Inc. Yakov is a licensed clinical psychologist, professor of psychology at Rutgers University, and director of the Rutgers Center for Mathematics, Science, and Computer Education. He serves as director of counseling services for IVF New Jersey. He is a member of the executive board of the International Council on Infertility Information Dissemination (INCIID). Helane and Yakov were the 1997 recipients of the Heather Bruce Thierman Online Angel Award from INCIID and Ferring Pharmaceuticals for their work with the infertility community.